Angele Bayou

W9-CWK-001

CLINICAL COMPANION

for use with

First Canadian Edition

HEALTH ASSESSMENT
AND
PHYSICAL EXAMINATION

Mary Ellen Zator Estes

RN, MSN, FNP, APRN-BC, NP-C
Family Nurse Practitioner in Internal Medicine
Fairfax, Virginia
and
Clinical Faculty Nurse Practitioner Track School of Nursing
Ball State University
Muncie, Indiana

Madeleine Buck

RN, B.Sc.(N), M.Sc.(A)
School of Nursing
McGill University
and
Clinical Associate
McGill University Health Centre
Montreal, Quebec, Canada

NELSON EDUCATION

NELSON / EDUCATION

Clinical Companion for use with Health Assessment
and Physical Examination, First Canadian Edition

by Mary Ellen Zator Estes and Madeleine Buck

**Associate Vice President,
Editorial Director:**
Evelyn Veitch

**Editor-in-Chief,
Higher Education:**
Anne Williams

Senior Acquisitions Editor:
Kevin Smulan

Marketing Manager:
William de Villiers

**Senior Developmental
Editor:**
Rebecca Ryoji

**Photo Researcher/
Permissions Coordinator:**
Sandra Mark

Proofreader:
Liba Berry

Indexer:
Gillian Watts

**Senior Manufacturing
Coordinator:**
Charmaine Lee Wah

Design Director:
Ken Phipps

Managing Designer:
Katherine Strain

Interior Design:
Tammy Gay

Cover Design:
Peter Papayanakis

Cover Images:
Antony Nagelmann/
Getty Images (nurse)
Lawrence Lawry/Photodisc
(stethoscope)

Compositor:
Brenda Prangley

Printer:
R.R. Donnelley

NOTICE TO THE READER

Dedication

Dedicated to Betty Liduke and other members of the Highlands Hope Nurse-Counsellor Network for their commitment, courage, creativity, and perseverance in dealing with the HIV pandemic in Tanzania.

Madeleine M. Buck

Contents

vi   Contents

Contributors

Caroline E. Marchionni RN, MSc
Admin, MSc (A.)
Chapter 7, Nutrition

Mitzi Boilanger, RNC, MS
Clinical Nurse Specialist
Clarian Health Partners, Inc.
Indianapolis, Indiana
Chapter 23: Pregnant Patient

Tamera D. Cauthorne-Burnette,
RN, MSN, FNP, CS
Family Nurse Practitioner
Montpelier Family Practice
Montpelier, Virginia
and
Family Nurse Practitioner
James E. Jones, Jr., MD and Associates
Obstetrics and Gynecology
Richmond, Virginia
and
Graduate Clinical Faculty
Medical College of Virginia
Virginia Commonwealth University
School of Nursing
Richmond, Virginia
Chapter 10: Skin, Hair, and Nails
Chapter 14: Breasts and Regional Nodes
Chapter 20: Female Genitalia

Catherine Wilson Cox, RN, PhD,
CCRN, CEN, CCNS
Assistant Professor
School of Nursing & Health Studies
Georgetown University
Washington, DC
Chapter 16: Heart and Peripheral
Vasculature

Jane L. Echols, RN, PhD
Professor of Nursing
School of Health Professions
Marymount University
Arlington, Virginia
Chapter 4: Developmental Assessment
Chapter 5: Cultural Assessment

Barbara Springer Edwards,
RN, BSN, MTS
Former Director
Cardiac Surgical Unit
Alexandria Hospital
Alexandria, Virginia
Chapter 6: Spiritual Assessment

Joseph Haymore, RN, MS, CNRN,
CCRN, ACNP
Nurse Practitioner
Montgomery Neurosurgery-P.A.
Silver Spring, Maryland
and
Adjunct Clinical Faculty
School of Nursing & Health Studies
Georgetown University
Washington, DC
Chapter 19: Mental Status and
Neurological Techniques

Randie R. McLaughlin, MS, CRNP
Certified Adult and Geriatric Nurse
Practitioner
Urology Private Practice
Frederick, Maryland
Chapter 21: Male Genitalia
Chapter 22: Anus, Rectum, and
Prostate

Kathy Murphy, RN, MSN, CS
Clinical Nurse Specialist
Children's Healthcare of Atlanta
Sibley Heart Center
Atlanta, Georgia
Chapter 24: Pediatric Patient

JoAnne Peach, RN, MSN, FNP
Family Nurse Practitioner
Forest Lakes Family Medicine
Charlottesville, Virginia
Chapter 11: Head, Neck, and Regional
Lymphatics
Chapter 12: Eyes
Chapter 13: Ears, Nose, Mouth,
and Throat

Susan Abbott Rogge, RN, NP
Department of Obstetrics and Gynecology
University of California, Davis
Sacramento, California
and
Private Practice
Sacramento, California
  Chapter 23: Pregnant Patient

Bonnie R. Sakallaris, RN, MSN
Director, Cardiac Services
Washington Hospital Center
Washington, DC
  Chapter 19: Mental Status and Neurological
  Techniques

Preface

Health assessment forms the foundation of all nursing care. Whether the patient is young or old, well or ill, assessment is an ongoing process of evaluating the whole person—the person as a physical, psychosocial, functional being. *Clinical Companion for use with Health Assessment and Physical Examination*, First Canadian Edition, provides a fresh and innovative approach to the process of holistic assessment, including physical assessment skills, clinical examination techniques and patient teaching guidelines.

CONCEPTUAL APPROACH

Clinical Companion for use with Health Assessment and Physical Examination, First Canadian Edition, is developed from a parent text, *Health Assessment and Physical Examination,* First Canadian Edition, by Mary Ellen Zator Estes and Madeleine Buck. It is designed to be used in the clinical setting, both in conjunction with the parent text and as a stand-alone product. *Clinical Companion for use with Health Assessment and Physical Examination*, First Canadian Edition, takes a user-friendly approach to delivering a wealth of information. The consistent, easy-to-follow format with recurring pedagogical features is based on two frameworks:

1. The IPPA method of examination (inspection, palpation, percussion, auscultation) is applied to body systems in describing complete, detailed physical assessment.

2. The ENAP format (examination, normal findings, abnormal findings, pathophysiology) follows every IPPA technique, providing a useful, valuable source of information. In acknowledgment of the fact that nurses' clinical decisions must be based on scientific rationale, pathophysiology is included for each abnormal findings.

Readers of *Clinical Companion for use with Health Assessment and Physical Examination*, First Canadian Edition, must have an understanding of anatomy and physiology as well as familiarity with basic nursing skills and the nursing process.

ORGANIZATION

Clinical Companion for use with Health Assessment and Physical Examination, First Canadian Edition, comprises 25 chapters organized into five units.

Unit 1 lays the foundation for the entire assessment process by guiding the reader through the nursing process, the patient interview, and the health history.

Unit 2 highlights developmental, cultural, spiritual, and nutritional areas of assessment, emphasizing the holistic nature of the assessment process.

Unit 3 opens with a description of fundamental assessment techniques, including measuring vital signs, then details assessment procedures and findings for specific body systems. The format used for all applicable physical assessment chapters in this unit is as follows:

1. Anatomy and physiology overview
2. Modified health history
3. Physical assessment
   a. Inspection
   b. Palpation
   c. Percussion
   d. Auscultation

Because assessment techniques and findings for pregnant women and children may differ from those of nonpregnant women and adults, those populations are discussed in separate chapters in **Unit 4**.

Unit 5 helps the reader assimilate and synthesize the wealth and information presented in the text in order to perform a thorough, accurate, and efficient health assessment.

Features

- All chapters reflect Canadian realities in health assessment and clinical care. Health and physical assessment approaches and evaluation procedures reflect Canadian standards and guidelines, including provincial and territorial variations.

- Best practice guidelines, systematic reviews, and evidence-based approaches to a range of health and physical assessment areas have been incorporated throughout the Clinical Companion.
- All biochemistry and mathematical units are in metric units.
- Nursing Checklists offer an organizing framework for the assessment process or for approaching certain tasks.
- Nursing Tips help the reader apply basic knowledge to real-life situations and offer hints and shortcuts useful to new and experienced nurses alike.
- The index facilitates access to material and includes specific entries for tables and illustrations.
- A list of abbreviations includes and defines abbreviations and symbols frequently used in charting.

Selected Highlights

- *Eating Well with Canada's Food Guide* is added in Chapter 7.
- Canadian Hypertension Education Program recommendations for blood pressure measurement are integrated in Unit 3.
- Canadian Standards for Infection Prevention and Control are found in Unit 1.
- The Braden Scale for determining pressure ulcer risk is found in Chapter 10.
- Photos and illustrations are updated.
- Risk factors for prevalent Canadian illnesses have been added throughout.

Unit 1

Laying the Foundation

1

Critical Thinking and the Nursing Process

Critical thinking is a purposeful, goal-directed thinking process that uses clinical reasoning to resolve patient care issues. It combines logic, intuition, and creativity. Critical thinking encompasses many skills, including *interpretation, analysis, inference, explanation, evaluation,* and *self-regulation.*[1]

The nursing process provides a framework to ensure that the elements of critical thinking are followed. The five interrelated phases (or steps) of the nursing process are assessment, diagnosis, planning, implementation, and evaluation. Some of the steps in the nursing process can be labelled differently. For example, the North American Nursing Diagnosis Association (NANDA) classification system will use the term "Nursing Diagnosis" to formulate and document the results of the assessment phase. Institutions that do not use the NANDA classification system may use the term "nursing analysis," "nursing conclusions," "nursing hypotheses," or "nursing summary" to represent the "diagnosis."

The primary focus of this text is assessment.

ASSESSMENT

Assessment is the first step of the nursing process and involves the orderly collection of information concerning the patient's health status. The assessment process aims to identify the patient's current health status, actual and potential health issues or concerns, and areas for health promotion. The sources of information include the patient's health history, the physical assessment, and diagnostic and laboratory data.

Health History

The health history interview is a means of gathering subjective data, usually from the patient. The data collected are subjective in that the information cannot always be verified by an independent observer.

Relatives, neighbours, and friends of the patient can provide insightful data for the health history. The patient's past charts or medical records are additional sources of information, as are health care colleagues. The health history is discussed in Chapter 3.

Physical Assessment Findings

Physical assessment findings constitute a second source of information that is used in the assessment phase of the nursing process. Physical assessment findings constitute objective data, or information that is observable and measurable, that can be verified by more than one person. This text describes the systematic and comprehensive physical assessment techniques that will elicit objective data (see Chapters 8–24). The physical assessment data can be obtained in a body system (see Table 1-1), or head-to-toe, approach.

Diagnostic and Laboratory Data

The final element that contributes to the information gathering in the assessment phase of the nursing process is diagnostic and laboratory data. Results of blood and urine studies, cultures, X-rays, and diagnostic procedures constitute objective data about the patient's status.

TABLE 1-1	Body System Assessment

1. General survey, vital signs, and pain
2. Skin, hair, and nails
3. Head and neck
4. Eyes
5. Ears, nose, mouth, and throat
6. Breasts and regional nodes
7. Thorax and lungs
8. Heart and peripheral vasculature
9. Abdomen
10. Musculoskeletal system
11. Mental status and neurological techniques
12. Female or male genitalia
13. Rectum and prostate

The assessment phase of the nursing process is dynamic in that the nurse continuously adds to the database, validating the data, and interpreting the data. With these data the nurse can progress to the second phase of the nursing process, the nursing analysis.

DIAGNOSIS (NURSING ANALYSIS, NURSING CONCLUSIONS)

The NANDA defines a nursing diagnosis as "a clinical judgment about individual, family, or community responses to actual or potential health problems/life processes." Institutions that do not use the NANDA system may use the terms "nursing analysis," "nursing conclusions," or "nursing assessment." Regardless, the diagnosis is formulated after the assessment data are analyzed.

PLANNING

Planning represents the third step in the nursing process. The nurse prioritizes nursing diagnoses or analyses to formulate a goal and then tests the subsequent nursing interventions aimed toward achieving the goal. Once the nurse has formulated an analysis of the patient's situation, the nurse establishes patient goals, ideally in collaboration with the patient. The essence is that once the analysis of the situation has been outlined, including identification of factors or variables that are influencing the situation, a focus (or goal) to ensure ongoing health must be established. The goal must be identified, along with the strategies to be used to achieve that goal.

Prioritization

The nurse formulates all of the nursing diagnoses that are derived from the clustering of data. When there is more than one nursing diagnosis, the nurse must decide which problem(s) is the most vital to the patient's well-being at that particular time. Generally, the nurse determines the priorities based on the balance between the strengths, deficits, and risks in any given patient situation.

Intervention Selection

Interventions are planned strategies, based on scientific rationale, devised by the nurse to assist patients in meeting their health outcomes. Whenever possible, the patient, family, and significant others can assist in planning the interventions. As with prioritization, interventions are more likely to be accurate and relevant if they have been tailored to the unique characteristics of the patient and family.

The interventions can be independent nursing actions (those that the nurse implements) or collaborative actions (those that require other members of the health care team). A growing trend in health care is toward evidence-based practice. No longer are health care practices being done "because they have always been done that way," nor are they being done intuitively. Rather, evidence-based practice uses the outcomes of scientific studies to guide clinical decision making and clinical care. Systematic reviews are continually being released that address a range of health issues and the interventions that are used to address them. Best practice guidelines also help the nurse to determine the most relevant nursing interventions.

Implementation

In this phase the nurse executes the interventions that were devised during the planning stage to help the patient meet predetermined outcomes. The time frame of the implementation phase varies from patient to patient and from nursing diagnosis to nursing diagnosis.

Implementation is a dynamic process. Plans of care can be changed or eliminated altogether based on the continuous flow of information.

Evaluation

During evaluation, the patient's progress in achieving the goal(s) is determined. Even before the time frame for assessing outcomes is reached, the nurse is continually assessing the patient's progress toward the outcomes, making evaluation a continual and dynamic process. Each intervention should be evaluated. It is important to know which interventions helped and which ones had either no impact or a negative impact on the overall goal achievement. The outcome can be met, partially met, or not met.

REFERENCES

[1]Pesut, D. J., & Herman, J. (1999). *Clinical reasoning: The art and science of critical and creative thinking.* Clifton Park, NY: Thomson Delmar Learning.

2

The Patient Interview

The nursing health assessment interview is a purposeful, time-limited verbal interaction between the nurse and the patient to collect information regarding the patient's health status. Other purposes of the interview include validating appropriate health and illness information presented by the patient or found in the patient's record, and identifying the patient's knowledge of personal health and illness status.

THE PATIENT INTERVIEW

The interview includes an assessment of physical, mental, emotional, developmental, social, cultural, and spiritual aspects of the patient. Data are collected concerning the patient's present and past states of health, including the patient's family status and relationships, cultural background, lifestyle preferences, and developmental level.

The Role of the Nurse

The nurse is often the first person from the health care team to interact with the patient and frequently assumes the role of intermediary for the patient to the larger health care system. The climate and tone of the initial patient interview can influence all future interactions the patient has in the health care setting.

The nurse can foster an atmosphere of safety and comfort by approaching each patient with an accepting, respectful, and nonjudgmental attitude.

The Role of the Patient

The patient is an active and equal participant in the interview process and should feel free to openly communicate thoughts, feelings, perceptions, and factual information.

The Collaborative Partnership

The nurse and patient each bring a unique perspective to any health-related situation and, ideally, will enter into a collaborative partnership. Gottlieb and Feeley describe this relationship as "the pursuit of person-centered goals through a dynamic process that requires the active participation and agreement of all parties. The relationship is one of partnership and the way of working together is collaborative."[1] In this partnership, nurses and patients each bring their knowledge, experience, and expertise to the relationship.

FACTORS INFLUENCING THE INTERVIEW

Factors that can affect the patient's comfort level, and therefore the effectiveness of the interview, are discussed in the following sections.

Legal Considerations

As health professionals, nurses are accountable to the public to ensure that the highest standards of care are met. In all provinces and territories, nurses have professional and legal obligations to maintain their standard of practice, which is monitored by the regulatory nursing organization that granted the nurse a licence to practise. Nurses are also expected to practise within the legislated boundaries as set out in provincial and territorial government structures.

Ethical Considerations

All licensed health professionals across Canada are expected to practise with a high degree of professionalism that includes moral and ethical conduct. Although each nursing regulatory body has its own specific code of ethics or ethic standards, the following ethical principles guide nursing practice across the country:

- Autonomy: a patient's right to self-determination; to respect a patient's thoughts and actions as to what he or she thinks is best for herself or himself
- Beneficence: to do what is "good" for the patient
- Nonmaleficence: to do no harm to the patient
- Justice: to be fair and impartial to the patient
- Fidelity: to be faithful to the patient
- Veracity: to be truthful to the patient
- Utilitarianism: to perform the greatest good for the greatest number of people

Confidentiality

Confidentiality is one of the hallmarks of moral conduct for health professionals. It is essential in developing trust between nurse and patient. The patient's willingness to communicate private and personal health information is predicated on the assumption that the information will be used with discretion and for the benefit of the patient.

Privacy Protection of Personal Health Information

Because of its nature, there is an expectation that health information will be used only for the benefit of the individual who puts his or her trust in the health professional or health care facility.

Proximal Environment

The interview setting directly influences the amount and quality of information gathered. Whenever possible, the interview should be conducted in a private room with controlled lighting and temperature. If securing this type of setting is not possible, control the environment by minimizing distractions and interruptions and increasing the comfort level of the patient.

Approach

Before approaching the patient, gather all accessible patient information. Admission data and past medical records are often available and can significantly reduce the time needed for the interview.

Begin the interview with an introduction, stating your name and title. Call the patient by his or her formal name at first, and ask how the patient prefers to be addressed. Simple communication using appropriate names is respectful and helps identify patients as unique persons at a time when they may be feeling quite anxious. Giving recognition also helps to lower patient anxiety and increase patient comfort level. Explain to the patient what is to follow and give an approximate time frame for the interview.

Time, Length, Duration

When scheduling an interview, look at the patient's daily activities. Ask the patient what interview times would be least disruptive to his or her daily routine and try to accommodate the patient's request.

Biases and Preconceptions

Personal belief and value systems, attitudes, biases, and preconceptions of both nurse and patient influence the sending and receiving of messages. The cultural and family contexts of each serve as a lens for interpreting societal views on ethnicity, gender, and health care.

STAGES OF THE INTERVIEW PROCESS

The three stages in the interview process are the introduction or joining stage, the working stage, and the termination stage.

Stage I

The joining stage is the introduction stage of the interview process during which the nurse and the patient establish trust and get to know one another.

Stage II

The working stage of the interview process is the time during which the bulk of the patient data is collected.

Stage III

The termination stage is the last stage of the interview process during which information is summarized and validated, and plans for future interviews are discussed.

FACTORS AFFECTING COMMUNICATION

Listening

Active listening, or the act of perceiving what is said both verbally and nonverbally, is a critical factor in conducting a successful health assessment interview. The primary goal of active listening is to decode patient messages in order to understand the situation or problem as the other person sees it.

Nonverbal Cues

Nonverbal communication is conveying a message without speaking. Nonverbal behaviours effectively supplement the spoken word and provide information about both nurse and patient. Nonverbal cues such as body position, repetitive movements of the hands or legs, rapid blinking, lack of eye contact, yawning, fidgeting, excessive smiling or frowning, and frequent clearing of the throat may indicate that the patient is not comfortable discussing his or her health or feelings verbally.

Distance

The amount of space a person considers appropriate for interaction is a significant factor in the interview process and is determined in part by cultural influences. In Canada, distances are generally categorized as follows:

- Intimate distance is from the patient to approximately 0.5 metres.
- Personal distance is approximately 1 to 1.5 metres.
- Social distance is approximately 1.5 to 3.5 metres.
- Public distance is approximately 3.5 metres or more.

Intimate distance is the closest and involves some physical contact. Personal distance may also involve physical contact, which can ease communication such as in the case of hearing impairment. Social distance is considered appropriate for the interview process because it allows for good eye contact and for ease in hearing and in seeing the patient's nonverbal cues. Public distance is usually used in formal settings such as in a classroom where the teacher stands in front of the class.

Personal Space

Personal space is the area over which a person claims ownership. The patient may be very protective of this space and regard unauthorized use of it as an invasion of privacy.

EFFECTIVE INTERVIEWING TECHNIQUES

Effective interviewing techniques facilitate, support, and foster interactions between the nurse and the patient. The techniques encompass both verbal and nonverbal approaches.

Using Open-Ended Questions

Open-ended questions encourage the patient to give general rather than more focused information.

Example of an open-ended question:
"How do you typically deal with an asthma attack?"

Open-ended questions that begin with the words *how, what, where, when,* and *who* will usually elicit the greatest amount of information. Open-ended questions can be time-consuming and may not be appropriate in situations requiring quick access to information.

Using Closed Questions

Closed questions regulate or restrict patient response and are frequently answered with a "yes" or a "no." Closed questions help focus the interview, pinpoint specific areas of concern, and elicit valuable information quickly and efficiently.

Example of an effective closed question:
"Has this type of allergic reaction ever happened to you before?"

If used too frequently, closed questions can disrupt communication because they limit patient responses and interaction.

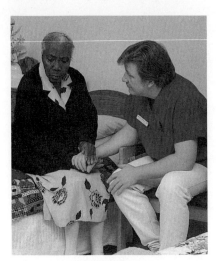

FIGURE 2-1 The nurse can facilitate the interview by displaying empathy and encouraging the patient to continue talking.

Facilitating

Periods may occur when patients stop talking because of anxiety, uncertainty, or embarrassment. Saying "go on" or "uh-huh," simply repeating key words the patient has spoken, or even nodding your head or touching the patient's hand prompts the patient to resume speaking.

Using Silence

Periods of silence help structure and pace the interview, convey respect and acceptance, and, in many cases, prompt additional patient data. Silence on the part of the patient may indicate feelings of anxiety, confusion, or embarrassment, or simply a lack of understanding about the question asked or an inability to speak the language.

Grouping Communication Techniques

Applying communication techniques often seems mechanical and artificial to the novice nurse; one way to diminish this reaction is to group or cluster the techniques according to their primary purposes. One simple method to group interview techniques is to divide them into two groups: listening responses and action responses.

Listening Responses

Listening responses are the nurse's attempts to accurately receive, process, and then respond to patient messages. The responses provide one way for the nurse to communicate empathy, concern, and attentiveness.

Making Observations

When making observations, the nurse verbalizes perceptions about the patient's behaviour, then shares them with the patient.

Example of making observations:
   "Talking about these symptoms seems to make you tense. I notice that you are clenching your fists and grimacing."

Restating

Restating is the act of repeating or rephrasing the main idea expressed by the patient; it informs the patient that you are paying attention.

Example of restating:
Patient: "I don't sleep well anymore. I find myself waking up frequently at night."
Nurse: "You're having difficulty sleeping?"

Reflecting

In reflecting, the nurse directs the patient's own questions, feelings, and ideas back to the patient, which allows the patient to reconsider or expand on what was just said.

Example of reflecting:
Patient: "Do you think I should tell the doctor I stopped taking my medication?"
Nurse: "What do you think about that?"
Patient: "Well, yes, I think that I probably should. Not taking my medication could be one of the reasons I'm feeling so rundown. But that medication just makes me so teary and agitated."
Nurse: "You sound a bit agitated now. It seems as if you've been thinking about this a lot."

Clarifying

Clarifying is a communication technique the nurse can use to verify something the patient has said, or to pinpoint the message when the patient's words and nonverbal behaviour do not match.

Example of a clarifying response:

Patient: "During certain activities, I have the most awful pain in my back."

Nurse: "Tell me what you mean by awful."

Interpreting

Interpreting means that the nurse shares with the patient the inferences or conclusions gathered from the interview.

Example of interpreting:

Nurse: "Your headaches seem to occur every time you eat nuts and chocolate."

Sequencing

To effectively assess patient needs, the nurse often requires knowledge of a time frame within which symptoms or problems developed or occurred. Getting at this information involves asking the patient to place a symptom, a problem, or an event in its proper sequence.

Example of sequencing:

"Did this sharp pain occur each time you had sexual intercourse or only when you didn't empty your bladder first?"

Encouraging Comparisons

Encouraging comparisons is a technique that enables the nurse and the patient to become more aware of related patterns or themes, or specific symptomatology, in the patient's life.

Example of encouraging comparisons:

"In what way was your reaction to this medication similar to or different from your reaction to other antibiotics you've taken before?"

Summarizing

Summarizations help patients (and the nurse) to organize their thinking. A brief, concise review of the important points covered helps the patient identify anything that has been left out and gives the nurse an opportunity to confirm that what he or she understood the patient to say is actually what was said.

Example of summarizing:

"During this past hour, you have shared with me several health concerns of which the most worrisome to you is your difficulty in losing weight. Is that correct?"

Action Responses

Action responses stimulate patients to make some change in their thinking and behaviour.

Focusing

Focusing allows the nurse to concentrate on or to track a specific point the patient has made.

Example of focusing:

"You've mentioned several times that your wife is concerned about your smoking. Let's go back to that."

Exploring

In exploring, the nurse attempts to develop, in more detail, a specific topic or patient concern.

Example of exploring:

"Tell me more about how you feel when you do not take your medication."

Presenting Reality

This technique is useful in the health assessment interview when the nurse is confronted with a patient who exaggerates or makes grandiose statements. Presenting reality encourages the patient to rethink a statement and perhaps modify it.

Example of presenting reality:

Patient: "I can never get an appointment at this clinic."

Nurse: "Mr. Jasper, I've seen you several times in the past four months."

Patient: "Well, yes, but I can never get an appointment at a time that is convenient for me."

Confronting

Confronting is a verbal response the nurse makes to a perceived discrepancy or incongruence between the patient's statements and behaviours.

Example of confronting:

Patient: "I have been working on lowering my risk for a heart attack. I take my cholesterol pill every day and have been watching my diet."

Nurse: "You say that you are working on reducing your cardiovascular risk;

however, I notice that you continue to smoke two packs of cigarettes every day and your triglycerides have doubled in the past three months. Perhaps we can discuss this a bit more?"

Informing

Providing the patient with essential information, such as explaining the nature of or the reasons for specific tests or procedures, is a nursing action that helps build trust and decreases patient anxiety.

Example of informing:
Patient: "Dr. Jones told me that I need to have my gallbladder taken out."
Nurse: "Did you understand what she told you about your gallbladder surgery?"
Patient: "No, I didn't understand what she said . . . something about a tube."
Nurse: "There is a relatively new technique where the surgeon inserts a tube in your abdomen to remove the gallbladder rather than making a large incision."
Patient: "Yes, that was it; please tell me more about that."

Limit-Setting

During the interview with a seductive, hostile, or talkative patient, the nurse may find it necessary to set specific limits on patient behaviour. Limit only the behaviour that is problematic or detrimental to the purpose of the interview.

Example of appropriate limit-setting:
"When you ask me questions about my sex life it makes me feel uncomfortable and I would like you to stop asking me such questions. You came to the clinic today because of a personal health reason, so please tell me about it so that I can know more how we can help you."

Normalizing

Normalizing allows the nurse to offer appropriate reassurance that the patient's response is quite common for the situation.

Example of normalizing:
"It is no wonder that you've been feeling shocked and overwhelmed since you first found that lump in your breast. Many women who have that experience react in a similar way."

INTERVIEWING THE PATIENT WITH SPECIAL NEEDS

The Patient Who Is Hearing Impaired

Some hearing-impaired patients can read lips, so it is important that the nurse remain within sight of the patient and face the patient while talking. If the patient uses a hearing device, make sure it is in working order and is turned on. Background noise should be minimized. Even if an intermediary (a liaison between the patient and a member of the health care team) assists in the interview, always face the patient and direct all communication to the patient. Nonverbal cues such as facial expressions and body movements can effectively convey the meaning of what is being said.

The Patient Who Is Visually Impaired

Look directly at the patient as if the patient were sighted. Because the visually impaired patient cannot rely on visual cues, the nurse's voice intonation, volume, and inflection become more important. It is common for those speaking to a visually impaired patient to speak loudly; this is not necessary and can hinder communication. Before touching the patient, be certain to inform the patient and ask permission to touch. Let the patient know when you are entering or leaving the room, and orient the patient to the immediate environment; use clock hours to indicate position of items in relation to the patient.

The Patient Who Is Speech Impaired or Aphasic

Ask simple questions that require yes or no answers and allow additional time for responses. Convert open-ended questions to closed questions. Repeat or rephrase any questions the patient has not understood. A written interview format, letter board, or yes/no cards are alternate methods of communication.

Dealing with Language Barriers

An interpreter may be necessary in situations where there is a language barrier. Often, information that is lost in the translation can be gained through nonverbal cues.

The Patient Who Has a Low Level of Understanding

The patient with a low level of intelligence requires time to process the interview questions, to formulate answers, and to clarify the meaning or intent of the interview.

The Patient Who Is Crying

Show empathy and allow the patient to cry. Offering tissues indicates to the patient that it is okay to cry and conveys a message of thoughtfulness.

The Patient Who Is Anxious and Angry

Allow the patient, family member, or significant other to express emotions. When interviewing an obviously angry person, recognize and acknowledge the emotion.

The Patient Who Is Hostile

Before beginning the interview, review any documentation that might alert you to people with a past history of violence or poor impulse control.

The risk of aggression can be minimized through nonthreatening interventions such as limit-setting and refocusing. Exploring the sources of the hostility may help to clarify and allay such feelings; however, if a negative tone continues and hostility increases, the nurse must consider his or her own safety. Positioning yourself near an accessible exit, keeping your face to the patient, leaving the door ajar, and alerting a colleague about a worrisome interview are ways to ensure personal safety.

The Patient Who Is Sexually Aggressive

It is important to set limits and to focus on tasks when dealing with sexually aggressive patients. The nurse can achieve this by defining appropriate boundaries, sharing personal reactions, and refocusing the patient; for example, by stating, "It makes me feel very uncomfortable when you stand this close to me. Let's get back to getting information to assist in your health care needs."

The Patient Who Is Very Ill

Collect pertinent data from the patient and defer the remainder of the interview for a later time. It may be necessary to interview a family member or significant other.

REFERENCES

[1]Gottlieb, L. N., & Feeley, N. & Dalton, C. (2006). The *collaborative partnership approach to care: A delicate balance* (p. 8). Toronto: Elsevier Canada.

3

The Complete Health History, Including Documentation

The health history interview is usually the first step of patient assessment. The health history provides information on a patient's social, emotional, physical, cultural, developmental, and spiritual identities. The patient's subjective information is combined with the physical assessment findings to guide the nurse in analyzing the strengths, deficits, and risks in any patient situation so that the most accurate and relevant plan of care can be developed.

The health history typically takes place before the physical assessment.

Analysis of the information obtained in the health history is the basis for planning the health care education needs of the patient and indicates the areas needing attention in the physical assessment.

DETERMINANTS OF HEALTH

For a health history to be relevant, it is important for the nurse to be aware of the multiple factors that influence health, often referred to as the determinants of health. Determinants of health represent a wide range of proximal and distal variables that can influence the patient's health.

Health Canada has identified 12 determinants of health: income and social status; social support networks; education; employment/working conditions; social environments; physical environments; personal health practices and coping skills; healthy child development; biology and genetic endowment; health services; gender; and culture.

TYPES OF HEALTH HISTORY

The four types of health history are complete, episodic, interval or follow-up, and emergency. The complete health history is a comprehensive history covering the many facets of the patient's past and present health status. The episodic health history is short and is specific to the patient's current reason for seeking health care. The interval or follow-up health history builds on a preceding visit to a health care facility. Finally, the emergency health history is elicited from the patient and other sources in an emergency situation.

PREPARING FOR THE HEALTH HISTORY

Conducting a health history interview may require 30 to 60 minutes. Inform the patient prior to the interview of the amount of time that will be required. If the history cannot be completed within the allotted period, continue the interview at another time to avoid patient fatigue. Some health care agencies request that the literate patient complete detailed health history forms prior to the interview; in this instance, the nurse can validate the responses during the health history.

IDENTIFYING INFORMATION

The patient usually completes the identifying information prior to the actual physical examination.

The following biographical data are usually requested for the patient record:

Patient name	Occupation
Address	Work address
Phone number	Work phone number
Date of birth	Usual source of health care
Birth place	Source of referral
Health care number	Emergency contact

THE COMPLETE HEALTH HISTORY ASSESSMENT TOOL

Source and Reliability of Information

It is usually the adult patient who is the historian. However, in some instances, such as in emergency situations, the historian may be someone other than the patient. Assess the reliability of the historian and note the name of the historian, as well as that person's relationship to the patient. It is also important to consider the mental state of the historian because emotions and certain medical conditions can influence the retelling of events. If an interpreter was used, note this in the record and supply the person's name.

Patient Profile

The patient profile includes a notation about age, gender, ethnicity, and a brief summary of how the patient appears (e.g., in distress, tired looking, calm).

Health Issue or Concern

The reasons patients seek health care can relate to general health issues that are normative, such as "I need a check up," or are anticipatory, such as, "I am approaching menopause so I want to learn about how to stay healthy." Such concerns involve health maintenance, illness prevention, or health promotion approaches. However, patients also may seek health care because of specific worries or concerns, such as a sign (objective finding) or symptom (subjective finding). The patient's issue or concern should be recorded as direct quotes in the chart.

When describing a patient's reason for seeking health care, some texts refer to the "Chief Complaint," which implies that a patient only presents with complaints. This text opts for more general terminology (e.g., health issue or concern) that encompasses health maintenance, health promotion, symptomatology, and developmental or situational issues/concerns that may arise across a patient's life span.

Present Health and History of Health Issue or Concern

If a patient seeks health promotion, the nurse should review the present health status. If the patient presents with a particular health issue or concern, then the nurse obtains the history of the health issue or concern in order to document the chronological account of the situation and the events surrounding it.

When a patient presents with a particular sign(s) or symptom(s), a thorough assessment of each health issue or concern must ensue. The 10 characteristics of a sign or symptom are:

1. Location
2. Radiation
3. Quality
4. Quantity
5. Associated manifestations
6. Aggravating factors
7. Alleviating factors
8. Setting
9. Timing
10. Meaning and impact

Note that not all signs or symptoms have all 10 characteristics; hoarseness, for example, may not be characterized by quantity.

Location

Location refers to the primary area where the sign or symptom occurs or originates.

Radiation

Radiation is the spreading of the symptom from its original location to another part of the body.

Quality

The quality of the sign or symptom experience describes the way it feels to the patient. Use the patient's own terms to describe the quality. If the patient is having difficulty describing pain, for example, suggest some quality terms, such as *gnawing, pounding, burning, stabbing, pinching, aching, throbbing,* and *crushing.*

Quantity

Quantity depicts the severity, volume, number, or extent of the presenting sign or symptom. The patient may use the terms *minor, moderate,* or *severe,* and *small, medium,* or *large.*

A variety of scales are available that measure symptoms, with the most well-known and most used scales relating to the assessment of pain. The quantity of pain is often measured using a Visual Analog Scale, a numerical scale that rates pain from 0 (no pain) to 10 (worst pain possible). Refer to Chapter 9 for additional pain-intensity scales.

Associated Manifestations

Associated manifestations are the signs and symptoms that accompany the principle sign or symptom. Frequently, a sign or a symptom is accompanied by other signs or symptoms. Positive findings are the associated manifestations that the patient has experienced along with the principle symptom. Negative findings, also called pertinent negatives, are manifestations expected in the patient with a suspected pathology but which the patient denies. If the patient does not mention specific signs or symptoms associated with the illness, ask the patient whether they are present. Document both positive findings and pertinent negatives;

both give clues to the patient's condition. For example, a patient with headaches may have nausea, vomiting, and diaphoresis as positive associated manifestations. Photophobia and nuchal rigidity are pertinent negatives because they might be present in a patient with headaches but absent in this patient at this time; lack of these associated manifestations may lead to a different diagnosis.

Aggravating Factors

Factors that worsen the severity of the principal sign or symptom are the aggravating factors.

Alleviating Factors

Alleviating factors are events that decrease the severity of the sign or symptom that is being assessed.

Setting

The setting in which the sign or symptom occurs can provide valuable information about its course. The setting can be the actual physical environment of the patient, the mental state of the patient, or can be an activity in which the patient was involved.

Timing

The timing used to describe a sign or symptom experience has three elements: onset, duration, and frequency. Onset refers to the time the experience began and is usually described as gradual or sudden. Duration depicts the amount of time the sign or symptom was present. *Continuous* and *intermittent* are terms that describe the duration of the experience. Frequency describes the number of times the experience occurs and how often it develops.

Meaning and Impact

The final information required in the assessment of the sign or symptom history is the meaning or significance of the symptom and the impact of the experience on the patient and his or her lifestyle.

Past Health History

The past health history (PHH) or past medical history (PMH) provides information on the patient's health status from birth to the present.

Medical History

The medical history comprises all medical problems and their sequelae (complications) that the patient has experienced, including chronic as well as serious episodic illnesses. Forward or reverse chronology can be used to describe the medical history.

"Have you ever been diagnosed as having an illness? What was it?"
"When was the illness diagnosed?"
"Who diagnosed this problem?"
"What is the current treatment for this problem?"
"Have you ever been hospitalized for this illness? Where? When? For what period of time? What was the treatment? What was your condition after the treatment?"
"Have you ever experienced any complications from this disease? What were they? How were they treated?"

Surgical History

Record each surgical procedure, both major and minor, including the year performed, the name of the hospital, and any sequelae, if known.

"Have you ever had surgery? What type? When and where was the surgery performed?"
"Were you hospitalized? For what period of time?"
"Were there any complications? How were they treated?"
"Are you currently receiving any treatment related to this surgery?"
"Have you ever had an adverse effect from anesthesia?"

Medications, Over-the-Counter, and Natural Health Products

Past and present consumption of prescribed medications and nonprescriptive over-the-counter (OTC) products, including natural health products (NHPs), can affect the patient's current health status. Ask the patient the following questions regarding medications.

Prescription Medication

"What prescription medications are you currently taking? Who prescribed them?" and
"What prescription medications have you taken in the past? Who prescribed them?"
"What is the dose? How often do you take this medication?"

"How do you take this medication (e.g., pills, drops, inhaler, ointment, injection)?"
"How long have you been taking this medication?"
"Have you ever experienced any side effects with this medication?"
"Have you ever had an allergic reaction to this medication? What happened?"
"Tell me the purpose of these medications."

Over-the-Counter and Natural Health Products

"Do you currently take any over-the-counter or natural health products? Which ones?"
"Why do you take these products?"
"Do you take any home remedies? Which ones? For what purpose?"
Repeat all but the first and last questions from the *Prescription Medication* section.
"Do you ever take Aspirin, acetaminophen, ibuprofen, antacids, calcium supplements, nutritional or herbal supplements, vitamins, or laxatives? Do you douche? Administer enemas? Do you take allergy pills or cold medications?"

Communicable Diseases

Communicable diseases can have a grave impact on the individual as well as on society. Some communicable diseases generate enough of a concern to the community that they must be reported to the public health department.

Sexually transmitted infections (STIs) are a type of communicable disease. Health Canada recommends use of the STI Risk Assessment Questionnaire (see Figure 3-1) when assessing for STIs. There is substantial value in asking the patient about possible remote exposure to communicable diseases because pathology may only manifest itself many years after exposure, such as in the case of AIDS.

Allergies

Carefully explore all patient allergies, including medications, animals, insect bites, foods, and environmental allergens. Allergies should be written down in red ink in a conspicuous location on the patient's chart as an alert.

"Are you allergic to any medications? Latex? Animals? Foods? Insect bites? Bee stings? Anything in the environment?"

Category and elements	Important questions to guide your assessment
Relationship	
• Present situation	• Do you have a regular sexual partner?
• Identify concerns	• If yes, how long have you been with this person?
	• Do you have any concerns about your relationship?
	• If yes what are they? (e.g., violence, abuse, coercion)
Sexual risk behaviour	
• Number of partners	• When was your last sexual contact? Was that contact with your regular partner or with a different partner?
• Sexual preference, orientation	• How many different sexual partners have you had in the past 2 months? In the past year?
	• Are your partners, men, women or both?
• Sexual activities	• Do you perform oral sex (i.e., kiss your partner on the genitals or anus)?
	• Do you receive oral sex?
	• Do you have intercourse (i.e., Do you penetrate your partners in the vagina or anus [bum]? Or do your partners penetrate your vagina or anus [bum])?
• Personal risk evaluation	• Have any of your sexual encounters been with people from a country other than Canada? If yes, where and when?
	• How do you meet your sexual partners (when travelling, bathhouse, Internet)?
	• Do you use condoms, all the time, some of the time, never?
	• What influences your choice to use protection or not?
	• If you had to rate your risk for STI, would you say that you are at no risk, low risk, medium risk or high risk? Why?
STI history	
• Previous STI screening	• Have you ever been tested for STI/HIV? If yes, what was your last screening date?
• Previous STI	• Have you ever had an STI in the past? If yes, what and when?
• Current concern	• When was your sexual contact of concern?
	• If symptomatic, how long have you had the symptoms that you are experiencing?
Reproductive health history	
• Contraception	• Do you and your partner use contraception? If yes, what? Any problems? If no, is there a reason?
• Known reproductive problems	• Have you had any reproductive health problems? If yes, when? What?
• Pap test	• Have you ever had an abnormal Pap test? If yes, when? Result if known.
• Pregnancy	• Have you ever been pregnant? If yes, how many times? Outcome: number of live births, abortions, miscarriages.

FIGURE 3-1 STI Questionnaire.

STI = sexually transmitted infection

Source: http://www.phac-aspc.gc.ca/std-mts/sti_2006/pdf/primary_care-soins_primaires_e%20.pdf. Public Health Agency of Canada (2006). Reproduced with permission of the Minister of Public Works and Government Services Canada, 2006.

Category and elements	Important questions to guide your assessment
Substance use	
• Share equipment for injection	• Do you use alcohol? Drugs? If yes, frequency and type?
	• If injection drug use, have you ever shared equipment? If yes, last sharing date.
• Sex under influence	• Have you had sex while intoxicated? If yes, how often?
	• Have you had sex while under the influence of alcohol or other substances? What were the consequences?
	• Do you feel that you need help because of your substance use?
• Percutaneous risk other than drug injection	• Do you have tattoos or piercings? If yes, were they done using sterile equipment (i.e., professionally)?
Psychosocial history	
• Sex trade worker or client	• Have you ever traded sex for money, drugs or shelter?
	• Have you ever paid for sex? If yes, frequency, duration and last event.
• Abuse	• Have you ever been forced to have sex? If yes, when and by whom?
	• Have you ever been sexually abused? Have you ever been physically or mentally abused? If yes, when and by whom?
• Housing	• Do you have a home? If no, where do you sleep?
	• Do you live with anyone?

FIGURE 3-1 STI Questionnaire. *continued*

Injuries and Accidents

A patient's injury and accident history can reveal a pattern that is amenable to health promotion.

"Have you ever been involved in an accident?" or "Have you ever been injured in any way?"

"What occurred? Did you require treatment or hospitalization? Were there any complications or long-term effects from this injury/accident? What were they?"

"Have you ever had a broken bone? Stitches? Burns?"

"Have you ever been assaulted? Raped? Shot? Stabbed?"

Special Needs

The awareness of any cognitive, physical, or psychosocial disability is essential to the individualized health care of a patient.

"Do you have any disability or special need(s)? Describe."

"What type of limitations does this disability/special need place on you?"

Blood Transfusions

Here are a few questions about blood transfusions that the nurse can ask the patient.

"Have you ever received a blood transfusion (whole blood or any of its components)? When?"

"Why did you receive this blood product? What quantity did you receive?"

"Did you experience any reaction to this blood product? What was it?"

Childhood Illnesses

Use of both medical and lay terminology helps to ensure an accurate history is obtained.

"Have you ever had any of the following illnesses: varicella (chickenpox), diphtheria, pertussis (whooping cough), measles, mumps, rubella, rheumatic fever, or scarlet fever?" (Eliminate this question if it was previously asked during the communicable diseases section.)

"Were there any complications? What were they?"

Immunizations

Table 3-1 lists the National Guidelines for Childhood Immunizations recommended by the National Advisory Committee on Immunization. Table 3-2 outlines the immunization schedule for children younger than 7 years who were not immunized in early infancy. Table 3-3 outlines the immunization schedule for children 7 years and older who were not immunized in early infancy. Table 3-4 outlines the routine immunization requirements for adults. There may be minor variations in the implementation of these schedules among provinces and territories, so it is important to verify local recommendations.

"What immunizations have you received since birth? When?"

"Have you received any immunizations as an adult: varicella (chickenpox), hepatitis A, hepatitis B, influenza, tetanus, pneumococcal, meningococcal?"

"Did you experience any allergic reactions to the immunizations? Were there any complications?"

TABLE 3-1   National Advisory Committee on Immunization (NACI) Recommended Immunization Schedule for Infants, Children and Youth

AGE AT VACCINATION	DTAP -IPV	HIB	MMR	VAR	HEP B	PNEU-C	MEN-C	DTAP	FLU
Birth					Infant 3 doses ★				
2 months	O	✳				◈	▶		
4 months	O	✳				◈	▶		
6 months	O	✳				◈	▶ or		6-23 months
12 months			■	❖	or	◈ 12-15 months	▶ if not yet given		◈ 1-2 doses
18 months	O	✳	■ or						
4-6 years	O		■		Pre-teen/ teen 2-3 doses if not yet given				
14-16 years							▶ if not yet given	♦	

O   **DTaP-IPV**   Diphtheria, Tetanus, acellular Pertussis, and inactivated Polio virus vaccine

✳   **Hib**   Haemophilus influenzae type b conjugate vaccine

■   **MMR**   Measles, Mumps and Rubella vaccine

❖   **Var**   Varicella vaccine

★   **Hep B**   Hepatitis B vaccine

◈   **Pneu-C**   Pneumococcal conjugate vaccine

▶   **Men-C**   Meningococcal C conjugate vaccine

♦   **dTap**   Diphtheria, Tetanus, acellular Pertussis vaccine (adult formulation)

◈   **Flu**   Influenza Vaccine

Source: http://www.phac-aspc.gc.ca/naci-ccni/is-si/recimmsche-icy_e.html. Reproduced with the permission of the Minister of Public Works and Goverment Services Canada, 2006.

TABLE 3-2	Routine Immunization Schedule for Children < 7 Years of Age Not Immunized in Early Infancy

TIMING	DTaP[1]	IPV	HiB	MMR	Td[3] OR dTap[10]	HEP B[4] (3 DOSES)	V	P	M
First visit	X	X	X[11]	X[12]		X	X[7]	X[8]	X[9]
2 months later	X	X	X	(X)[6]		X		(X)	(X)
2 months later	X	(X)[5]						(X)	
6-12 months later	X	X	(X)[11]			X			
4-6 years of age13	X	X							
14-16 Years of age					X				

P Pneumococcal vaccine   M Meningococcal vaccine

Source: http://www.phac-aspc.gc.ca/publicat/cig-gci/pdf/part2-cdn_immuniz_guide-2002-6.pdf, Table 2. Reproduced with the permission of the Minister of Public Works and Government Services Canada, 2006.

TABLE 3-3	Routine Immunization Schedule for Children ≥ 7 Years of Age Not Immunized in Early Infancy

TIMING	dTap[10]	IPV	MMR	HEP B[4] (3 DOSES)	V	M
First visit	X	X	X	X	X	X[9]
2 months later	X	X	X[6]	X	(X)[7]	
6-12 months later	X	X		X		
10 years later	X					

M Meningococcal vaccine

Notes for Tables 3-2 and 3-3:

1. DTaP (diphtheria, tetanus, acellular or component pertussis) vaccine is the preferred vaccine for all doses in the vaccination series, including completion of the series in children who have received ≥ 1 dose of DPT (whole cell) vaccine.
2. Hib schedule shown is for PRP-T or HbOC vaccine. If PRP-OMP is used, give at 2, 4 and 12 months of age.
3. Td (tetanus and diphtheria toxoid), a combined adsorbed "adult type" preparation for use in people ≥ 7 years of age, contains less diphtheria toxoid than preparations given to younger children and is less likely to cause reactions in older people.
4. Hepatitis B vaccine can be routinely given to infants or preadolescents, depending on the provincial/territorial policy; three doses at 0, 1 and 6 month intervals are preferred. The second dose should be administered at least 1 month after the first dose, and the third at least 2 months after the second dose. A two-dose schedule for adolescents is also possible (see original document for further details).
5. This dose is not needed routinely, but can be included for convenience.
6. A second dose of MMR is recommended, at least 1 month after the first dose for the purpose of better measles protection. For convenience, options include giving it with the next scheduled vaccination at 18 months of age or with school entry (4-6 years) vaccinations (depending on the provincial/territorial policy), or at any intervening age that is

practicable. The need for a second dose of mumps and rubella vaccine is not established but may benefit (given for convenience as MMR). The second dose of MMR should be given at the same visit as DTaP IPV (± Hib) to ensure high uptake rates.

7. Children aged 12 months to 12 years should receive one dose of varicella vaccine. Individuals ≥ 13 years of age should receive two doses at least 28 days apart.
8. Recommended schedule, number of doses and subsequent use of 23 valent polysaccharide pneumococcal vaccine depend on the age of the child when vaccination is begun (see original document for specific recommendations).
9. Recommended schedule and number of doses of meningococcal vaccine depends on the age of the child (see original document for specific recommendations).
10. dTap adult formulation with reduced diphtheria toxoid and pertussis component.
11. Recommended schedule and number of doses depend on the product used and age of the child when vaccination is begun (see original document for specific recommendations). Not required past age 5.
12. Delay until subsequent visit if child is < 12 months of age.
13. Omit these doses if the previous doses of DTaP and polio were given after the fourth birthday.

Source: http://www.phac-aspc.gc.ca/publicat/cig-gci/pdf/part2-cdn_immuniz_guide-2002-6.pdf, Table 3.
Reproduced with the permission of the minister of Public Works and Government Services Canada, 2006,

TABLE 3-4   Routine Immunization of Adults

VACCINE OR TOXOID	INDICATION	FURTHER DOSES
Diphtheria (adult preparation)	All adults	Every 10 years, preferably given with tetanus toxoid (Td)
Tetanus	All adults	Every 10 years, preferably given as Td
Influenza	Adults ≥ 65 years; adults < 65 years at high risk of influenza-related complications and other select groups	Every year using current vaccine formulation
Pneumococcal	Adults ≥ 65 years; conditions with increased risk of pneumococcal diseases	See NACI original document
Measles	All adults born in 1970 or later who are susceptible to measles	May be given as MMR
Rubella	Susceptible women of childbearing age and health care workers	May be given as MMR
Mumps	Adults born in 1970 or later with no history of mumps	May be given as MMR

Source: http://www.phac-aspc.gc.ca/publicat/cig-gci/pdf/part2-cdn_immuniz_guide-2002-6.pdf, Table 4.
Reproduced with permission of the Minister of Public Works and Government Services Canada, 2006.

"(If born outside Canada or from Northern Canada) have you received the Bacillus Calmette-Guerin (BCG) vaccine (against TB)?"

"Have you ever received any other immunizations (cholera, typhoid fever, yellow fever), perhaps prior to visiting a specific geographical region?"

Family Health History

The family health history (FHH) records the health status of the patient as well as the health status of immediate blood relatives. At a minimum, the FHH should contain the age and health status of the patient, spouse/partner, children, siblings, and the patient's parents. Ideally, the patient's grandparents, aunts, and uncles

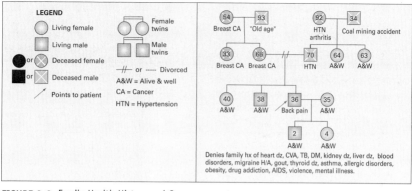

FIGURE 3-2 Family Health History and Genogram.

should be incorporated into the history as well. It is helpful to draw the FHH genogram while the patient is describing the family history to you because it can be completed much more quickly than narrative documentation. Documenting this information is done in two parts: the genogram, and a list of familial or genetic diseases, including pertinent negatives (e.g., no history of heart disease or diabetes). Figure 3-2 demonstrates the appropriate method for constructing the genogram.

"Tell me about the members of your family: spouse/partner, children, siblings, and parents. How old are they?"

"Do any of these individuals have any medical illnesses or diseases? What are they?"

"Have there been any deaths in your immediate family? What was the cause of death? How old was this person at the time of death?"

Social History

The social history (SH) explores information about the patient's lifestyle that can affect health.

Alcohol Use

"How much and what type of alcohol do you drink in an average week?"

"How often do you drink?"

"What quantity do you usually consume at one time?"

"Has your drinking pattern changed? In what way?"

"When did you first start to drink?"

"How long have you been drinking the amount that you are currently consuming?"

"Have you ever lost consciousness or blacked out after drinking?"

"Have you ever forgotten what happened when you were drinking?"

"Do you drive after drinking?"

"Did you ever drink during pregnancy? (for women) How much?"

"Do you think you have a drinking problem?"

"Do you ever feel bullied or pressured into drinking? How do you handle this situation?"

Drug Use

The questions about use of drugs in the SH section of the complete health history should not be confused with the medication section under the PHH. The latter includes the use and abuse of prescription medications, OTC, and NHPs, whereas the former refers to the use of illegal substances.

"Do you use or have you ever used marijuana, amphetamines, uppers, downers, cocaine, crack, heroin, PCP, inhalants, or other recreational or street drugs?"

"When did you first start to use drugs?"

"What amount do you use?"

"How often do you use this drug?"

"Has this amount changed? In what way?"

"In what form do you use the drug (pill, needle, snort, other)?"

"Describe how you inject the drug. Do you share needles? Do you clean needles between uses?"

"Have you experienced any health problems from the drug use?"

"Have you ever overdosed? What happened?"

"Have you ever been through a drug rehabilitation program? What was the outcome?"

"Do you think you have a drug problem?"

"Do you ever feel bullied or pressured into using drugs? How do you handle this situation?"

Tobacco Use

To calculate the pack/year history, multiply the number of packs of cigarettes smoked on a daily basis by the number of years that the patient has smoked: A patient who has smoked 2.5 packs a day for 30 years has a pack/year history of 75 (2.5 × 30 = 75).

"Do you use or have you ever used tobacco (filtered or nonfiltered cigarettes, pipes, cigars, chewing tobacco, snuff)?"

"At what age did you start to use tobacco?"

"What quantity do you use on a daily basis? Has this amount changed? In what way?"

"Have you ever tried to quit smoking? What method(s) did you use? What was the outcome?"

"How long ago did you quit?"

"Do you think you have a smoking (tobacco) problem?"

"Do you live with someone who smokes?"

"If you do not smoke, are you being pressured to start? How do you deal with these pressures?"

Domestic and Intimate Partner Violence

Domestic and intimate partner violence occurs within relationships based on kinship, intimacy, dependency, or trust and can include a range of abusive behaviours from psychological, emotional, and sexual, to financial abuse.

It is vital to be familiar with your provincial or territorial statutes regarding reporting actual and suspected violence and abuse, as well as the local resources available to help people in such situations.

Some clues that might alert the nurse to the possibility of domestic and intimate partner violence are:

- Frequent injuries, accidents, or burns
- Previous injuries for which the individual did not seek health care
- Injury is inconsistent with the patient's report of how it occurred
- Refusal of the patient to discuss the injury
- Significant other accompanies the patient to health care encounters, answers questions for patient, and refuses to leave the patient's side
- Significant other has a history of previous violence or substance abuse

Using the communication technique of normalizing, the nurse can screen for potential domestic and intimate partner violence. Some appropriate introductory comments might include:

"Many women experience domestic and intimate partner violence. Has this ever happened to you?"

"Domestic and intimate partner violence occur very frequently in our community.

Nursing Tip

The Four A's of Smoking Cessation

Ask: At every patient encounter the nurse asks the patient about his or her smoking habits: type, amount, duration.

Advise: The nurse strongly *advises* the patient that quitting smoking is in his or her best health interest.

Assist: The nurse assists the patient in selecting an appropriate nicotine withdrawal method (e.g., "cold turkey," patch, gum, nasal spray, prescription medication, acupuncture, or hypnosis). Advantages and disadvantages of each method are discussed to empower the patient to make an informed decision.

Arrange: The nurse *arranges* for a close follow-up with the patient once the smoking cessation is started. Studies demonstrate that patients who have a support mechanism (professional or nonprofessional) and encouragement have greater success in quitting smoking. The follow-up can be a scheduled appointment or successive phone calls during which the nurse inquires how the patient is doing in meeting the smoking cessation goals and if there are any questions about the chosen withdrawal method.

Nursing Tip

HITS Screening Tool

The HITS screening tool assesses for domestic and intimate partner violence. It is easily administered in a short period of time. The patient is asked how many times each incident has occurred in the past month or year.

H   Have you been physically **Hurt**?
I   Have you been **Insulted** or did someone talk down to you?
T   Have you been **Threatened** with physical harm?
S   Has someone **Screamed** at you or cursed you?

Keeping this in mind, I would like to ask you some questions."

A single broad question can also be used to screen for domestic and intimate partner violence:
"In the past year, have you been hit, kicked, punched, or hurt in other ways by someone close to you?"
"Have you been put down, ridiculed, taunted, or forced to engage in sexual acts that you did not feel comfortable engaging in by someone close to you?"

If the patient answers "yes" to any of these questions, you need to inquire whether or not the patient feels safe in his or her current environment or situation. It is imperative to document physical violence assessment findings concisely and accurately. Incorporate drawings of injury locations or use printed anatomical maps on which injuries can be documented. Many agencies photograph the injuries so that physical violence can be validated in the event of legal proceedings.

Sexual Practice

"What term would you use to describe your sexual orientation (heterosexual, homosexual, bisexual)?"
"At what age was your first sexual experience?"
"With how many partners are you currently involved? Has this changed?"
"What method of birth control do you use? Do you have any questions about it?"
"What measures do you use to prevent exchange of body fluids during sexual activity?"
"Do you engage in oral sex or anal intercourse?"

"Have you ever had a sexual partner who had a sexually transmitted disease?"
"Do you take any prescription or over-the-counter medications to help your sexual performance?"
"Do you use any sexual aid devices?"
"Are you satisfied with your sexual performance?"
"Are you being pressured to have sex when you do not want to? How do you deal with this pressure?"

Travel History

"Where within Canada have you travelled? Was this a rural or an urban environment? When?"
"Have you ever travelled outside of Canada? Where? When? How long were you away?"
"Did you receive any immunizations before you visited that area?"
"Did you need to take any medications before or while you were gone?"
"Were you ill when you were there? Was a diagnosis made? By whom? What was it?"
"What treatment did you receive? Were there any complications?"
"Since returning from this area, have you been ill or not feeling normal?"

Work Environment

"Are you exposed to excessive noise, vibration, radiation, or extremes of heat or cold in your work?"
"Do you work with any chemicals or raw materials?"
"How do you protect yourself from such work hazards?"

"Are material safety data sheets available to you? Do you follow the recommendations?"

"Do you work with any biological hazards such as viruses, insects, plants, animals?"

"Do you spend the majority of your workday sitting, standing, lifting, or doing repetitive work?"

"Do you enjoy your work?"

"Is your work mentally or emotionally demanding?"

"Do you experience any conflict, violence, or harassment in your workplace?"

"Do you feel secure in your work?"

"Have you had any work-related accidents or injuries?"

Home Environment
Physical Environment

"How old are your living quarters (i.e., house or apartment building)?"

"In what condition are your living quarters?"

"What is the temperature on your hot water heater?"

"From what source do you draw your water (e.g., well, reservoir)?"

"Do you have smoke detectors? Where? Are the batteries inspected on a regular basis?"

"Do you have a carbon monoxide detector?"

"Do you think your living space is adequate for the number of people who live with you?"

"How often do you have your fireplace or chimney cleaned?"

"How often do you replace the filter in your ventilation system?"

"What pets do you have? Do they live inside or outside?"

"Do you have easy access to a grocery store? Pharmacy? Health care facility?"

"Where do you store your medications, cleaning supplies, and other toxic substances? How are they secured?" (if children live in the living quarters)

"Do you have a gun in the house? Where is it stored? Where are the bullets stored?"

Psychosocial Environment

"Do you feel safe in your neighbourhood?"

"Does your neighbourhood have a crime watch prevention program?"

Hobbies and Leisure Activities

"What hobbies do you have?" or "What do you like to do in your spare time?"

"Have you ever felt sick during or after any leisure activities? What happened?"

"Have you ever had an injury from your hobby?"

"Are the hobbies and leisure activities relaxing?"

Stress

"What are the current stressors in your life?"

"What is your greatest stress at the present time?"

"Have you ever progressed from the point of being stressed to panic? What were the circumstances? How did you handle it?"

"Are you able to recognize when you become stressed?"

"How do you cope with stress?"

Education

"What was the highest level of education that you completed?"

"Do you have any plans to continue your education?"

Economic Status

"What are the sources of your income?"

"Are you able to meet food, medication, housing, clothing, and personal expenses for your needs?"

"Are you able to save any money?"

Religion and Spirituality

"Are you affiliated with a specific religion?"

"Do you currently practise this religion?"

"Do your religious/spiritual beliefs affect your health status? In what way?"

Ethnicity

"With what culture or ethnic group do you identify yourself?"

"What are common practices in your culture that might influence your health?"

Roles and Relationships

"Who lives with you?"

"What type of relationship do you have with these individuals?"

"What is your role within your family (e.g., caregiver, breadwinner, child, student)?"

"What responsibilities go along with this role?"

Characteristic Patterns of Daily Living and Functional Health Assessment

"Describe a typical day for you, starting from the time you wake up to the time you go to bed."

"Do you need assistance with any activities of daily living? (if yes) Is assistance readily available?"

"Do you socialize, meet, or talk with people outside your house on a daily basis?"

Health Maintenance Activities

Health maintenance activities (HMA) are practices a person incorporates into his or her lifestyle to promote healthy living. You can make the transition from the SH to HMA with a statement such as:

"There are many things you can do to promote your health and that of your family. I would like us to discuss some of those practices."

Sleep

"At what time do you usually go to bed? What time do you usually awake?"

"Is this an adequate amount of sleep for you? How do you feel when you awaken?"

"How long does it take you to fall asleep? Once asleep, do you have difficulty staying asleep? If you awaken, is it easy for you to fall back to sleep?"

"Have you ever been told that you snore loudly or excessively?"

"Do you ever have difficulty staying awake?" "Have you ever been told that you have sleep apnea or narcolepsy?"

Diet

Refer to Chapter 7 for a more thorough discussion of nutrition and diet history.

"Are you on any special therapeutic diet (low salt, low cholesterol, low fat, etc.)?"

"Do you follow any particular diet plan (vegetarian, liquid, Atkins diet, etc.)?"

"How many meals a day do you eat? At what times do you eat? Do you snack? When?"

"Has your weight fluctuated in the past year? Explain."

Exercise

"Do you participate in a formal or informal exercise program? (if yes) How long have you been doing this?"

"What type of exercise do you do?"
"How many times per week do you exercise?"
"How long do you exercise (in minutes)?"
"What is your resting heart rate?"
"Does your health pose any restrictions on your ability to exercise?"

Stress Management

"What do you do to help alleviate the stress when you become stressed?"

"When do you use this skill? Is it effective for you?"

"How many times per day do you use this technique? Per week?"

"Have you tried other ways to manage stress? How did they work?"

Use of Safety Devices

"Do you wear a seat belt when you are in an automobile?"

"Do you wear a helmet if playing hockey or riding a bicycle (motorcycle, skate board, etc.)?"

Health Check-ups

"When was the last time you had the following performed: pulse and blood pressure, complete physical examination, PAP or prostate exam (as indicated by sex), urinalysis, hematocrit, and blood chemistry, including blood glucose and cholesterol? What were the results?"

"How often do you see a dentist, an ophthalmologist? For what reason?

"Do you know how to perform breast self-examination? How often do you perform it? Do you have any questions about it? What was the date and the result of your last mammogram?" (for women)

"Do you know how to perform a testicular self-examination? How often do you perform it? Do you have any questions about it?" (for men)

"Do you have any other health care providers (psychiatrist, psychologist, podiatrist, occupational or physical therapist, chiropractor, shaman, etc.)? For what reason? How often do you see this person?"

Review of Systems

The review of systems (ROS) is the patient's subjective response to a series of body system–related questions and serves as a check that vital information is not overlooked. The ROS covers a broad base of clinical states, but it is by no means exhaustive. The review follows a head-to-toe or cephalocaudal approach and includes two types of questions: sign or symptom related and disease related. Remember to ask the questions in terms that are understood by the patient. The signs or symptoms and diseases are grouped according to physiological body parts and systems.

Both positive and pertinent negative findings are documented in the ROS. When a response is positive, ask the patient to describe it as completely as possible. Refer to the 10 characteristics of a health issue or concern when gathering more information about positive responses of signs and symptoms. Table 3-5 lists the symptoms and diseases that can be ascertained during the ROS.

TABLE 3-5	Review of Systems
General	Patient's perception of general state of health at the present, difference from usual state, vitality and energy levels, body odours, fever, chills, night sweats
Skin	Rashes, itching, changes in skin pigmentation, ecchymoses, change in colour or size of mole, sores, lumps, dry or moist skin, pruritus, change in skin texture, odours, excessive sweating, acne, warts, eczema, psoriasis, amount of time spent in the sun, use of sunscreen, skin cancer
Hair	Alopecia, excessive growth of hair or growth of hair in unusual locations (hirsutism), use of chemicals on hair, dandruff, pediculosis, scalp lesions
Nails	Change in nails, splitting, breaking, thickened, texture change, onychomycosis, use of chemicals, false nails
Eyes	Blurred vision, visual acuity, glasses, contacts, photophobia, excessive tearing, night blindness, diplopia, drainage, bloodshot eyes, pain, blind spots, flashing lights, halos around objects, floaters, glaucoma, cataracts, use of sunglasses, use of protective eyewear
Ears	Cleaning method, hearing deficits, hearing aid, pain, phonophobia, discharge, lightheadedness (vertigo), ringing in the ears (tinnitus), usual noise level, earaches, infection, piercings, use of ear protection, amount of cerumen
Nose and Sinuses	Number of colds per year, discharge, itching, hay fever, postnasal drip, stuffiness, sinus pain, sinusitis, polyps, obstruction, epistaxis, change in sense of smell, allergies, snoring
Mouth	Dental habits (brushing, flossing, mouth rinses), toothache, tooth abscess, dentures, bleeding or swollen gums, difficulty chewing, sore tongue, change in taste, lesions, change in salivation, bad breath, caries, teeth extractions, orthodontics
Throat and Neck	Hoarseness, change in voice, frequent sore throats, dysphagia, pain or stiffness, enlarged thyroid (goiter), lymphadenopathy, tonsillectomy, adenoidectomy
Breasts and Axilla	Pain, tenderness, discharge, lumps, change in size, dimpling, rash, benign breast disease, breast cancer, results of recent mammogram

Respiratory	Dyspnea on exertion, shortness of breath, sputum, cough, sneezing, wheezing, hemoptysis, frequent upper respiratory tract infections, pneumonia, emphysema, asthma, tuberculosis, tuberculosis exposure, result of last chest X-ray or PPD
Cardiovascular and Peripheral Vasculature	Paroxysmal nocturnal dyspnea, chest pain, cyanosis, heart murmur, palpitations, syncope, orthopnea (state number of pillows used), edema, cold or discoloured hands or feet, leg cramps, myocardial infarction, hypertension, valvular disease, intermittent claudication, varicose veins, thrombophlebitis, deep vein thrombosis, use of support hose, anemia, result of last ECG
Gastrointestinal	Change in appetite, nausea, vomiting, diarrhea, constipation, usual bowel habits, melena, rectal bleeding, hematemesis, change in stool colour, flatulence, belching, regurgitation, heartburn, dysphagia, abdominal pain, jaundice, ascites, hemorrhoids, hepatitis, peptic ulcers, gallstones, gastroesophageal reflux disease, appendicitis, ulcerative colitis, Crohn's disease, diverticulitis, hernia
Urinary	Change in urine colour, voiding habits, dysuria, hesitancy, urgency, frequency, nocturia, polyuria, dribbling, loss in force of stream, bedwetting, change in urine volume, incontinence, urinary retention, suprapubic pain, flank pain, kidney stones, urinary tract infections
Musculoskeletal	Joint stiffness, muscle pain, cramps, back pain, limitation of movement, redness, swelling, weakness, bony deformity, broken bones, dislocations, sprains, crepitus, gout, arthritis, osteoporosis, herniated disc
Neurological	Headache, change in balance, incoordination, loss of movement, change in sensory perception or feeling in an extremity, change in speech, change in smell, syncope, loss of memory, tremors, involuntary movement, loss of consciousness, seizures, weakness, head injury, vertigo, tic, paralysis, stroke, spasm
Psychological	Irritability, nervousness, tension, increased stress, difficulty concentrating, mood changes, suicidal thoughts, depression, anxiety, sleep disturbances
Female Reproductive	Vaginal discharge, change in libido, infertility, sterility, pelvic pain, pain during intercourse, postcoital bleeding; menses: last menstrual period (LMP), menarche, regularity, duration, amount of bleeding, premenstrual symptoms, intermenstrual bleeding, dysmenorrhea, menorrhagia, fibroids; menopause: age of onset, duration, symptoms, bleeding; obstetrical: number of pregnancies, number of miscarriages or abortions, number of children, type of delivery, complications; type of birth control, hormone replacement therapy
Male Reproductive	Change in libido, infertility, sterility, impotence, pain during intercourse, age at onset of puberty, testicular or penile pain, penile discharge, erections, emissions, hernias, enlarged prostate, type of birth control
Nutrition	Present weight, usual weight, desired weight, food intolerances, food likes and dislikes, where meals are eaten, caffeine intake

Endocrine	Exophthalmos, fatigue, change in size of head, hands, or feet, weight change, heat and cold intolerances, excessive sweating, polydipsia, polyphagia, polyuria, increased hunger, change in body hair distribution, goiter, diabetes mellitus
Lymph Nodes	Enlargement, tenderness
Hematological	Easy bruising or bleeding, anemia, sickle cell anemia, blood type, exposure to radiation

CONCLUDING THE HEALTH HISTORY

After completing the ROS, ask the patient if there is any additional information to discuss. At the conclusion of the interview, thank the patient for the time spent in gathering the health history. Inform the patient what the next step will be; for example, physical assessment, diagnostic tests, and treatment, and when to expect it.

Unit 2

Special Assessments

4

Developmental Assessment

All individuals, from birth to death, pass through identifiable, cyclical stages of growth and development that determine who and what they are and can become. Growth refers to an increase in body size and function to the point of optimum maturity. Development refers to patterned and predictable increases in the physical, cognitive, socioemotional, and moral capacities of individuals that enable them to successfully adapt to their environments.

DEVELOPMENTAL THEORIES

A variety of theories have been developed that depict and predict growth and development. The traditional theories are the "ages and stages" theories of Jean Piaget, Sigmund Freud, Erik Erickson, and Lawrence Kohlberg. The ages and stages developmental theories are based on the premise that individuals experience similar sequential physical, cognitive, socioemotional, and moral changes during the same age periods, each of which is termed a developmental stage. During each developmental stage, specific physical and psychosocial skills known as developmental tasks must be achieved. An individual's readiness for each new developmental task is dependent on successfully achieving prior developmental tasks in an appropriate environment. If prior developmental tasks have not been achieved or if the appropriate environment was not available, the individual's capacity to successfully adapt to the environment and develop new skills may be reduced.

Life event or transitional developmental theories are based on the premise that development occurs in response to specific life events,

such as new roles (e.g., parenthood) and life transitions (e.g., career changes), events that may require individuals to change their life patterns. Life events and transitions, which can occur singly or together and may cause positive or negative stress, are not tied to a specific time or stage in the life span. Each event, however, does have certain tasks associated with it that must be achieved.

Ages and Stages Developmental Theories

The major tenets of Piaget, Freud, Erikson, and Kohlberg are discussed next; these are summarized in Table 4-1.

Piaget's Theory of Cognitive Development

Piaget's theory of cognitive development depicts age-related, sequential stages through which all developing children must progress to learn to think, reason, exercise judgment, and implement the cognitive skills (e.g., language development, problem solving, decision making, critical thinking, and oral and written communication) needed to successfully adapt to their environments.[1] Cognitive development is influenced by innate intellectual capacity, maturation of the nervous and endocrine systems, and environmental interactions during which sensory and motor input is experienced and processed. Piaget divides cognitive development into four periods: sensorimotor stage, preoperational stage, concrete operations stage, and formal operational stage.

TABLE 4-1	Summary of Ages and Stages Developmental Theories			
STAGE/AGE	**PIAGET'S COGNITIVE STAGES**	**FREUD'S PSYCHOSEXUAL STAGES**	**ERIKSON'S PSYCHOSOCIAL STAGES**	**KOHLBERG'S MORAL JUDGMENT STAGES**
1. Infancy Birth to 1 year	**Sensorimotor** (birth to 2 years): begins to acquire language Task: Object permanence	**Oral:** pleasure from exploration with mouth and through sucking Task: Weaning	**Trust vs. Mistrust** Task: Trust Socializing agent: Mothering person Central process: Mutuality Ego quality: Hope	**Preconventional Level:** **1. Morality Stage:** Avoid punishment by not breaking rules of authority figures
2. Toddler 1 to 3 years	**Sensorimotor:** continues **Preoperational** (2 to 7 years) begins: use of representational thought Task: Use language and mental images to think and communicate	**Anal:** control of elimination Task: Toilet training	**Autonomy vs. Shame and Doubt** Task: Autonomy Socializing agent: Parents Central process: Imitation Ego quality: Self-control and willpower	
3. Preschool 3 to 6 years	**Preoperational:** continues	**Phallic:** attracted to opposite-sex parent Task: Resolve Oedipus/Electra complex	**Initiative vs. Guilt** Task: Initiative and moral Socializing agents: Parents Central process: Identification Ego quality: Direction, purpose, and conscience, responsibility	**2. Individualism, Instrumental Purpose, and Exchange Stage:** "Right" is relative, follow rules when in own interest
4. School Age 6 to 12 years	**Preoperational:** continues **Concrete Operations** (7 to 12 years) begins: engage in inductive reasoning and concrete problem solving Task: Learn concepts of conservation and reversibility	**Latency:** identification with same-sex parent Task: Identify with same-sex parent, and test and compare own capabilities with peer norms	**Industry vs. Inferiority** Task: Industry, self-assurance, self-esteem Socializing agents: Teachers and peers Central process: Education Ego quality: Competence	**Conventional Level:** **3. Mutual Expectations, Relationships, and Conformity to Moral Norms Stage:** Need to be "good" in own and others' eyes, believe in rules and regulations

TABLE 4-1 Summary of Ages and Stages Developmental Theories *continued*

STAGE/AGE	PIAGET'S COGNITIVE STAGES	FREUD'S PSYCHOSEXUAL STAGES	ERIKSON'S PSYCHOSOCIAL STAGES	KOHLBERG'S MORAL JUDGMENT STAGES
5. Adolescence 12 to 18 years	**Formal Operations** (12 years to adulthood): engage in abstract reasoning and analytical problem solving Task: Develop a workable philosophy of life	**Genital:** develop sexual relationships Task: Establish meaningful relationship for lifelong pairing	**Identity vs. Role Confusion** Task: Self-identity and concept Socializing agents: Society of peers	**4. Social System and Conscience Stage:** Uphold laws because they are fixed social duties Central process: Role experimentation and peer pressure; Ego quality: Fidelity and devotion to others, personal and sociocultural values
6. Young Adult 18 to 30 years	**Formal Operations:** continues		**Intimacy vs. Isolation** Task: Intimacy Socializing agent: Close friends, partners, lovers, spouse Central process: Mutuality among peers Ego quality: Intimate affiliation and love	**Postconventional Level: 5. Social Contract or Utility and Individual Rights Stage:** Uphold laws in the interest of the greatest good for the greatest number; uphold laws that protect universal rights

TABLE 4-1   Summary of Ages and Stages Developmental Theories *continued*

STAGE/AGE	PIAGET'S COGNITIVE STAGES	FREUD'S PSYCHOSEXUAL STAGES	ERIKSON'S PSYCHOSOCIAL STAGES	KOHLBERG'S MORAL JUDGMENT STAGES
7. Early Middle Age 30 to 50 years			**Generativity vs. Stagnation** (30 to 65 years) Task: Generativity Socializing agent: Spouse, partner, children, sociocultural norms Central process: Creativity and person-environment fit Ego quality: Productivity, perseverance, charity, and consideration	6. **Universal Ethical Principles Stage:** Support universal moral principles regardless of the price for doing so
8. Late Middle Age 50 to 70 years			**Generativity vs. Stagnation** continues	
9. Late Adult 70 years to death			Ego Integrity vs. Despair (65 years to death) Task: Ego integrity Socializing agent: Significant others Central process: Introspection Ego quality: Wisdom	

Freud's Psychoanalytic Theory of Personality Development

Sigmund Freud contended that human behaviour is motivated by psychodynamic forces within an individual's unconscious mind.[2] Driven to act by these internal forces, individuals repeatedly interact with the external environment to develop their personality and psychosexual identity.

Personality

Personality, according to Freud, consists of three components with distinctly separate functions: id, ego, and superego. The id, evident at birth, is inborn, unconscious, and driven by biological instincts and urges to seek immediate gratification of needs such as hunger, thirst, and physical comfort. The ego is conscious, rational, and emerges during the first year of life as infants begin to test the limits of the world around them. The ego seeks realistic and acceptable ways to meet needs. The superego, appearing in early childhood, is the internalization of the moral values formed as children interact with their parents and significant others.

Freud believed individuals experience an ongoing struggle among the id, ego, and superego. Achieving a balance among the three, however, is prerequisite to the development of socially acceptable behaviour and an integrated personality.

Psychosexual Stages

Freud perceived the desire to satisfy biological needs, primarily sexual, as the major drive governing human behaviour. At different psychosexual developmental stages, individuals experience tension in a specific body region that prompts them to seek gratification and to resolve associated conflicts. If an individual's needs are met during a given stage and conflicts are resolved, development proceeds to the next stage, and healthy integration of the developing personality will occur. If resolution of the conflict does not occur, however, the individual will become fixated at that stage, and personality and psychosexual identity will be arrested or impaired. Freud identified five psychosexual stages of development: oral, anal, phallic, latency, and genital.

Erikson's Epigenetic Theory of Personality

The most frequently used theory of personality development is Erik Erikson's epigenetic theory, which is based on the biological concept that all growing organisms have an inherent plan of development.[3] Each part of a growing entity has a designated time of ascendancy and forms the basis for growth of the next part until the functional whole is fully developed. Erikson's theory was built on Freud's theory of personality but goes beyond it by depicting personality development as a passage through eight sequential stages of ego development from infancy through old age.

According to Erikson, individuals must master and resolve, to some extent, a core conflict/crisis during each stage by integrating their needs and skills with the social and cultural demands and expectations of their environment. Moving on to another stage is dependent on the resolution of the core conflict of the preceding stage. No core conflict is ever completely mastered; rather, a conflict can present itself in a new form, which provides new opportunities to resolve the core conflict. Thus, the potential for further development and refinement always exists. The eight stages are trust versus mistrust, autonomy versus shame and doubt, initiative versus guilt, industry versus inferiority, identity versus role confusion, intimacy versus isolation, generativity versus stagnation, and ego integrity versus despair.

Kohlberg's Theory of Moral Development

The basic premise of Kohlberg's theory of moral development is that when a conflict occurs among any of several universal values (e.g., punishment, affection, authority, truth, law, life, liberty, and justice), the moral choice that must be made and justified requires cognitive and systematic problem-solving capabilities, which constitute moral reasoning.[4] The individual's moral reasoning and associated behaviours parallel the development of cognitive behaviour primarily. According to Kohlberg, moral development is contingent upon children's ability to learn and internalize parental and societal rules and standards, to develop the ability to empathize with others' responses, and to form their own standards of conduct. Moral development progresses through three levels, with two distinct stages per level for a total of six stages.

DEVELOPMENTAL STAGES, TASKS, AND LIFE EVENTS

The following section gives a composite sketch of the developmental tasks, life events, and transitions for each major theory of development.

Developmental Tasks of Infants (Birth to 1 Year)

Infancy is a period of dramatic and rapid physical, motor, cognitive, emotional, and social growth, which marks it as one of the most critical periods of growth and development. During the first year of life, infants change from totally helpless, dependent newborns to unique individuals who actively interact with their environments and form meaningful relationships with significant others. A list of key gross and fine motor, language, and sensory milestones associated with this period can be found in Table 4-2. Developmental tasks that must be achieved during infancy are to develop:

1. A basic, relative sense of trust.
2. A sense of self as dependent but separate from others, particularly the mother.
3. A desire for affection and a response from others, particularly the mother.
4. A preverbal communication system, including emotional expression, to communicate needs and desires.
5. Conceptual abilities and a language system.
6. Fine and gross motor skills, particularly eye-hand coordination and balance.
7. A need to explore and recognize the immediate environment.
8. Object permanence.

Developmental Tasks of Toddlers (1 to 3 Years)

The toddler period is one of steadily increasing motor development and control, intense activity and discovery, rapid language development, increasingly independent behaviours, and marked personality development. Key gross and fine motor, language, and sensory milestones associated with the toddler period can be found in Table 4-3. The principal developmental tasks that must be mastered during the toddler stage are to:

1. Interact with others less egocentrically.
2. Acquire socially acceptable behaviours.
3. Differentiate self from others.

4. Tolerate separation from key socializing agents such as the parent(s) or caregiver(s).
5. Develop increasing verbal communication skills.
6. Tolerate delayed gratification of wants and desires.
7. Control bodily functions (toilet training) and begin self-care (feed and dress self almost completely).

Developmental Tasks of Preschoolers (3 to 6 Years)

During the preschool period, children are focused on developing initiative and purpose. Play provides the means for physical, mental, and social development and becomes the "work" of children as they begin to understand, adjust to, and work out experiences with their environment. Key gross and fine motor, language, and sensory milestones associated with the preschool period can be found in Table 4-4. Among the principal developmental tasks that must be mastered during the preschool stage are to:

1. Develop a sense of separateness as an individual.
2. Develop a sense of initiative.
3. Use language for increasing social interaction.
4. Interact in socially acceptable ways with others.
5. Develop a conscience.
6. Identify sex role and function.
7. Develop readiness for school.

Developmental Tasks of School-Age Children (6 to 12 Years)

With a well-developed sense of trust, autonomy, and initiative, school-age children increasingly reduce their dependency on the family as their primary socializing agents and move to the broader world of peers (primarily same-sex peers) in their neighbourhoods and schools, as well as to teachers and adult leaders of social, sports, and religious groups. Key gross and fine motor, language, and sensory milestones associated with this period can be found in Table 4-5.

The principal developmental tasks that must be mastered during the school-age stage are to:

1. Become a more active, cooperative, and responsible family member.

TABLE 4-2 Growth and Development During Infancy

AGE	GROSS MOTOR	FINE MOTOR	LANGUAGE	SENSORY
Birth to 1 Month	• Assumes tonic neck posture • When prone lifts and turns head	• Holds hands in fist • Draws arms and legs to body	• Cries	• Comforts with holding and touch • Looks at faces • Follows objects when in line of vision • Alert to high-pitched voices • Smiles
2 to 4 Months	• Can raise head and shoulders when prone to 45°–90°; supports self on forearms • Rolls from back to side	• Hands mostly open • Looks at and plays with fingers • Grasps and tries to reach objects	• Vocalizes when talked to; coos, babbles • Laughs aloud • Squeals	• Smiles • Follows objects 180° • Turns head when hears voices or sounds
4 to 6 Months	• Turns from stomach to back and then back to stomach • When pulled to sitting, almost no head lag • By 6 months can sit on floor with hands forward for support	• Can hold feet and put in mouth • Can hold bottle • Can grasp rattle and other small objects • Puts objects in mouth	• Squeals	• Watches a falling object • Responds to sounds

TABLE 4-2	Growth and Development During Infancy *continued*			
AGE	**GROSS MOTOR**	**FINE MOTOR**	**LANGUAGE**	**SENSORY**
6 to 8 Months	• Puts full weight on legs when held in standing position • Can sit without support • Bounces when held in a standing position	• Transfers objects from one hand to the other • Can feed self a cookie • Can bang two objects together	• Babbles vowel-like sounds, "ooh" or "aah" • Imitation of speech sounds ("mama," "dada") beginning • Laughs aloud	• Responds by looking and smiling • Recognizes own name
8 to 10 Months	• Crawls on all fours or uses arms to pull body along floor • Can pull self to sitting • Can pull self to standing	• Beginning to use thumb-finger grasp • Dominant hand use • Has good hand-mouth coordination	• Responds to verbal commands • May say one word in addition to "mama" and "dada"	• Recognizes sounds
10 to 12 Months	• Can sit down from standing • Walks around room holding onto objects • Can stand alone	• Picks up and drops objects • Can put small objects into toys or containers through holes • Turns many pages in a book at one time • Picks up small objects	• Understands "no" and other simple commands • Learns one or two other words • Imitates speech sounds • Speaks gibberish	• Follows fast-moving objects • Indicates wants • Likes to play imitative games such as patty cake and peek-a-boo

TABLE 4-3 Growth and Development During Toddlerhood

AGE	GROSS MOTOR	FINE MOTOR	LANGUAGE	SENSORY
12 to 15 Months	• Can walk alone well • Can crawl up stairs	• Can feed self with cup and spoon • Puts raisins into a bottle • May hold crayon or pencil and scribble • Builds a tower of two cubes	• Says four to six words	• Binocular vision is developed • Visual acuity 20/40
18 Months	• Runs, falling often • Can jump in place • Can walk up stairs holding on • Plays with push and pull toys	• Can build a tower of three to four cubes • Can use a spoon	• Says 10 or more words • Points to objects or body parts when asked	
24 Months	• Can walk up and down stairs • Can kick a ball • Can ride a tricycle	• Can draw a circle • Tries to dress self	• Talks a lot • Approximately 300-word vocabulary • Understands commands • Knows first name, refers to self • Verbalizes toilet needs	
30 Months	• Throws a ball • Jumps with both feet • Can stand on one foot for a few minutes	• Can build a tower of eight blocks • Can use crayons • Learning to use scissors	• Knows first and last name • Knows the name of one colour • Can sing • Expresses needs • Uses pronouns appropriately	

2. Learn the rules and norms of a widening social, religious, and cultural environment.
3. Increase psychomotor and cognitive skills needed for participation in games and working with others.
4. Master concepts of time, conservation, and reversibility, as well as oral and written communication skills.
5. Win approval from peers and adults.
6. Obtain a place in a peer group.
7. Build a sense of industry, accomplishment, self-assurance, and self-esteem.
8. Develop a positive self-concept.
9. Exchange affection with family and friends without seeking an immediate payback.
10. Adopt moral standards for behaviour.

Developmental Tasks of Adolescents (12 to 18 Years)

The adolescent period is one of struggle and sometimes turmoil as the adolescent strives to develop a personal identity and achieve a successful transition from childhood to adulthood. The biological, social, cognitive, and psychological changes associated with adolescence are the most complex and profound of any developmental period. Physical and sexual maturity are reached during adolescence, with girls experiencing puberty and a growth spurt earlier than boys. In addition, adolescents develop increasingly sophisticated cognitive and interpersonal skills, test out adult roles and behaviours, and begin to explore educational and occupational opportunities for their future. Key gross and fine motor, language, and sensory milestones associated with this period can be found in Table 4-6.

The principal developmental tasks that must be mastered during the adolescent stage are to:

1. Develop self-identity and appreciate own achievements and worth.
2. Form close relationships with peers.
3. Gradually grow independent from parents.
4. Evolve own value system and integrate self-concept and values with those of peers and society.
5. Develop academic and vocational skills and related social, work, and civic sensitivities.
6. Develop analytic thinking.
7. Adjust to rapid physical and sexual changes.
8. Develop a sexual identity and role.

9. Develop skill in relating to people from different backgrounds.
10. Consider and possibly choose a career.

Developmental Tasks of Young Adults (18 to 30 Years)

Young adulthood is a time of separation and independence from the family and of new commitments, responsibilities, and accountability in social, work, and home relationships and roles. Individuals are exposed to more diverse people, situations, and values and, in recent decades, to a more rapidly changing socioeconomic and technological environment than ever before.

Among the developmental tasks that the young adult must achieve are to:

1. Establish friendships and a social group.
2. Grow independent of parental care and home.
3. Set up and manage one's own household.
4. Form an intimate affiliation with another and choose a mate.
5. Learn to love, cooperate with, and commit to a life partner.
6. Develop a personal style of living (e.g., shared or single).
7. Choose and begin to establish a career or vocation.
8. Assume roles and responsibility in professional, political, religious, and civic organizations.
9. Learn to manage life stresses accompanying change.
10. Develop a realistic outlook and acceptance of cultural, religious, social, and political diversity.
11. Form a meaningful philosophy of life and implement it in home, employment, and community settings.
12. Begin a parental role for one's own or life partner's children, or for young people in a broader social framework; for example, teaching, health care, or volunteer work.

Developmental Tasks of Early Middle Adulthood (30 to 50 Years)

Middle age, spanning the ages of 30 to 70 years, is the longest stage of the life cycle and is now often divided into early and late middle adulthood.

TABLE 4-4	Growth and Development During Preschool Years		
AGE	**GROSS MOTOR**	**FINE MOTOR**	**LANGUAGE**
3 to 6 Years	• Can ride a bike with training wheels • Can throw a ball overhand • Skips and hops on one foot • Can climb well • Can jump rope	• Can draw a six-part person • Can use scissors • Can draw a circle, square, or cross • Likes art projects, likes to paste and string beads • Can button • Learns to tie and buckle shoes • Can brush teeth	• Language skills are well developed with the child able to understand and speak clearly • Vocabulary grows to over 2,000 words • Talks endlessly and asks questions
			SENSORY • Visual acuity is well developed • Focused on learning letters and numbers

TABLE 4-5	Growth and Development During School-Age Years		
AGE	**GROSS MOTOR**	**FINE MOTOR**	**LANGUAGE**
6 to 12 Years	• Can use in-line skates or ice skates • Able to ride two-wheeler • Plays baseball	• Can put models together • Likes crafts • Enjoys board games, plays cards	• Vocabulary increases • Language abilities continue to develop
			SENSORY • Reading • Able to concentrate on activities for longer periods

TABLE 4-6	Growth and Development During Adolescence		
AGE	**GROSS MOTOR**	**FINE MOTOR**	**LANGUAGE**
12 to 19 Years	• Muscles continue to develop • At times awkward, with some lack of coordination	• Well-developed skills	• Vocabulary is fully developed
			SENSORY • Development is complete

During early middle adulthood, individuals experience relatively good physical and mental health; settle into their careers, lifestyles, relationships (married, parental, partnered, single), political, civic, social, professional, and religious activities; and achieve maximum influence over themselves and their environments. Individuals also experience a need to contribute to the next generation, such as raising children or producing something socially useful to others.

Among the developmental tasks that must be achieved during early middle adulthood are to:

1. Attain a desired level of achievement and status in career.
2. Review, evaluate, refine, and redirect career goals consistent with one's personal value system.
3. Learn and refine competencies in personal and career interests.
4. Manage life stresses accompanying change.
5. Develop mature relationships with life partner and significant others.
6. Participate in social, professional, political, religious, and civic activities.
7. Cope with an empty nest and possibly a refilled nest.
8. Adjust to aging parents and help plan for when they will need assistance.
9. Enjoy hobbies and leisure activities and develop ones for postretirement.
10. Plan for personal, financial, and social aspects of retirement.

Developmental Tasks of Late Middle Adulthood (50 to 70 Years)

Many individuals during late middle adulthood may be diagnosed with a chronic health problem, such as arthritis, cardiovascular disease, cancer, diabetes, or asthma. In addition, women generally experience a decrease in estrogen and progesterone production and undergo menopause during their late 40s or early 50s. Changes also occur during late middle adulthood in work, family, social, and civic areas.

A variety of developmental tasks must be achieved by individuals during late middle adulthood. Among these tasks are to:

1. Manage life stresses accompanying change.
2. Maintain interest in current political, cultural, and scientific advances, trends, and issues.

3. Maintain affiliations with social, religious, professional, civic, or political organizations.
4. Adapt to health status changes that accompany aging.
5. Continue current activities and develop new interests and leisure activities that can be pursued consistent with changing abilities.
6. Adjust to increased interaction and time spent with life partner without the presence of children.
7. Develop supportive, interdependent relationships with adult children.
8. Help elderly parents and relatives cope with lifestyle changes (may include providing a home for them).
9. Adjust to possible or actual loss of parents, life partner, elder family members, and friends through death or their decreasing abilities to maintain independent living and self-care.
10. Prepare for and adjust to changes in roles, finances, or lifestyles resulting from retirement.

Developmental Tasks of Late Adulthood (70 Years to Death)

Individuals in late adulthood widely diverge in how they physically and emotionally age and how they confront and adjust to the changes associated with this stage. People who have accomplished the developmental tasks of middle adulthood are comfortable with the achievement of their life goals and the independence from the workplace, and also welcome the time to pursue leisure activities. Although there is an inevitable loss of work-related status and social outlets, and a decrease in income, in physical or cognitive capabilities, in resistance to illness, and in recuperative powers, most individuals adjust to these changes with equanimity. Indeed, a high percentage manage their activities of daily living independently and in their own homes, enjoying new roles and giving advice and moral support to members of younger generations, and sharing leisure activities with friends in their own age group.

Conducting a life review is an important developmental task during late adulthood. This task entails reviewing the experiences, relationships, and events of your life as a whole, viewing successes and failures from the perspective of age, and accepting your life choices and their outcomes. Individuals who successfully complete the life review task feel that they have been a meaningful part of human history, have integrity, and are able to face death with equanimity. If individuals fail to achieve the life review developmental task, a sense of hopelessness, resentment, futility, despair, fear of death, and clinical depression may result. Among the developmental tasks that must be achieved during late adulthood are to:

1. Accept and adjust to changes in health status.
2. Maintain and develop new activities that contribute to a continuing sense of usefulness and self-worth, enhance self-image, and help retain functional capacities.
3. Develop new roles in family as eldest member.
4. Establish affiliation with own age group.
5. Accept and adjust to social, financial, and lifestyle changes.
6. Adapt to loss of life partner, family members, and friends.
7. Work on life review.
8. Prepare for inevitability of own death.

REFERENCES

[1] Piaget, J. (1952). *The origins of intelligence in children.* New York: International Universities Press.
[2] Freud, S. (1946). *The ego and the mechanism of defense.* New York: International Universities Press.
[3] Erikson, E. (1974). *Dimensions of a new identity.* New York: W. W. Norton.
[4] Kohlberg, L. (1981). *The philosophy of moral development: Moral stages and the idea of justice.* New York: Harper & Row.

5

Cultural Assessment

Canada is known around the world as a multicultural society whose ethnocultural makeup has been shaped by years of immigration. In addition to Aboriginal people (First Nations, Inuit, and Métis), waves of new peoples arriving from a range of countries have helped populate this vast country from coast to coast. Nurses working anywhere in Canada will need to be culturally competent and will benefit from the many rewards of working with clients from diverse cultural backgrounds.

CULTURALLY COMPETENT CARE

The Canadian Nurses Association espouses cultural competence and defines it as "the application of knowledge, skill, attitudes and personal attributes required by nurses to provide appropriate care and services in relation to cultural characteristics of their clients (individuals, families, groups, and the population at large). Cultural competence includes valuing diversity, knowing about cultural mores and traditions of the population being served and being sensitive to these while caring for the individual."[1] Nurses who are culturally competent will deliver care that is characterized by cultural safety— care that is based on recognition and respect rather than on power inequities, or individual or institutional discrimination.

The Canadian health care system is one of cultural diversity, consisting of patients and health care providers from different combinations of ethnic (e.g., Arabic), racial (e.g., Caucasian), national (e.g., Swiss), religious (e.g., Sikh), generational (e.g., grandparent), marital status (e.g., single), socioeconomic (e.g., middle class), occupational (e.g., accountant), preference in life partner (e.g., heterosexual), health status (e.g., handicapped), and cultural orientations coexisting in a given location. Cultural diversity should be viewed as an opportunity for health care professionals to experience the benefits of exchange and cooperation across cultures.

Culturally competent nursing care is provided by nurses who use research and cross-cultural nursing care models (nursing care provided within the cultural context of patients who are members of a culture or subculture different from that of the nurse) to identify patients' health care needs. The process of culturally competent nursing care consists of: (1) eliciting patient statements of cultural values and beliefs so that culturally sensitive approaches to care can be provided; (2) recognizing and understanding the behaviours and responses of different cultural groups to health and illness; (3) obtaining information on ethnic variations and on normal racial growth patterns to assist in identifying abnormal patterns and designing appropriate interventions; and (4) using the ethic of cultural relativism, which is the belief that no culture is either inferior or superior to another, that behaviour must be evaluated in relation to the cultural context in which it occurs, and that respect, equality, and justice are basic rights for all racial, ethnic, subcultural, and cultural groups.

BASIC CONCEPTS ASSOCIATED WITH CULTURALLY COMPETENT ASSESSMENTS

Culture and Subculture

Culture is a learned and socially transmitted orientation and way of life of a group of people.

Subculture refers to membership in a smaller group within a larger culture. These smaller groups possess many of the values, beliefs, and customs of the larger culture but have unique characteristics in relation to age, education, marital status, preference in life partner, generational placement, occupation, socioeconomic level, health status, or religion.

Racial Groups and Ethnic Groups

Race classifies individuals based on the shared traits of skin tone, facial features, and body build, all of which are inherited from biological ancestors and are usually sufficiently obvious to warrant a member as being part of a specific racial group.

Ethnic group members share a unique national or regional origin and social, cultural, and linguistic heritage.

Minority Groups

Minority group members are individuals who are considered by themselves or by others to be members of a minority because they have a different racial, cultural, ethnic, gender, sexual orientation, or different socioeconomic level than do members of the dominant cultural group.

Values, Norms, and Value Orientations

Cultures and subcultures have a fundamental set of principles, known as values, that govern how each group member thinks, acts, and responds to the internal and external environment. Cultural values tend to be acquired subconsciously during the process of enculturation and are usually a fundamental, often unchanging, set of principles that serve to build an individual's beliefs, customs, goals, and aspirations.

Cultural norms are the often unwritten but generally understood prescriptions for acceptable behaviour in the various situations that group members encounter in their daily lives.

All cultures have a fundamental set of values and concurrent value orientations; that is, patterned principles that provide order and direction to individuals' thoughts and behaviours and help solve commonly occurring human problems.

Beliefs

Cultural beliefs consist of the explanatory ideas and knowledge that members of a culture have about various aspects of the world, based on the group's cultural values and norms.

Customs and Rituals

Customs are frequent or common practices carried out by tradition and include communication patterns, family and kinship relations, work patterns, dietary and religious practices, and health behaviours. Cultural rituals are highly structured and prescribed patterns of behaviour used by a cultural group to respond to or in anticipation of specific life events such as birth, death, illness, healing, marriage, and worship.

Cultural Assessment

To guide your cultural health assessment of patients and families, refer to Table 5-1.

TABLE 5-1 Echols-Armstrong Cultural Assessment Tool (EACAT)

Directions: The questions in bold print are recommended for use during the initial contact with the patient. The remaining items can be used if time permits or if examples are needed to prompt the patient's replies. If a long-term health care relationship or prolonged hospitalization and/or home care is anticipated, it is advisable to complete all remaining questions during subsequent encounters.

1. **ETHNIC GROUP AFFILIATION AND RACIAL BACKGROUND**
   a. **Would you tell me how long you have lived here in _____?**

| TABLE 5-1 | Echols-Armstrong Cultural Assessment Tool (EACAT) *continued* |

    b. Where are you from originally? (or Where were you born? or Where were your parents or grandparents born and raised?)

    c. With which particular ethnic group would you say you identify? (Chinese, Vietnamese, Arab, Black, Filipino, Aboriginal, etc.) **How closely do you identify with this ethnic group or combination of ethnic groups?**

    d. Where have you lived and when? What health problems did you experience or were you exposed to when you lived in each place? What helped you recover from each of the health problems identified?

2. **MAJOR BELIEFS AND VALUES**

    a. What is your primary **time orientation:** past, present, or future? What do you believe is the **basic nature of human beings:** basically good; evil but can be perfected; good and evil requiring self-control; or neither good nor evil? What is the primary **purpose of life:** just to be whatever one is; to be who one is while striving for self-improvement; or to exist to be constantly active and achieving, striving for excellence? What is the **purpose of human relations?** Whose goals should take precedence: the family, the community, or the individual? What should be the **relationship between human beings and nature:** humans dominate and control nature; live in harmony with nature; or be subjugated to nature with no control over it?

    b. Do you practise any special activities that are part of your cultural traditions?

    c. What are your values, beliefs, customs, and practices related to education, work, and leisure?

3. **HEALTH BELIEFS AND PRACTICES**

    a. What does being healthy mean to you?

    b. What do you believe promotes being healthy?

    c. What do you do to help you stay healthy? (hygiene, immunizations, self-care practices such as OTC drugs, herbal drinks, special foods, wearing charms)

    d. What does being ill or sick mean to you?

    e. What do you believe causes illness? What do you believe caused your illness?

    f. What do you usually do when you are sick or not feeling well? (self-care and home remedies, herbal remedies, healing rituals, wearing medals or charms, prayers, rely on folk healers)

    g. When you are sick or not feeling well, who do you go to for help? How helpful are they and for what type of problems?

    h. Who determines when you are and when you are not sick? Who cares for you at home when you are sick? **Who do you want to be with when you are sick?** Who do you want to be with you when you are in the hospital?

    i. Who in your family is primarily responsible for making health care decisions (such as when to go to someone outside the family for help, where to go, who to see, what help to accept), **who should be taught how to deal with your** (or your loved one's) **specific health problems** (or what can be taught about how to prevent problems)?

TABLE 5-1   Echols-Armstrong Cultural Assessment Tool (EACAT) *continued*

    j. What do you believe about mental illness, chronic disease, handicapping conditions, pain, dying, and death?

    k. Are there any cultural or ethnic sanctions or restrictions (related to the expression of emotions and feelings, privacy, exposure of body parts, response to illness, certain types of surgery, or certain types of medical treatments) **that you want to or must observe?**

    l. By whom do you prefer to have your health and medical care provided: a nurse, physician, or other health care provider? Do you prefer they have the same cultural background (or be the same age) **or gender as your own?**

4. LANGUAGE BARRIERS AND COMMUNICATION STYLES

    a. What language(s) or dialect(s) do you speak or read? Which one do you speak most frequently? Where? (home, work, with friends) **In which language are you most comfortable communicating?**

    b. How well do you understand spoken and written English? French? **Do you need an interpreter when discussing health care information and treatments?** Is there a relative or friend you would prefer to have interpret? Is there anyone you do not want to interpret?

    c. Are there special ways of showing respect or disrespect in your culture?

    d. Are there any cultural preferences or restrictions related to touching, social distance, making eye contact, or other verbal or nonverbal behaviours when communicating?

    e. Are there culturally appropriate forms of greeting, parting, initiating or terminating an exchange, topic restrictions, or times to visit?

5. ROLE OF THE FAMILY, SPOUSAL RELATIONSHIP, AND PARENTING STYLES

    a. What is the composition of your family? Who is considered to be a member of your family? (Include a genogram and an ecomap if needed.)

    b. With what ethnic group(s) does your family as a whole (parents, aunts, uncles, cousins) **identify?** How do their ethnic identity and traditions affect the decision-making processes of your own family? **How does their ethnic identity, and which of their ethnic traditions, do you think most affect their health status?**

    c. Which of your relatives live nearby? With which of your family members and relatives do you interact the most often?

    d. How do each of your family members, relatives, and you and your significant other interact in relation to chores, mealtimes, child care, recreation, and other family-oriented responsibilities? Are you satisfied with these interactional patterns?

    e. What are the major events that are most important to your family (marriage, birth, holidays, religious ceremonies), and how are they celebrated?

    f. What are your family's goals for the health and well-being of the family as a group? What dreams do they have for the family's future? Do they work together as a family unit or individually to achieve these goals and dreams? What barriers do they see that might inhibit the accomplishment of these goals and dreams?

TABLE 5-1	**Echols-Armstrong Cultural Assessment Tool (EACAT)** *continued*

g. **In what ways do your family members believe the nurse, physician, and other health care practitioners can help the family members achieve their goals and dreams for health and well-being of the family?**

h. **With what social (church, community, work, recreation) groups does your family interact, and what is the nature of their social contact and social support?**

i. Are there special beliefs and customs practised by your family related to marriage, conception, pregnancy, childbirth, breast feeding, baptism, child care (including attitude toward children, discipline, showing affection), puberty, separation, divorce, health, illness, and death?

j. **What are the family members' health and social history, including health habits, recent major stress events, work patterns, participation in religion, community activities, and recreation patterns?**

6. **RELIGIOUS INFLUENCES OR SPECIAL RITUALS (See Chapter 6).**

7. **DIETARY PRACTICES (Chapter 7).**

REFERENCES

[1]Canadian Nurses Association. *Position statement: Promoting culturally competent care.* Retrieved June 11, 2006, from http://www.cna-nurses.ca/CNA/documents/pdf/publications/PS73_Promoting_Culturally_Competent_Care_March_2004_e.pdf

6

Spiritual Assessment

Nursing assessment of the spiritual aspects of health and illness is an important element of providing care that is accurate and relevant in any patient care situation. There are many proposed links between spirituality and such outcomes as quality of life, general health status, abilities to find meaning and to cope with difficult situations, and dealing with death and dying issues.

SPIRITUALITY AND RELIGION

There is a range of definitions of spirituality; however, most involve a relationship to something that is intensely personal and goes beyond the physiological and psychological to the existential search for meaning and purpose of life and all of its complexities. Spirituality generally integrates values and ultimate concern with oneself, one's relationship with a higher power, and the surrounding environment. Spirituality involves the search for the sacred, such as a divine being, or the ultimate reality or truth.

By contrast, religion is an organized system of beliefs usually centred around the worship of a supernatural force or being, which in turn defines the self and the self's purpose in life. Religion exists in group form over time and is a tradition of shared beliefs. Although many variances may exist among believers within any given religion, there are common threads uniting the followers.

HOLISTIC HEALTH AND SPIRITUALITY

Nurses meet people from a range of religions, each having their specific spiritual tenets, rites and rituals, and views on health and illness. Table 6-1 illustrates how certain religions view a range of events from birth to death. *These descriptions provide context and are in no way meant to be prescriptive and do not represent the actual practices and beliefs of any particular person.*

ROLE OF THE NURSE IN SPIRITUAL CARE

Nurses have a vital role to play in the spiritual care of patients by:

1. Performing a spiritual assessment. (It is impossible to know if a patient is in a state of spiritual distress or spiritual well-being unless an assessment is done.)
2. Establishing priorities based on the assessment.
3. Planning, implementing, and evaluating appropriate strategies for spiritual care.

Spiritual Assessment

The purpose of a spiritual history is to collect information in order to understand the patient's religious or spiritual beliefs and practices, if any.

1. The spiritual assessment should obtain the following information: the nature of the patient's spiritual beliefs; the nature of the patient's spiritual support, how the patient's spiritual beliefs affect the treatment of health and illness, the patient's state of spiritual well-being or spiritual distress.
2. Begin the interview with the physical history of the patient. Move on to the psychological history and end with spiritual history.

TABLE 6-1	Religions and Health Care				
RELIGION	**JUDAISM**	**ISLAM**	**ROMAN CATHOLIC/ORTHODOX**		**PROTESTANT**
Description	A monotheistic religion that believes that God (Yahweh) has chosen the Jewish people and made a covenant with them to protect and preserve them if they follow God's law.	A monotheistic religion following the teachings of the Prophet Mohammed.	A monotheistic religion and an offshoot of Judaism. Catholics believe that Jesus is the son of God, that Jesus died on the cross to serve as a sacrifice for the sins of humanity, that Jesus was resurrected from the dead, and that God exists in three forms: God (Father), Jesus (Son), and the Holy Spirit.		A monotheistic religion emphasizing the Bible and the individual's interpretation of it.
Religious Leaders	Rabbi; cantor; mohel	Imam	Pope; bishop; priest; monk; nun		Priest; minister; pastor
Holy Books	Torah; Bible	Koran	Bible		Bible
Holy Day of the Week	Friday from sundown until Saturday at sundown	Friday	Sunday		Sunday
Dietary Restrictions	Dietary rules are complex. Kosher food is prepared according to strict dietary laws, which prohibit pork and any other meat of an animal with a cloven hoof that chews a cud, as well as shellfish. Meat and dairy products must not be taken together.	Pork and products made from pork are forbidden. Alcohol and street drugs are also forbidden.	There is a tradition of not eating meat on Friday during Lent.		None.

TABLE 6-1 Religions and Health Care *continued*

RELIGION	JUDAISM	ISLAM	ROMAN CATHOLIC/ORTHODOX	PROTESTANT
Medical Treatment	Encouraged to seek medical care and treatment when needed as part of the religious obligation to take care of oneself.	Seeking medical treatment for illness is encouraged.	Medical treatment is encouraged, even obligated, as part of the obligation to care for oneself.	Same as Roman Catholicism although some sects may emphasize prayer and spiritual healing over medical treatment.
Birth Control	Birth control is allowed within marriage.	Teachings on birth control are contradictory, but in general, the use of birth control within marriage to control family size or to protect the health of the wife is permitted.	Birth control is forbidden. Natural family planning is permitted.	Birth control is permitted.
Abortion	Reluctantly permits abortion to preserve the life or welfare of the mother.	Forbidden after the fetus is "ensouled," either at 40 or 120 days of pregnancy. The father must give permission.	Abortion is prohibited.	Reluctantly allows abortion to preserve the health of the mother.
Observances at Birth	Circumcision is performed on all males, traditionally at the age of 8 days.	Upon birth, the baby's father, nearest male relative, or the mother whispers the central tenet of Islam into the baby's ear.	Baptism is a sacrament that should be performed shortly after birth.	Prayers and blessings are customary at the time of birth.

TABLE 6-1 Religions and Health Care *continued*

RELIGION	JUDAISM	ISLAM	ROMAN CATHOLIC/ORTHODOX	PROTESTANT
Withdrawal of Life Support	Active euthanasia and assisted suicide are forbidden. The withdrawal of life support is allowed only to reduce suffering.	Active euthanasia and assisted suicide are forbidden. The withdrawal of life support is allowd only to reduce suffering.	Suicide and active euthanasia are forbidden. The withdrawal of life support is allowed only to reduce suffering.	Suicide and active euthanasia are forbidden. The withdrawal of life support is allowed only to reduce suffering.
Death	Autopsies are controversial but permitted. Burial should be within 24 hr of death, though this may be extended to 48 hr in special circumstances. Cremation is forbidden.	There may be an expectation for the patient to say, or for a person to whisper, into the ear of the patient, "There is no God but Allah, and Mohammed is His Prophet." Men wash a man's body, and women wash a woman's body. Autopsies are permitted. Burial should be done without delay.	Prayers are common. Autopsies are permitted.	Prayers are common. Annointing the sick and laying on of hands may be practised. Bible readings are important to the dying person and the family.
Organ Donation	Organ donation and receiving transplanted organs are permitted.	Organ donation and receiving transplanted organs are permitted.	Organ donation is permitted.	Organ donation and receiving transplanted organs are permitted.

TABLE 6-1	Religions and Health Care *continued*	
RELIGION	**BUDDHISM**	**HINDUISM**
Description	A varied, intellectual, and psychological religion originating with the teachings of Siddhartha Gautama (Buddha).	A complex religion that embraces a variety of gods, practices, and spiritual paths.
Religious Leaders	Monk; nun	Priest; guru; sadhu; yogi
Holy Books	*The Tibetan Book of the Dead. The Buddha Dharma.*	*The Vedas; Upanishads; Bhagavad Gita.*
Holy Day of the Week	Every day is a holy day.	No particular holy day.
Dietary Restrictions	Some Buddhists, but not all, are vegetarians.	No beef is eaten, though milk and milk products, particularly yogurt, are staples.
Medical Treatment	Medical treatment that may enhance life is approved of.	Taking care of the body is an obligation. Medical treatment is encouraged when needed.
Birth Control	Birth control is discouraged.	Birth control is discouraged.
Abortion	Permission for abortion is circumstantial.	Abortion is discouraged.
Observances at Birth	From 1 month to 100 days of age, the parents of a new baby give thanks to the Buddha and dedicate the child to Buddha.	A naming ceremony is performed on the 10th to 11th day after birth.
Withdrawal of Life Support	Withdrawal of life support is permitted to reduce suffering.	Withdrawal of life support is permitted to reduce suffering.
Death	Cremation is common. After death, the body should not be disturbed with movement, talking, or crying.	Holy water is poured into the mouth of the dying person. The body should lie under a white sheet and be disturbed as little as possible. Embalming is forbidden. Autopsies are discouraged.
Organ Donation	Organ donation is controversial.	Traditional Hindu thought is against receiving organ donations.

3. Ask the patient whether he or she has an advance directive (such as a living will or durable medical power of attorney), which states what should be done if the patient is too ill to self-direct medical care.
4. Ask the patient whether he or she has signed an organ donor card or given any thought to donating organs or tissue after death.
5. Ask the patient if there are any spiritual or religious beliefs that will affect the health care received.
6. Observe the patient for clues about spiritual or religious beliefs. Does the patient have religious reading material, such as a Koran or religious pamphlets?
7. Ask the patient who should be notified in the event that there is a change in his or her condition. After noting this, ask if the patient also wants you to notify a place of worship or a specific religious leader.
8. If the patient is experiencing any threat to his or her health, ask whether the patient is thinking spiritually about the change.

Planning and Implementation

Once priorities have been established, you can plan and implement nursing interventions for the patient. The following interventions are appropriate for spiritual nursing care:

1. Listen actively.
2. Project an empathetic and warm response to the patient's concerns.
3. Display respect for the patient's spiritual beliefs by demonstrating tolerance for the patient's religious and spiritual beliefs.
4. Ensure patients are able to practise their religion or spirituality as much as possible.
5. Make appropriate referrals to the hospital chaplain or the patient's own spiritual or religious leader.

Evaluation

Evaluate the effect of your nursing interventions by observing the patient. Signs that the patient's spiritual distress has decreased include:

1. Acceptance of spiritual support from the source with which the patient feels most comfortable.

2. Decrease in crying, restlessness, and sleeplessness. There may even be a decrease in complaints of pain or the severity of pain.
3. Decrease in statements of worthlessness and hopelessness.
4. Verbalization of satisfaction with spiritual beliefs and the support and comfort they provide.

7

Nutritional Assessment

Nutrition, or the processes by which the body metabolizes and utilizes nutrients, affects every system in the body. Health care providers must also understand how the body digests and absorbs nutrients, the importance of meeting daily nutritional requirements, and how to assess the causes and results of an imbalance of nutrients. Psychological, social, environmental, financial, and cultural issues should also be considered during a nutritional assessment.

HEALTHY EATING IN CANADA— EATING WELL WITH CANADA'S FOOD GUIDE

Eating Well with Canada's Food Guide (Figure 7-1) provides Canadians with guidelines about the amount and type of food needed to meet nutrient requirements across the lifespan.

Canada's Food Guide emphasizes healthy eating "patterns" of food consumption over time rather than food choices made at any given meal. The guide includes key directional statements:

- Have vegetables and fruit more often than juice
- Eat at least one dark green and one orange vegetable every day (such as broccoli and carrots)
- Have at least half of daily grain products intake from whole grain
- Have meat alternatives such as beans, lentils, and tofu often
- Eat at least two Food Guide servings of fish every week
- Satisfy thirst with water
- Drink skim, 1% or 2% milk each day—drink fortified soy beverages if you do not drink milk

- Reduce the total amount of fat in the diet, especially saturated and trans fats, however, a small amount of unsaturated fat is recommended each day (30–45 ml for an adult)
- Lower salt and sugar intake
- Achieve and maintain a healthy body weight by enjoying regular physical activity—adults should get 30 to 60 minutes of moderate physical activity every day and children should get 90 minutes
- All women who could become pregnant should take 400 μg (0.4 mg) of folic acid a day to avoid neural tube defects in the unborn fetus
- All adults over 50 years of age should, in addition to following the Food Guide, take a daily vitamin D supplement of 10 μg (400 IU) a day

Eating Well with Canada's Food Guide does not make specific recommendations about the amount of calories that should be consumed per person per day. An individual who follows the guide will consume between 1800 and 3200 calories per day depending on the size and number of food portions eaten.

NUTRIENTS

Nutrients are the substances found in food that are nourishing and useful to the body. Carbohydrates, proteins, fats, vitamins, minerals, and water are the nutrients essential for life.

Carbohydrates, proteins, and fats supply the body with energy, which is measured in units called kilocalories (kcal), or calories. A calorie is the amount of heat required to raise 1g of water 1° centigrade. Health Canada does not stipulate

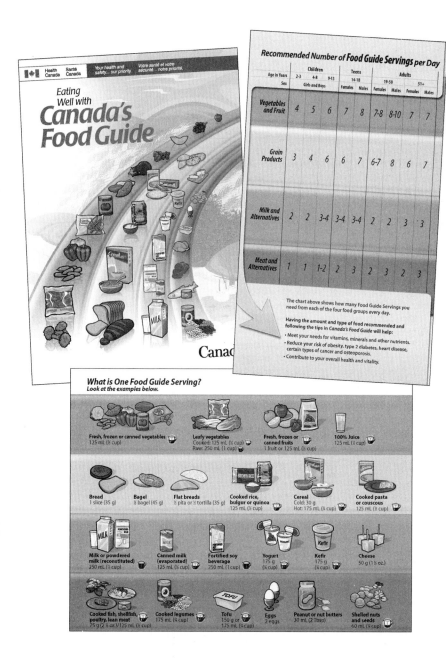

FIGURE 7-1 Eating Well with Canada's Food Guide, 2007

Source: http://www.hc-sc.gc.ca/fn-an/food-guide-aliment/hist/fg_history-histoire_ga_e.html#food, Health Canada, 2007. Reproduced with the permission of the Minister of Public Works and Government Services Canada, 2007.

daily calorie counts per se, but instead focuses on the portions and portion sizes.

Carbohydrates

The major source of energy for the various functions of the body is carbohydrates. Each gram of carbohydrates contains four calories. Adults require 45–65% of their daily caloric intake in the form of carbohydrates to prevent ketosis and protein breakdown of muscles.

Carbohydrates help form adenosine triphosphate (ATP), which is needed to transfer energy within the cells. Carbohydrates supply fibre and assist in the utilization of fat. The primary sources of carbohydrates are bread, potatoes, pasta, corn, rice, dried beans, and fruits.

Proteins

There are four calories in every gram of protein, but foods usually are a combination of protein and fat (meats, milk), or protein and carbohydrates (legumes).

Canada's Food Guide recommends that adults obtain 10–35% of their total daily caloric intake from protein. Protein is needed to manufacture and repair body tissue; it helps to maintain osmotic pressure within the cells, is a component of antibodies, and is ultimately a source of energy. The major sources of protein are meat, poultry, fish, eggs, tofu, cheese, and milk. Legumes (dried beans and peas) also are a good source of protein when eaten with corn or wheat.

Fats

Lipids, or fats, contain nine calories per gram. The Heart and Stroke Foundation of Canada recommends that fat consumption be reduced to 20–35% of total calories (about 45–75 g/day for a woman and about 60–105 g/day for a man).[1] Fats supply the essential fatty acids that form a part of the structure of all cells and help to lower serum cholesterol. The food sources of fat are animal fat (butter, shortening, lard) and vegetable fat (vegetable oil, margarine, and nuts). Saturated fats, which have been found to raise cholesterol levels, come from animal sources (butter, lard, fatty meats) and vegetable sources (coconut, palm, and partially hydrogenated oils that occur in some processed foods). Monounsaturated fats (olive and canola oils, avocado, nuts) help reduce low-density lipoproteins (LDLs) but do not reduce high-

density lipoproteins (HDLs). Cholesterol is a lipid contained only in animal products. Health Canada recommends the consumption of more polyunsaturated fat, especially Omega-3 fatty acids, monounsaturated fat, and lower amounts of saturated and trans fatty acids.

Triglycerides account for most of the lipids stored in the body's tissues. In the bloodstream, triglycerides produce energy for the body. An elevated triglyceride level occurs in hyperlipidemia, a risk factor for CAD.

Trans Fatty Acids (Trans Fats)

Trans fats are created when an unsaturated fat is hydrogenated to convert a liquid vegetable oil into a solid such as in the manufacturing of margarine. Health Canada has recognized that the consumption of trans fats can increase the risk of heart disease.[2]

Vitamins

Vitamins are organic substances needed to maintain the function of the body. They are not supplied by the body in sufficient amounts and must be obtained from dietary sources. Fat-soluble vitamins (vitamins A, D, E, and K) are stored in dietary fat and absorbed in the fat portions of the body's cells. Water-soluble vitamins include C, thiamine (B_1), riboflavin (B_2), niacin, pyridoxine (B_6), folacin (folate), cobalamin (B_{12}), pantothenic acid, and biotin. These vitamins are not stored in the body and are excreted in the urine. Various disease conditions occur when a vitamin source is lacking.

Minerals

Minerals are inorganic elements that help build body tissue and regulate body processes such as fluid and acid-base balance, nerve cell transmission, vitamin absorption, enzyme and hormonal activity, and muscle contractions. Minerals are divided into two classifications. Macrominerals, or major minerals, are needed by the body in large amounts (>100 mg/day). Microminerals, or trace minerals, are needed in smaller amounts by the body (<15 mg/day).

Water

Water accounts for 50–60% of the body's weight. The daily amount needed depends on the size of the person, the climate, and the amount of activity. The average adult needs six to eight 240 mL glasses of water a day.

VEGETARIAN DIETS

More and more Canadians are choosing vegetarian diets for health and ethical considerations. Some vegetarians may include dairy products and eggs in their diets (lacto-ovo-vegetarians) whereas others exclude eggs (lacto-vegetarians). Total vegetarians (vegans) eat only nonanimal products. All vegetarian diets include the following food groups: fats; fruits; vegetables; grains; calcium-rich foods; and legumes, nuts, and other protein-rich foods. Access to a wide range of soy products, tofu, cheese, and meat analogs has made it easier for vegetarians to meet their daily nutritional requirements than in the past when such products were not readily available.

NUTRITION THROUGH THE LIFE CYCLE

Nutritional needs change throughout the life cycle and are affected by both physical and developmental changes.

Children

Recommended daily nutritional requirements for children change with each age group. An understanding of development with regard to physical, cognitive, and psychosocial changes is needed to properly assess the nutritional needs of children. Educating the caregiver about these changes before they occur helps families to have more realistic expectations and to understand what is within the normal range and what should be cause for concern.

Nursing Tip

Infant Feeding Guidelines

The Canadian Pediatrics Society Nutrition Committee, Dieticians of Canada, and Health Canada recommend that breast milk be the sole form of feeding for the first 6 months of life.[3]

Birth to 6 months: breast milk or infant formula only. Increase gradually to 800–950 mL per day by the third to fourth month of life. Infants should receive a daily 400 IU vitamin D supplement until they reach 12 months of age.

Transition to Solid Foods

6 to 9 months: add iron-fortified cereals. Rice cereal is the least allergenic and is usually introduced first. Wheat cereals are usually not added until after 6 months of age. Iron-fortified formulas should be selected over cow's milk until the infant is 9 to 12 months old. Pasteurized whole cow's milk can be introduced after this time and continued until the child is at least 2 years old. It is important to help the infant adjust to spoon-feeding. Offer only one new food every 3 or 4 days to observe for signs of allergic reactions. Do not use mixed foods that may have other ingredients added.

5 to 8 months: fruits and vegetables. Encourage parents to read the labels of all foods to determine what has been added. Noncitrus fruit juices may be introduced but limited to 120 mL/day. It is helpful to use a cup because it prevents infants from associating sweet fruit juices with a bottle and also limits the amount they ingest. Do not add sugar or seasoning to foods. Introduce egg yolks, then gradually introduce meats.

9 to 10 months: finger foods may be introduced. Bite-size pieces that are cooked, mashed, and soft will allow the child independence and will provide increased texture that requires chewing. Gradually increase foods with texture as the child's chewing skills improve and teeth emerge.

Infants

Infants grow more during the first 6 to 12 months of life than at any other time. This is also the time when there is rapid neurological development, which indicates a need for proper nutrients. If the infant cannot be breast-fed for the full 6-month minimum recommendation, nurses should inform parents that even a few weeks of breast-feeding can be beneficial, except in cases where the mother is HIV-positive (HIV infection can be transmitted via breast milk).

Toddlers

Toddlers have unique nutritional needs as their physical growth slows. Toddlers' increased independence and control over their bodies is demonstrated in their eating patterns, such as refusing to eat or desiring only certain foods. Instruct parents to offer small portions of foods that the toddler can self-feed, and to provide only one new food at a time. Encourage routine mealtimes that are enjoyed with the family together, which provides toddlers with role models for developing good eating habits.

Preschoolers

Preschoolers have food dislikes and may become picky eaters. Giving them choices, serving small amounts of foods they can eat easily (finger foods), and providing a routine and enjoyable eating environment helps to foster good eating habits.

Nursing Tip

DASH Diet for Hypertension

The Dietary Approaches to Stop Hypertension (DASH) diet and reduced dietary sodium help hypertensive patients eat a nutritionally sound diet while lowering the effects of their diet on their blood pressure. The DASH diet is low in total fat, cholesterol, saturated fats, red meats, sweets, and sugar-containing beverages, and it is rich in vegetables, fruits, and low-fat dairy products. The DASH diet may not be appropriate for patients with advanced renal disease because it contains too much potassium and protein.

Preschoolers often have smaller appetites, which can be caused by drinking too many beverages (milk, juice, fruit punch) and by their slower increase in growth. Discuss the need to provide healthy snacks.

School-Age Children

School-age children tend to have erratic growth patterns that are reflected in their equally erratic eating patterns. Encourage families to maintain a balanced diet and to limit foods high in sugar. Caregivers should be advised to teach children proper nutrition and to show them how to read nutrition and ingredient labels. Monitor for childhood obesity.

Adolescents

Adolescents experience rapid growth and change and their nutritional needs fluctuate accordingly. They are concerned with body image and often compare their bodies to those of their peers in an attempt to fit into an acceptable identity. A poor body image can lead to eating disorders such as anorexia nervosa, bulimia nervosa, and obesity.

Young and Middle-Aged Adults

Growth and caloric needs usually stabilize in young and middle-aged adults. Eating habits may be altered by changes in activity levels and by the effects of work and life stressors. Obesity is frequently seen in young and middle-aged adults.

Pregnant and Lactating Women

It is important to assess and counsel the pregnant woman about proper nutrition—to promote a healthy pregnancy and to ensure the development of a healthy infant. If the woman does not gain adequate weight, the infant has an increased risk of being small for gestational age and may be prone to developmental delay, neonatal mortality, and other illnesses. However, the mother is at risk for gestational diabetes, hypertension, prolonged labour, birth trauma, and cesarean section if the weight gain is excessive. A woman with a BMI of <20 should gain 12.5 to 18.0 kg. If her BMI is 20–27, then the gain should be less (11.5 to 16.0 kg). If a woman has a BMI of >27, weight gain should be limited to 7.0 to 11.5 kg. Assessment includes a general knowledge of physical changes and their relationships to nutrition. Some of the common complaints experienced during pregnancy (e.g., heartburn, constipation, nausea, and vomiting) can be alleviated by dietary changes, such as small frequent meals, increased fluid intake, and a well-balanced diet.

Iron supplements and prenatal vitamins are given routinely during pregnancy because diet alone is often not adequate in meeting the body's requirements. There is evidence that folic acid helps to reduce the risk of neural tube defects, especially when instituted three months prior to pregnancy. Health Canada recommends an additional 100 calories per day in the first trimester, 300 calories in the second or third trimester, and an increase in milk consumption, which increases both protein and caloric intake. Pregnant women should also be encouraged to drink 6 to 8 glasses of fluid daily (water, fruit juices, and milk); lactating women need additional fluids, ranging from 2 to 3 litres daily.

Older Adults

Good eating habits and nutrition established early in life will benefit adults as they age, whereas poor eating habits may contribute to disease processes (e.g., hypertension, diabetes mellitus, and CAD). Caloric needs decrease as a person ages due to the reduction in basal metabolic rate, so health teaching should focus on modifications in portion size.

Assess any problems the elderly may have with difficulty chewing (oral problems) or swallowing (possible stroke or Parkinson's disease), decreased appetite, decreased taste and smell, and decreased ability to self-feed (musculoskeletal diseases, such as osteoarthritis; and degenerative neurological disorders). The older adult should eat in a sitting position to avoid aspiration. Constipation is a common problem that can be alleviated through adequate fluid intake and by eating foods high in fibre.

EQUIPMENT

- Wall-mounted unit (stadiometer), rod attached to the scale that has a right-angle headboard
- Tape measure
- Scale (preferably a balance-beam scale or electronic scale)
- Skinfold calipers (ideally one with a spring-loaded lever)

NUTRITIONAL ASSESSMENT

Table 7-1 illustrates a comprehensive nutritional assessment that includes the nutritional history, physical assessment, anthropometric measurements, laboratory data, and diagnostic data.

The Nutritional History

Specific diet information may be obtained in a variety ways via the Diet History (Table 7-2).

Physical Assessment

Certain physical signs may indicate poor nutrition. See Table 7-3 for a list of signs and symptoms of poor nutritional status.

Anthropometric Measurements

Anthropometric measurements are the various measurements of the human body, including height, weight, and body proportions.

Height

A standing height is obtained for patients 3 years and older.

E 1. Have the patient stand erect with back and heels against the wall or measuring device.
  2. Place the headboard at a right angle to the wall and along the crown of the patient's head.
  3. Record height to the nearest mm.
N Compare to standardized charts. Bear in mind that patients will reflect familial growth patterns.
A Insufficient growth.
P Chronic malnutrition.
A Excessive growth.
P Hormone abnormalities (acromegaly, gigantism, precocious puberty).
A Decreased height.
P Osteoporosis.

Weight

  1. Have patient stand on scale, facing weights.
  2. Slide weight until balanced.
  3. Read and record to the nearest 100 g (10 g for infants).

| E Examination | N Normal Findings | A Abnormal Findings | P Pathophysiology |

TABLE 7-1	Comprehensive Nutritional Assessment

NUTRITIONAL HISTORY

Physical Assessment	1. General appearance 2. Skin 3. Nails 4. Hair 5. Eyes 6. Mouth 7. Head and neck 8. Heart and peripheral vasculature 9. Abdomen 10. Musculoskeletal system 11. Neurological system 12. Female genitalia
Anthropometric Measurements	Weight: _____ kg Height: _____ cm BMI: _____ Waist to hip ratio: _____ % Usual Body Weight: _____ % Weight Change: _____ Triceps Skinfold: _____ mm Mid-Arm Circumference: _____ cm Mid-Arm Muscle Circumference: _____ cm
Laboratory Data	Hematocrit (Hct): _____ Hemoglobin (Hgb): _____ g/L Cholesterol: _____ mmol/L HDL-C: _____ mmol/L LDL-C: _____ mmol/L Total cholesterol: _____ HDL-C ratio Triglycerides: _____ mmol/L Transferrin: _____ g/L TIBC: _____ μmol/L Iron: _____ μmol/L Total Lymphocyte Count: _____ 10^9 cells/L Prealbumin: _____ mg/L Albumin: _____ g/L Glucose: _____ mmol/L Antigen Skin Testing: _____ Creatinine Height Index: _____ % Nitrogen Balance: _____ g Blood Urea Nitrogen: _____ mmol/L
Diagnostic Data	DEXA Scan _____ X-rays _____

TABLE 7-2	Diet History

PART 1: GENERAL DIET INFORMATION

Do you follow a particular diet?

What are your food likes and dislikes?

Do you have any especially strong cravings?

How often do you eat fast foods?

How often do you eat at restaurants?

Do you have adequate financial resources to purchase your food?

How do you obtain, store, and prepare your food?

Do you eat alone or with a family member or other person?

In the last 12 months have you

- experienced any change in weight?
- had a change in your appetite?
- had a change in your diet?
- experienced nausea, vomiting, or diarrhea from your diet?
- changed your diet because of difficulty in feeding yourself, eating, chewing, or swallowing?

PART 2: FOOD INTAKE HISTORY (24-HOUR RECALL, 3-DAY DIARY, DIRECT OBSERVATION)

Time	Food/Drink	Amount	Method of Preparation	Eating Location

4. Calculate percentage of ideal body weight (IBW), using the formula:

$$\% \text{ IBW} = \frac{\text{Current Weight}}{\text{IBW}^*} \times 100$$

5. Calculate the percentage of usual body weight, using the formula:

$$\% \text{ Usual Body Weight} = \frac{\text{Current Weight}}{\text{Ususal Body Weight}} \times 100$$

6. Calculate the percentage of weight change, using the formula:

$$\% \text{ Weight Change} = \frac{\text{Usual Weight} - \text{Current Weight}}{\text{Ususal Weight}} \times 100$$

Note: In Canada, BMI, waist circumference (WC), and waist-to-hip ratio are generally used to determine an individual's weight status rather than IBW. However, IBW calculations are provided because some agencies and/or patients may prefer this approach.

N A person's weight is compared to the theoretical ideal for their height. An IBW between 90 and 109 is adequate.

A Mild obesity occurs when the patient is 20–40% above the IBW; moderate obesity occurs when the patient is 40–100% above the IBW; and morbid obesity occurs when a patient is more than 100% above the IBW.

E Examination	N Normal Findings	A Abnormal Findings	P Pathophysiology

TABLE 7-3	Physical Signs and Symptoms of Poor Nutritional Status

	SUBJECTIVE	OBJECTIVE
1. General appearance	Fatigue, poor sleep, change in weight, frequent infections	Dull affect, apathetic, increased weight, decreased weight
2. Skin	Pruritus, swelling, delayed wound healing	Dry, rough, scaling, flaky, edema, lesions, decreased turgor, changes in color (pallor, jaundice), petechiae, ecchymoses, xanthomas (slightly elevated yellow nodules)
3. Nails	Brittle	Dry, splinter hemorrhages, spoon-shaped, pale
4. Hair	Easily falls out, brittle	Less shiny, dry, changes in color pigment
5. Eyes	Vision changes, night blindness, eye discharge	Hardening and scaling of cornea, conjunctiva pale or red
6. Mouth	Mouth sores	Lips: cracked, dry, swollen, fissures around corners Gums: recessed, swollen, bleeding, spongy Tongue: smooth, beefy red, magenta, pale, fissures, sores, increased or decreased in size, increased or decreased papillae Teeth: missing, caries
7. Head and neck	Headaches, decreased hearing	Xanthelasma, irritation and crusting of nares, swollen cheeks (parotid gland enlargement), goiter
8. Heart and peripheral vasculature	Palpitations, swelling	Cardiac enlargement, changes in blood pressure, tachycardia, heart murmur, edema
9. Abdomen	Tender, changes in appetite, nausea, changes in bowel habits	Edema, hepatosplenomegaly, vomiting, diarrhea
10. Musculoskeletal	Weakness, pain, cramping, frequent fractures	Muscle tone is decreased, flabby muscles, muscle system wasting, bowing of lower extremities
11. Neurological system	Irritable, changes in mood, numbness, paresthesia	Slurred speech, unsteady gait, tremors, decreased deep tendon reflexes, loss of position and vibratory sense, paresthesia, decreased coordination
12. Female genitalia	Changes in menstrual pattern	None

P Increased food intake, decreased activity level, medications (e.g., steroids), hypothyroidism.

A A weight under 90% of IBW is termed undernutrition. A weight between 80 and 90% of the IBW is mild undernutrition; between 70 and 80% is moderate under-nutrition; and below 70% is severe under-nutrition.

P Decreased food intake may occur with dental problems, depression, medications, alcoholism, anorexia nervosa, poverty;

E Examination	N Normal Findings	A Abnormal Findings	P Pathophysiology

impaired absorption, as in malabsorption diseases (e.g., celiac disease), AIDS, and small bowel disease; loss of nutrients with diarrhea, vomiting, and diabetes mellitus; increased demand for nutrients may be present in malignancies, fever, burns, hyperthyroidism.

Body Mass Index

Body Mass Index (BMI) is a measurement that reflects body composition. BMI is related to increased mortality when it is very high or very low. BMI is an index of weight-to-height. It does not reflect the actual distribution of fat on the body. Health Canada recommends the use of waist circumference (WC) measurements in addition to BMI. The formula to determine BMI is:

$$BMI = \frac{weight\ (in\ kg)}{m^2}$$

BMI can be difficult to calculate because many Canadians continue to report their weight in pounds and their height in feet and inches. Thus, two methods of BMI calculations are provided:

E
1. Determine the BMI measurement by using the BMI nomogram (Figure 7-3) (ideal method), OR (less ideal method):
1. Multiply the weight in pounds by 703.
2. Multiply the height in inches by the height in inches.
3. Divide the first number in 2 by the second number in 3.
4. The answer is the BMI.

For example: weight = 107 lbs, height = 60 inches

107 × 703 = 75221
60 × 60 = 3600
75221/3600 = 20.9 or 21

N   A BMI of 18.5–24.9 is considered within normal limits.

A   A BMI of 25.0–29.9 is considered overweight. A BMI of 30.0–34.9 is considered Obese (Class I), 35–39.9 is moderately obese (Obese Class II), and greater than 40 is extremely obese (Obese Class III).

P   A BMI greater than 25 is associated with an increased morbidity and mortality from cardiovascular disease, cancer, and other diseases.

A   A BMI less than 18.5.

P   Underweight, associated with possible malnutrition; self-induced (e.g., anorexia nervosa, bulimia), caused by illness (e.g., cancer, AIDS); or from a lack of adequate nutrition.

Waist-to-Hip Ratio and Waist Circumference

Body fat distribution is linked to morbidity and mortality. Fat distribution gives rise to two predominant body shapes: gynoid (pear shaped) and android (apple shaped). Women tend to deposit fat more in their hips and buttocks, giving them a pear-shaped appearance. Men, on the other hand, tend to deposit fat around the abdominal midline, thus giving them an apple appearance. Abdominal fat includes fat located under the skin (subcutaneous) and fat that surrounds organs (visceral fat). Waist circumference is a good indicator of abdominal fat. Excess abdominal fat, especially excess visceral fat, has been linked to the development of type 2 diabetes mellitus, CAD, and hypertension.

E
1. Stand beside the person. The patient's feet should be 25–30 cm apart. Measure the waist in centimetres at the part of the trunk located midway between the lower costal margin (bottom of lower rib) and the iliac crest (top of the pelvic bone). Fit the measuring tape snugly without compressing abdominal tissue. Measure to the nearest 0.5 cm *at the end of expiration.*
2. Measure the hips at the widest point.
3. Divide the waist measurement by the hip measurement to obtain the waist-to-hip ratio. For example: waist = 63.5 cm, hips = 88.9 cm
63.5/88.9 = 0.71

N   For men, a WC between 80 and 99 cm is normal, and for women, a WC between

E Examination   N Normal Findings   A Abnormal Findings   P Pathophysiology

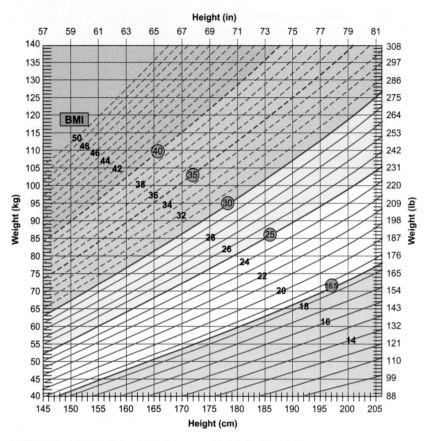

FIGURE 7-3 Body Mass Index (BMI) Nomogram (Health Canada, 2003)

Source: http://www.hc-sc.gc.ca/home-accueil/important_e.html. Reproduced with the permission of the Minister of Public Works and Government Services Canada, 2006.

70 and 88 is normal. A waist-to-hip ratio <0.8 is normal in women and <1.0 is normal in men. See Figure 7-4

A A WC for men ≥ 102 cm, for premenopausal woman ≥ 88 cm, and postmenopausal women ≥ 110 cm is associated with an increased risk of developing health problems. A waist-to-hip ratio greater than 0.8 in women and 1.0 in men is abnormal.

P These measurements are associated with the adverse morbidity and mortality of obesity.

Skinfold Thickness

Skinfold thickness is used to determine body fat stores and nutritional status. It is a more reliable indicator of body fat than is weight because more than half of the body's total fat is located in the subcutaneous tissue. The most common measurement site is the triceps skinfold (TSF). Measurements can also be performed in subscapular and suprailiac skinfolds.

E 1. Place the patient in a sitting or standing position.

E **Examination**   N **Normal Findings**   A **Abnormal Findings**   P **Pathophysiology**

	BMI		
	Normal (18.5–24.9)	Overweight (25.0–29.9)	Obese Class 1(30.0–34.9)
< 102 cm (males)	Least Risk	Increased Risk	High Risk
WC < 88 cm (females)			
≥ 102 cm (males)	Increased Risk	High Risk	Very High Risk
≥ 88 cm (females)			

FIGURE 7-4 Relative Risk Based on Waist Circumference and BMI.

Source: Adapted from: National Institutes of Health (1998). *Clinical guidelines on the identification, evaluation and treatment of overweight and obesity in adults: The evidence report.* Washington, DC: NIH, p. 17. Courtesy of National Institutes of Health.

2. Take the measurements on the nondominant arm, with the patient in a relaxed position.
3. Make a mark on the posterior portion of the upper arm midway between the acromion process and the olecranon process.
4. Using your nondominant hand, grasp the skin and pull it free from the muscle.
5. Apply the caliper with your dominant hand and align the markers.
6. Note the measurement to the nearest 0.5 mm.
7. Release the skin and repeat two or three times.
8. Average the findings to determine the TSF.

N Normal measurements fall between the 5th and 95th percentiles of standard charts.
A See abnormal findings and pathophysiology under mid-arm and mid-arm muscle circumference.

Mid-Arm and Mid-Arm Muscle Circumferences

The mid-arm circumference (MAC) provides information on skeletal muscle mass. This measurement alone is not of great significance but it is used to calculate the mid-arm muscle circumference (MAMC).

E
1. Instruct patient to flex the arm at the elbow.
2. Measure the circumference of the upper arm (MAC) midway between the acromion process and the olecranon process.
3. Calculate MAMC using the formula:

$$\text{MAMC (cm)} = \text{MAC (cm)} - [3.14 - \text{TSE* (cm)}]$$

N Normal measurements fall between the 5th and 95th percentiles of standard charts.
A Results less than the 3rd percentile on the standard charts are abnormal.
P Malnutrition.
A Results greater than the 97th percentile.
P Obesity.

Laboratory Data

Laboratory analysis is used to screen for potential nutritional problems and to assist with diagnosis when problems are suspected after a thorough history and physical are conducted.

Hematocrit and Hemoglobin

Hematocrit is the proportion of red cells to volume of whole blood. Hemoglobin is the iron component of the blood that transports oxygen. Both values are obtained from a venous blood sample.

---

*The TSF is measured in mm. You need to convert the TSF from mm to cm in order to calculate the MAMC.

E **Examination**	N **Normal Findings**	A **Abnormal Findings**	P **Pathophysiology**

N Hemoglobin and hematocrit results should fall within expected values as shown in Table 7-4. Increased hematocrit and hemoglobin may normally occur with people living in high altitudes due to the decrease in partial pressure of oxygen in those areas.

A Decreased hematocrit and hemoglobin.

P Anemia, leukemia, cirrhosis, hyperthyroidism, hemorrhage, hemodilution, hemolytic reactions.

P Increased hematocrit and hemoglobin.

P Chronic hypoxia, severe dehydration.

Lipids

In 2003, the Working Group on Hypercholesterolemia and Other Dyslipidemias published revised guidelines to assist health care providers in assessing and managing hyperlipidemia. The Working Group determined target *LDL-C levels and **total cholesterol: HDL-C ratio for patients based on their 10-year risk of coronary artery disease.

*LDL Cholesterol (LDL-C) (mmol/L)
<2.5 Target level for patients at high risk of CAD
<3.5 Target level for patients at moderate risk of CAD
<4.5 Target level for patients at low risk of CAD

HDL Cholesterol (HDL-C) (mmol/L)
<1.04 Very low (undesirable)
1.04–1.29 Low (less desirable)
1.30–1.54 Acceptable
>1.55 Desirable

Total Cholesterol (mmol/L)
<5.19 Desirable
5.2–6.19 Borderline high
>6.20 High
>7.21 Extremely high

**Total Cholesterol: HDL-C ratio
<4.0 Target level for patients at high risk of CAD
<5.0 Target level for patients at moderate risk of CAD
<6.0 Target level for patients at low risk of CAD

TABLE 7-4	Normal Values for Hematocrit and Hemoglobin	
	NORMAL VALUES	
Age	Hematocrit	Hemoglobin g/L
1 mo	0.38–0.52	107–171
12 mo	0.37–0.41	113–141
1–2 yr	0.32–0.40	110–140
9–14 yr	0.36–0.42	120–144
18–44 yr		
Female	0.38–0.44	117–155
Male	0.43–0.49	132–173
65–74 yr		
Female	0.38–0.44	117–161
Male	0.37–0.51	126–174

Triglycerides (mmol/L)
<1.70 Optimal
1.70–2.25 Borderline high
2.26–5.64 High
>5.65 Very high

A Elevated total cholesterol: HDL-C ratio, LDL-C, and triglycerides above desirable range are abnormal. HDL-C less than 1.04 mmol/L is undesirable in adults.

P Increased fat intake, genetics, medications (e.g., steroids, estrogens, cyclosporin).

Transferrin, Total Iron-Binding Capacity, and Iron

Transferrin is a protein that regulates iron absorption. Transferrin can be measured by the total iron-binding capacity (TIBC), the amount of iron with which it can bind. Serum iron is the amount of transferrin-bound iron. Serum transferrin can be calculated using the following formula: Transferrin = $(0.8 \times TIBC) - 43$.

N Normal adult levels are:
Transferrin
Male 2.2–3.6 g/L
Female 2.5–3.8 g/L
TIBC
45–63 μmol/L

E **Examination** N **Normal Findings** A **Abnormal Findings** P **Pathophysiology**

Serum iron
   Male   13.2−31.3 μmol/L
   Female   11.6−29.6 μmol/L

A An increase in transferrin.

P Inadequate dietary iron, iron-deficiency anemia, hepatitis, oral contraceptive use.

A Decreased levels of transferrin.

P Pernicious anemia, sickle cell anemia, anemia associated with infection or chronic diseases, cancer, malnutrition.

A Increases in serum iron levels.

P Hemolytic anemia, lead poisoning.

A Decreases in serum iron levels.

P Iron deficiency, chronic diseases, third-trimester pregnancy, severe physiological stress.

Total Lymphocyte Count

Total lymphocyte count (TLC) is measured in the complete blood count with differential and measures immune function and visceral protein status. When the white blood cell (WBC) count is abnormally high (bacterial infections) or low (AIDS), the TLC is not always a reliable indicator of nutritional status.

N Normal adult levels are 1.5–1.8 × 10^9.

A A decrease in the TLC of less than 1.5 indicates moderate protein deficiency; a count of less than 0.9 indicates severe protein deficiency.

P Malnourished state.

Antigen Skin Testing

Antigen skin testing is another test of immune function. Intradermal injections of various antigens can be used, such as with PPD tuberculin skin tests, mumps virus, *Candida albicans*, streptokinase, *Streptococcus, coccidioidin,* and *Trichophyton*. Results are read at 24 and 48 hours postinjection.

N A negative skin reaction (no induration or erythema) after being tested with various antigens is normal. These are antigens to which most people have been exposed and have developed an antibody response.

A A positive reaction to antigens placed intradermally, which is indicated by a red area or induration 5 mm or more around the test site 24 hours or more after the injection. A negative reaction to only one of the antigens tested or a delayed positive reaction may occur with malnutrition.

P Poor antibody response occurs in patients who are immunocompromised. Protein malnutrition has been shown to decrease immune function. This diminished reaction to antigens is called anergy.

Prealbumin

Prealbumin (also called thyroxine-binding prealbumin) is the transport protein for thyroxine and retinol-binding protein. The half-life is 24 to 48 hours so it is an excellent value to monitor the effects of recent nutritional support and changes in nutritional status.

N See Table 7-5, Prealbumin and Albumin Values, for normal values.

A Liver disease, such as cirrhosis and hepatitis, as well as severe stress from infection, burn injury, and sepsis, prolonged surgery, hyperthyroidism, and cystic fibrosis can all lead to decreased prealbumin levels.

P Severe acute conditions where severe catabolism occurs tend to lower the prealbumin level. In the case of liver disease, the levels are lower because of decreased hepatic synthesis of proteins.

TABLE 7-5	Prealbumin and Albumin Values
Albumin	
Normal value	38–45 g/L
Mild depletion	30–37 g/L
Moderate depletion	25–29 g/L
Severe depletion	<25 g/L
Prealbumin	
Normal value	200 mg/L
Mild depletion	100–150 mg/L
Moderate depletion	50–100 mg/L
Severe depletion	<50 mg/L

E Examination   **N** Normal Findings   **A** Abnormal Findings   **P** Pathophysiology

Albumin

Albumin is formed in the liver. It transports nutrients, blood, and hormones, and helps maintain osmotic pressure. Albumin must have functioning liver cells and an adequate amount of amino acids to be synthesized. It is an indicator of visceral protein status. Because albumin has a long half-life (about 20 days), it is not an indicator that detects subtle or early changes in nutritional status. It is measured from a venous blood sample.

N See Table 7-5, Prealbumin and Albumin Values, for normal values.
A Less than 38 g/L.
P Malnutrition, massive hemorrhage, burns, kidney disease.

Glucose

Serum glucose tests the body's ability to metabolize glucose. It is best assessed after a fasting period.

N The normal glucose levels are:
Adult: FPG (no caloric intake for at least 8 hr) 3.6 – 5.5 mmol/L
A An increase in glucose level.
P Diabetes mellitus, impaired glucose tolerance, vitamin B_1 deficiency, convulsive states.
A A decrease in serum glucose level.
P Pancreatic disorders, liver disease, insulin overdose.

Creatinine Height Index

Creatinine is a substance normally excreted in the urine; it is dependent on the amount of skeletal muscle mass and measures the amount of protein reserves. Urine creatinine is tested after collecting a 24-hour urine sample. An ideal urine creatinine level by height table is used to establish the denominator in the equation used to calculate Creatinine Height Index (CHI). Use the following equation to calculate CHI:

$$CHI = \frac{\text{actual 24-hour creatinine excretion}}{\text{ideal 24-hour creatinine excretion}} \times 100$$

N Normal values for creatinine, collected with a 24-hour urine sample, are 0.13–0.22 mmol/kg/day. For CHI, where values are compared to an ideal urine creatinine by height table, normal CHI values are greater than 90%.
A CHI between 80% and 90% indicates mild protein deficiency.
CHI between 70% and 80% indicates moderate protein deficiency.
CHI of less than 70% indicates severe protein deficiency.
P Protein malnutrition may be indicated by the loss of lean body mass, which can occur in severe trauma, prolonged fever, and stress.

Nursing Alert

Diagnosis of Diabetes

Any patient with one of the following indicators of diabetes mellitus must be referred to the appropriate health care professional.

FPG ≥ 7.0 mmol/L

or

Casual plasma glucose ≥ 11.1 mmol/L + symptoms of diabetes
Casual plasma glucose is taken at any time of the day, without regard to the interval since the last meal. Classic symptoms of diabetes = polyuria, polydipsia, and unexplained weight loss

or

2h plasma glucose with a 75 g OGTT ≥ 11.1 mmol/L

E Examination   N Normal Findings   A Abnormal Findings   P Pathophysiology

Nitrogen Balance

Nitrogen is one of the compounds of amino acids; it is incorporated into protein from food sources and is excreted in urine and feces. The balance of intake of nitrogen to output of nitrogen is compared, usually with a 24-hour urine sample. The nitrogen balance can be calculated using this formula:

$$\text{Nitrogen Balance} = \frac{\substack{\text{grams of protein} \\ \text{eaten in 24 hours}}}{6.25} - (\text{UNN*} + 4)$$

- **N** A zero balance is normal. A positive balance indicates tissue formation, found in growing children and in pregnant women.
- **A** A negative nitrogen balance.
- **P** Malnutrition, catabolic states (burns, severe stress, trauma, surgery).

Diagnostic Data

Radiographic studies are used to determine bone formation and to assess development. Rickets and scurvy are examples of long-term nutritional deficiencies that have radiographic manifestations. Rickets is a deficiency of vitamin D, and scurvy is a deficiency of vitamin C; both are characterized by softening and deformities of the bones. A bone density, or dual-energy X-ray absorptiometry (DEXA), scan is a low-radiation, noninvasive test that assesses the hip, spine, and wrist for osteoporosis. Although osteoporosis can result from many variables, nutrition is one of the leading etiologies in various age groups.

*UNN = 24-hour urine urea nitrogen (in grams).

REFERENCES

[1]Heart and Stroke Foundation of Canada. *Position Statement. Trans fatty acids "trans fats" and heart disease and stroke.* Retrieved October 12, 2006, from http://ww2.heartandstroke.ca/images/English /TransFat-ENGLISH-APR04.pdf

[2]Health Canada—Food and Nutrition. *Trans fats.* Retrieved October 12, 2006, from http://www.hc-sc.gc.ca/fn-an/nutrition/gras-trans-fats/index_e.html

[3]Canadian Paediatric Society, Dietitians of Canada, and Health Canada. (2005). *Nutrition for healthy term infants.* Ottawa: Minister of Public Works and Government Services.

[4]Genest, J., Frohlich, J., Fodor, G., & McPherson, R. (2003). Recommendations for the management of dyslipidemia and the prevention of cardiovascular disease: Summary of the 2003 update. Reprinted from *Canadian Medical Association Journal, 169*(9), 921–24, October 28, 2003. Used with permission of the publisher.

| E **Examination** | N **Normal Findings** | A **Abnormal Findings** | P **Pathophysiology** |

Unit 3

Physical Assessment

8

Physical Assessment Techniques

Inspection, palpation, percussion, and auscultation are the techniques used to assess the patient during a physical examination. This chapter introduces the assessment techniques and equipment used to conduct physical examinations.

ASPECTS OF PHYSICAL ASSESSMENT

Physical assessment can serve many purposes:

1. Screening of general well-being. The findings will serve as baseline information for future assessments.
2. Validation of the health issues or concerns that brought the patient to seek health care.
3. Detection of pathology in situations when the patient does not present with a health issue or concern but variations in health are detected by virtue of the systematic approach of physical assessment.
4. Monitoring of current health problems for amelioration or deterioration and determining appropriate referral if necessary.
5. Formulation of nursing analyses that will help determine care and treatment plans, including education and anticipatory guidance needs of the patient and family.

Role of the Nurse

The nurse plays a vital role in the health and physical assessment of the patient. The knowledge base of nursing is broad and includes an understanding of the many health and illness issues that can arise across the life span, the role of the family in health and illness events, and the nature of coping with normative and non-normative events. Nurses assess the biological, psychological, social, and spiritual nature of patient situations to gain a holistic understanding of the situation. Nurses are trusted members of the health care team and have a significant presence in the health care system. People may disclose health issues or concerns to nurses either formally (such as during a well-baby clinic visit) or informally (such as the teenager who meets the nurse in the school hallway and says "My friend thinks she is pregnant"). Nurses are often the entry point into the health care system—they often play a "triage" role in community and hospital clinics, provide

---

Nursing Alert

Latex Allergies

In accordance with routine practices, nurses frequently use gloves when dealing with patients' body fluids. Be alert to the possibility that you, as well as your patients, may have latex allergies. Reactions range from eczematous contact dermatitis to anaphylactic shock. Before touching patients while wearing latex gloves or using other latex products, ask them if they have any known allergy to latex products. Many hospitals and clinics, especially those dealing with the pediatric population and people with chronic illness, are moving toward latex-free environments.

telephone information services to help people determine if a health issue or concern needs further assessment, act as case managers to coordinate care, and may be the only health care professional available in remote settings. Nurses provide care to hospitalized patients as well as those in long-term and palliative care facilities—their round-the-clock presence ensures ongoing assessment for responses to illness situations. By conducting a systematic health and physical assessment, a nurse can determine the relevance of health issues or concerns that patients present with as well as establish the most accurate therapeutic plan to address the uniqueness of the patient situation.

Routine Practices and Transmission-Based Precautions

The transmission of infectious illnesses such as hepatitis and human immunodeficiency virus (HIV), and the increasing prevalence of antibiotic-resistant organisms, such as methicillin-resistant staphylococcus aureus (MRSA) and vancomycin-resistant enterococcus (VRE), among other potential infections, is a primary concern for health care professionals and for patients. On the one hand, health care workers must protect themselves and other patients from transmissible illnesses carried by a particular patient; on the other hand, the patient must be protected from any contamination by health care workers or the environment in which care is delivered.

Routine practices, formerly known as universal precautions, were developed by Health Canada's Laboratory Centre for Disease Control to protect health care professionals and patients. Routine practices should be used with every patient throughout the entire encounter. Figure 8-1 illustrates the routine practices recommended by Health Canada. Complete guidelines for acute care, ambulatory care, home care, and long-term care facilities are also available.[1] Figure 8-2 summarizes the recommended procedure for washing hands.

Another level of precaution called transmission-based precautions is to be used in conjunction with routine practices. Routes of transmission of microorganisms have been classified as contact (includes direct contact, indirect contact, and droplet transmission), airborne, common vehicle, and vectorborne. Direct contact transmission occurs when microorganisms are transferred

Nursing Alert

Gloves are not a substitute for hand washing; rather, they provide an additional measure of protection, particularly from blood and moist body substances. Hands can become contaminated through gloves or during their removal.

from direct physical contact between an infected or colonized person and a susceptible host, such as in the transmission of impetigo, scabies, and varicella zoster virus. Indirect contact transmission occurs when passive transfer of microorganisms via a contaminated intermediate object such as unwashed hands or contaminated stethoscopes occurs. Droplet transmission is a form of contact transmission and refers to large droplets, ≥ 5 μm in diameter, that arise from the respiratory tract during coughing, sneezing, or invasive procedures (e.g., suctioning). Pertussis and *Haemophilus influenzae* are examples of this mode of transmission. Droplet transmission occurs at a distance of <1 metre. Airborne transmission spreads microorganisms <5 μm by air currents and inhalation. They can also be passed through ventilation systems. Measles and the varicella virus as well as the tuberculosis bacterium can spread by this mode. Common vehicle transmission refers to a single contaminated source, such as food, medication, intravenous fluid, or an insulin vial. Vectorborne transmission refers to transmission by insect vectors, such as the tsetse fly, spreading malaria in African countries. Vectorborne transmission has not been reported in Canada.

ASSESSMENT TECHNIQUES

Physical assessment findings, or objective data, are obtained through the use of four specific techniques that are usually performed in this order: inspection, palpation, percussion, and auscultation. An exception is in the assessment of the abdomen, when auscultation is performed prior to percussion and palpation, as the latter two can alter bowel sounds. These four techniques when used systematically can validate information provided by a patient in the health

ROUTINE PRACTICES

(for complete recommendations, see Health Canada Infection Control Guidelines[1])

HAND WASHING	Performed before and after any direct hand contact with a patient (including the skin, body fluids, blood, secretions and excretions and wound exudates) or contaminated items (e.g., urinal, wound dressing).
	Plain soap is used for routine hand washing; antiseptic hand rinse is used before performing invasive procedures or when caring for an immunocompromised person.
	Waterless antiseptic hand rinses are an alternative to hand washing, especially when access to sinks is limited. Hand washing with soap and water before using waterless antiseptic hand rinses is necessary when there is visible soiling.
GLOVES	Not required for routine care that is limited to contact with the patient's intact skin.
	Clean, non-sterile gloves are worn for contact with blood, body fluids, secretions and excretions, mucous membranes, draining wounds or non-intact skin.
	Used in addition to, not as a substitute for, hand washing. Wash hands before and after wearing gloves.
	Remove gloves immediately after care to avoid environmental contamination.
MASK, EYE PROTECTION, FACE SHIELD	These are worn during patient care activities and procedures that are likely to generate splashes or sprays of blood, body fluids, secretions, or excretions.
GOWNS	Used when soiling of clothing or uncovered skin is a risk such as during procedures or care activities that can generate splashes or sprays of blood, body fluids, secretions, or excretions.
ACCOMMODATION	Single patient rooms are not required for routine patient care in the acute care setting; transmission based precautions can call for a single room or negative pressure room for certain airborne or contact transmitted microorganisms.
PATIENT CARE EQUIPMENT	Needles and sharp instruments must be disposed of puncture-resistant containers.
	In acute care settings, reusable equipment that has been in direct contact with the patient must be cleansed before use with another patient.
	In the ambulatory setting, items that are only in contact with intact skin must be cleansed on a routine basis if cleaning between patient use is not feasible. A barrier, such as a sheet or paper, on the examination table will prevent contamination between patients.
ENVIRONMENTAL CONTROL	In the acute care setting, cleaning and disinfection of environmental surfaces and patient furniture must be completed on a routine basis

FIGURE 8-1 Routine Practices.

Source: Excerpted from Health Canada Infection Control Guidelines.

Procedure	Rationale
Remove jewelry before hand wash procedure.	
Rinse hands under warm running water.	This allows for suspension and washing away of the loosened microorganisms.
Lather with soap and, using friction cover all surfaces of the hands and fingers.	The minimum duration for this step is 10 seconds: more time may be required if hands are visibly soiled.
	For antiseptic agents 3–5 mL are required.
	Frequently missed areas are thumbs, undernails, backs of fingers and hands.
Rinse under warm running water.	To wash off microorganisms and residual hand washing agent.
Dry hands thoroughly with single-use towel or forced air dryer.	Drying achieves a further reduction in number of microorganisms.
	Reusable towels are avoided because of the potential for microbial contamination.
Turn off faucet without recontaminating hands.	To avoid recontaminating hands.
Do not use fingernail polish or artificial nails.	Artificial nails or chipped nail polish may increase bacterial load and impede visualization of soil under nails.

FIGURE 8-2 How to Wash Hands.

Source: Health Canada Infection Control Guidelines, *How to Wash Hands*, from http://www.phac-aspc.gc.ca/publicat/ccdr-rmtc/98pdf/cdr24s8e.pdf. Reproduced with the permission of the Minister of Public Works and Government Services Canada, 2006.

history, can verify a suspected diagnosis, and can ensure comprehensive assessment. In addition, a health issue may be discovered that was not originally identified by the patient as a concern, such as when palpation of the abdomen yields abnormal findings when there were no subjective symptoms of pathology.

Inspection

Inspection is an ongoing process that uses the nurse's senses of vision and smell to consciously observe the patient throughout the entire physical assessment.

Vision

Use of sight can reveal many facts about a patient. Visual inspection of a patient's respira-

tory status, for example, might reveal a rate of 38 breaths per minute and cyanotic nailbeds. In this case, the patient is tachypneic and possibly hypoxic and would need a more thorough respiratory assessment. The process of visual inspection necessitates full exposure of the body part being inspected, adequate overhead lighting, and, when necessary, tangential lighting (light that is shone at an angle on the patient to accentuate shadows and highlight subtle findings).

Smell

The nurse's olfactory sense also provides vital information about a patient's health status. The patient may have a fruity breath odour characteristic of diabetic ketoacidosis; the smell of urine or feces may indicate difficulties with self-care.

Palpation

The second assessment technique is palpation, which is the act of touching a patient in a therapeutic manner to elicit specific information. Prior to palpating a patient, some basic principles need to be observed. The nurse should have short fingernails to avoid hurting the patient. Hands should be warmed prior to placing them on the patient; cold hands can make a patient's muscles tense, thus distorting assessment findings. Encourage the patient to breathe normally throughout the palpation and discontinue immediately if pain is experienced. Most significantly, the patient needs to be informed where, when, and how the touch will occur, especially when he or she cannot see what is happening. The patient is therefore aware of what to expect in the assessment process.

Different sections of the hands are used for assessing certain areas of the body. The dorsum of the hand is most sensitive to temperature changes in the body. Therefore, placing the dorsum of the hand on a patient's forehead to assess body temperature is more accurate than using the palmar surface of the hand. The palmar surface of the fingers at the metacarpophalangeal joints, the ball of the hand, and the ulnar surface of the hand best discriminate vibrations, such as a cardiac thrill and fremitus. The finger pads of the hand are used most frequently in palpation to assess fine tactile discrimination, skin moisture, and texture; the presence of masses, pulsations, edema, and crepitation, and the shape, size, position, mobility, and consistency of organs.

Gloves must be worn when examining any open wounds, skin lesions, a body part with discharge, as well as internal body parts such as the mouth and rectum.

There are two distinct types of palpation techniques: light and deep palpation.

Light Palpation

Light palpation is done more frequently than deep palpation and is always performed before deep palpation. As the name implies, light palpation is superficial, delicate, and gentle. The finger pads are used to gain information on the patient's skin surface to a depth of approximately 1 cm below the surface. Light palpation reveals information on skin texture and moisture; overt, large, or superficial masses; and fluid, muscle guarding, and superficial tenderness. To perform light palpation:

1. Keeping the fingers of the dominant hand together, place the finger pads lightly on the skin over the area that is to be palpated. The hand and forearm will be on a plane parallel to the area being assessed.
2. Depress the skin 1 cm in light, gentle, circular motions.
3. Keeping the finger pads on the skin, let the depressed body surface rebound to its natural position.
4. If the patient is ticklish, lift your hand off the skin before moving it to another area.
5. Using a systematic approach, move the fingers to an adjacent area and repeat the process.
6. Continue to move the finger pads until the entire area being examined has been palpated.
7. If the patient has complained of tenderness in any area, palpate this area last. Figure 8-3 shows how light palpation is performed.

Deep Palpation

Deep palpation can reveal information about the position of organs and masses, as well as their size, shape, mobility, consistency, and areas of discomfort. Use your hands to explore the patient's internal structures to a depth of 4 or 5 cm, or more (Figure 8-4). This technique is most often used for the abdominal and male and female reproductive assessments. Variations in this technique are single-handed and bimanual palpation, which are discussed in Chapter 17.

Percussion

Percussion is the technique of striking one object against another to cause vibrations that produce sound. The density of underlying structures produces characteristic sounds that can be indicative of normal and abnormal findings. The presence of air, fluid, and solids can be confirmed, as can organ size, shape, and position. Any part of the body can be percussed, but only limited information can be obtained in specific areas such as the heart. The thorax and abdomen are the most frequently percussed locations.

Percussion sound can be analyzed according to its intensity, duration, pitch (frequency), quality, and location. Intensity refers to the relative

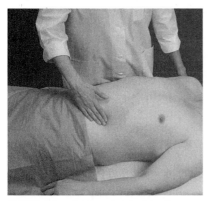

FIGURE 8-3 Technique of Light Palpation.

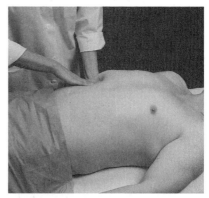

FIGURE 8-4 Technique of Deep Palpation.

loudness or softness (also called the amplitude) of the sound. Duration of percussed sound describes the time period over which a sound is heard when elicited. Frequency describes the concept of pitch and is caused by the sound's vibrations, or the highness or lowness of a sound. More rapidly occurring vibrations have a pitch that is higher than that of slower vibrations. The quality of a sound is its timbre, or how a person perceives it musically. Location of sound refers to the area where the sound is produced and heard.

The process of percussion can produce five distinct sounds in the body: flatness, dullness, resonance, hyperresonance, and tympany. Therefore, when an unexpected sound is heard in a particular area of the body, the cause must be further investigated.

Table 8-1 illustrates each of the five percussion sounds in relation to its respective intensity, duration, pitch, quality, location, and relative density. In addition, examples are provided of normal and abnormal locations of percussed sounds.

Sound waves are better conducted through a solid medium than through an air-filled medium because of the increased concentration of molecules. The basic premises underlying the sounds that are percussed are:

1. The more solid a structure, the higher its pitch, the softer its intensity, and the shorter its duration.
2. The more air-filled a structure, the lower its pitch, the louder its intensity, and the longer its duration.

There are four types of percussion techniques: immediate, mediate, direct fist percussion, and indirect fist percussion. It is important to keep in mind that the sounds produced from percussion are generated from body tissue up to 5 cm below the surface of the skin. If the abdomen is to be percussed, the patient should have the opportunity to void before the assessment.

Immediate Percussion

Immediate or direct percussion is the striking of an area of the body directly. To perform immediate percussion:

1. Spread the index or middle finger of the dominant hand slightly apart from the rest of the fingers.
2. Make a light tapping motion with the finger pad of the index finger against the body part being percussed.
3. Note what sound is produced.

Percussion of the sinuses (Figure 8-5) illustrates the use of immediate percussion in the physical assessment.

Mediate Percussion

Mediate, or indirect, percussion is a skill that takes time and practice to develop and to use effectively. Most sounds are produced using mediate percussion. Follow these steps to perform mediate percussion (Figure 8-6):

1. Place the nondominant hand lightly on the surface to be percussed.
2. Extend the middle finger of this hand, known as the pleximeter, and press its

TABLE 8-1 Characteristics of Percussion Sounds

SOUND	INTENSITY	DURATION	PITCH	QUALITY	NORMAL LOCATION	ABNORMAL LOCATION	DENSITY
Flatness	Soft	Short	High	Flat	Muscle (thigh) or bone	Lungs (severe pneumonia)	Most dense
Dullness	Moderate	Moderate	High	Thud	Organs (liver)	Lungs (atelectasis)	→
Resonance	Loud	Moderate-long	Low	Hollow	Normal lungs	No abnormal location	
Hyperresonance	Very loud	Long	Very low	Boom	No normal location in adults; normal lungs in children	Lungs (emphysema)	
Tympany	Loud	Long	High	Drum	Gastric air bubble	Lungs (large pneumothorax)	Least dense

distal phalanx and distal interphalangeal joint firmly on the location where percussion is to begin. The pleximeter will remain stationary while percussion is performed in this location.

3. Spread the other fingers of the nondominant hand apart and raise them slightly off the surface. This prevents interference and, thus, dampening of vibrations during the actual percussion.

4. Flex the middle finger of the dominant hand, called the plexor. The fingernail of the plexor finger should be very short to prevent undue discomfort and injury to the nurse. The other fingers on this hand should be fanned.

5. Flex the wrist of the dominant hand and place the hand directly over the pleximeter finger of the nondominant hand.

6. With a sharp, crisp, rapid movement from the wrist of the dominant hand, strike the pleximeter with the plexor. At this point, the plexor should be perpendicular to the pleximeter. The blow to the pleximeter should be between the distal interphalangeal joint and the fingernail. Use the finger pad rather than the fingertip of the plexor to deliver the blow. Concentrate on the movement to create the striking action from the dominant wrist only.

7. As soon as the plexor strikes the pleximeter, withdraw the plexor to avoid dampening the resulting vibrations. Do not move the pleximeter finger.

8. Note the sound produced from the percussion.

9. Repeat the percussion process one or two times in this location to confirm the sound.

10. Move the pleximeter to a second location, preferably the contralateral location from where the previous percussion was performed. Repeat the percussion process in this manner until the entire body surface area being assessed has been percussed.

Recognizing Percussion Sound

When using mediate and immediate percussion, the change from resonance to dullness is more easily recognized by the human ear than is the change from dullness to resonance. It is often helpful to close your eyes and concentrate on the sound in order to distinguish if a change in sounds occurs. This concept has implica-

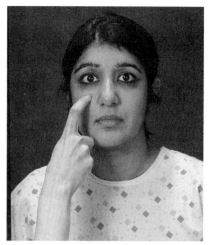

FIGURE 8-5 Technique of Immediate Percussion.

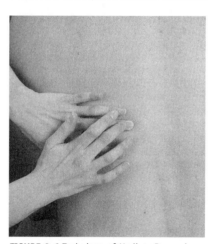

FIGURE 8-6 Technique of Mediate Percussion.

tions for patterns of percussion in areas of the body where known locations have distinct percussible sounds. For example, the techniques of diaphragmatic excursion and liver border percussion can proceed in a more defined pattern because percussion can be performed from an area of resonance to an area of dullness. Another helpful hint is to validate the change in sounds by percussing back and forth between the two areas where a change is noted.

Direct Fist Percussion

Direct fist percussion is used to assess the presence of tenderness and pain in internal organs,

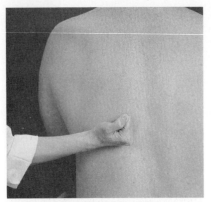

FIGURE 8-7 Technique of Direct Fist Percussion: Left Kidney.

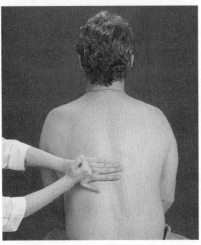

FIGURE 8-8 Technique of Indirect Fist Percussion: Left Kidney.

such as the liver or the kidneys. To perform direct fist percussion (Figure 8-7):

1. Explain this technique thoroughly so the patient does not think you are hitting him or her.
2. Make a fist with your dominant hand.
3. With the ulnar aspect of the closed fist, directly hit the area where the organ is located. The strike should be of moderate force, and it may take some practice to achieve the right intensity.

The presence of pain in conjunction with direct fist percussion may indicate inflamma-

tion of that organ or a strike that was too high in intensity.

Indirect Fist Percussion

Indirect fist percussion has the same purpose as the direct method and is preferred over the direct method. It is performed in the following manner (Figure 8-8):

1. Place the palmar side of the nondominant hand on the skin's surface over the organ to be examined. Place the fingers adjacent to one another and in straight alignment with the palm.
2. Make a fist with your dominant hand.
3. With the ulnar aspect of the closed fist, use moderate intensity to hit the outstretched nondominant hand on the dorsum.

The nondominant hand will absorb some of the force of the striking hand. The resulting intensity should be of sufficient force to produce pain in the patient if organ inflammation is present.

Auscultation

Auscultation is the act of actively listening to body organs, including sounds that are produced voluntarily and involuntarily. A deep inspiration a patient takes during the lung assessment illustrates a voluntary sound; heart sounds are involuntary sounds. Auscultation requires a quiet environment, with sounds analyzed in relation to their relative intensity, pitch, duration, quality, and location. There are two types of auscultation: direct and indirect.

Direct Auscultation

Direct or immediate auscultation is the process of listening with the unaided ear. This can be done by listening to the patient from some distance away or by placing your ear directly on the patient's skin surface. An example of immediate auscultation is the wheezing that is audible to the unassisted ear in a person having a severe asthmatic attack.

Indirect Auscultation

Indirect or mediate auscultation is the process of listening with an amplification or mechanical device. The nurse most often performs mediate auscultation with an acoustic stethoscope, which does not amplify the body sounds, but instead the earpieces block out environmental sounds. The earpieces come in various sizes; choose an earpiece that fits snugly in the ear canal without causing pain. Angling the earpieces and binaurals toward the nose permits the natural direction of the ear canal to be accessed. In this manner, sounds will be directed toward the adult tympanic membrane. The length of the rubber or plastic tubing should be between 30.5 and 40 cm. Stethoscopes with longer tubing will diminish the body sounds that are auscultated.

The acoustic stethoscope has two listening heads: the bell and the diaphragm. The bell is a concave cup that transmits low-pitched sounds; the diaphragm is flat and transmits high-pitched sounds. Breath sounds and normal heart sounds are examples of high-pitched sounds. Bruits and some heart murmurs are examples of low-pitched sounds. Another commonly used stethoscope has a single-sided, dual-frequency listening head with a single chest piece. The nurse applies different pressures on the chest piece to auscultate high- and low-pitched sounds.

Prior to auscultation, any dangling necklaces or bracelets must be removed as they can cause false noises. Warm the headpieces of the stethoscope in your hands before use, because shivering and movement can obscure assessment findings. When using the diaphragm, place it firmly against the skin surface to be auscultated. If the patient has a large quantity of hair in an area, it may be necessary to wet the hair to prevent it from interfering with the auscultated sounds. Otherwise, a grating sound may be heard. The bell is placed lightly on the skin surface that is to be auscultated. The bell will stretch the skin and act like a diaphragm and transmit high-pitched sounds if it is pressed too firmly on the skin. Auscultation requires a great deal of concentration so closing your eyes during the auscultation process may help to isolate the sound. Sometimes more than one sound is heard in a given location. If this occurs, each sound must be assessed separately. The stethoscope can act as a vector in the transmission of pathogens and therefore must be cleaned after each patient.

Amplification of body sounds can also be achieved with the use of a Doppler ultrasonic stethoscope. Water-soluble gel is placed on the body part being assessed, and the stethoscope is placed directly on the patient. Fetal heart tones and unpalpable peripheral pulses are frequently assessed via the Doppler ultrasonic stethoscope.

EQUIPMENT

The equipment needed to perform a complete physical examination of the adult patient includes:

- Pen and paper
- Marking pen
- Tape measure
- Clean gloves
- Penlight or flashlight
- Scale (the patient will need to walk to a central location if a scale cannot be brought to the patient's room.)
- Thermometer
- Sphygmomanometer
- Gooseneck lamp
- Tongue depressor
- Stethoscope
- Otoscope
- Nasal speculum
- Ophthalmoscope
- Transilluminator
- Visual acuity charts
- Tuning fork
- Reflex hammer
- Sterile needle
- Cotton balls
- Odours for cranial nerve assessment (coffee, lemon, flowers, etc.)
- Small objects for neurological assessment (paper clip, key, cotton ball, pen, etc.)
- Lubricant
- Various sizes of vaginal speculums
- Cervical brush
- Cotton-tip applicator
- Cervical spatula
- Slide and fixative
- Occult blood test material
- Specimen cup
- Goniometer

The use of these items is discussed in the chapters describing the assessments for which they are used.

◄ NURSING CHECKLIST ►

Preparing for a Physical Assessment

- Always dress in a clean, professional manner; ensure that your name pin or workplace identification is visible.
- Remove all bracelets, necklaces, or earrings that can interfere with the physical assessment.
- Fingernails must be short and hands warmed for maximum patient comfort.
- Hair must not fall forward and obstruct vision or touch the patient.
- The room should be well lit, warm, and provide privacy.
- Necessary equipment should be ready for use and within reach.
- Introduce yourself to the patient: "My name is Veronica Rojas. I am the nurse who is caring for you today and will be performing your physical assessment."
- Clarify with the patient how he or she wishes to be addressed: Miss Jones, José, Mr. Casy, Rev. Grimes, etc.
- Explain what you plan to do and how long it will take; allow the patient to ask questions.
- Instruct the patient to undress (the undergarments can be left on until the end of the assessment); provide a gown and drape for the patient and explain how to use them.
- Allow the patient to undress privately; inform the patient when you will return to start the assessment.
- Have the patient void prior to the assessment.
- Wash your hands in front of the patient to show your concern for cleanliness.
- Observe routine practices and transmission-based precautions, as indicated.
- Ensure that the patient is accessible from both sides of the examining bed or table.
- If a bed is used, raise the height so that you do not have to bend over to perform the assessment.
- Position the patient as dictated by the body system being assessed; see Figure 8-9 for positioning and draping techniques.
- Enlist the patient's cooperation by explaining what is to be done, where it will be done, and how it may feel.
- Warm all instruments prior to their use (use your hands or warm water).
- Examine the unaffected body part or side first if a patient's complaint is unilateral.
- Explain to the patient why you may be spending a long time performing one particular skill: "Listening to the heart requires concentration and time."
- If the patient complains of fatigue, continue the assessment later (if possible).
- Be cognizant of your facial expression when dealing with patients who are unkempt or with disturbing findings (infected wounds, disfigurement, etc.).
- Conduct the assessment in a systematic fashion every time to avoid forgetting a particular assessment.
- Thank the patient when the physical assessment is concluded and inform the patient what will happen next.
- Document assessment findings in the appropriate section of the patient record.

POSITION	SYSTEM ASSESSED
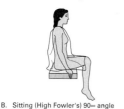 A. Semi-Fowler's 45∞ angle	Skin, head, and neck; eyes, ears, nose, mouth, and throat; thorax and lungs; heart and peripheral vasculature; musculoskeletal; neurological; patients who cannot tolerate sitting up at a 90° angle
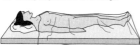 B. Sitting (High Fowler's) 90∞ angle	Skin, head, and neck; eyes, ears, nose, mouth, and throat; back; posterior thorax and lungs; anterior thorax and lungs; breast; axillae; heart; peripheral vasculature; musculoskeletal; neurological
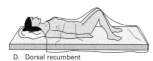 C. Horizontal recumbent (supine)	Breasts; heart and peripheral vasculature; abdomen; musculoskeletal
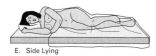 D. Dorsal recumbent	Female genitalia; patients who cannot tolerate knee flexion
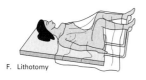 E. Side Lying	Skin; thorax and lungs; bedridden patients who cannot sit up
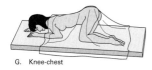 F. Lithotomy	Female genitalia and rectum
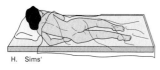 G. Knee-chest	Rectum and prostate
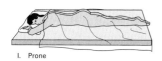 H. Sims'	Rectum and female genitalia
I. Prone	Skin; posterior thorax and lungs; hips

FIGURE 8-9 Positioning and Draping Techniques.

REFERENCES

[1]Health Canada. (1999). Infection control guidelines: Routine practices and additional precautions for preventing the transmission of infection in health care. *Canada Communicable Disease Report 1999*, 25S4, 1–155. Retrieved October 15, 2006, from http://www.phac-aspc.gc.ca/publicat/ ccdr-rmtc/99pdf/ cdr25s4e.pdf.

[2]Health Canada. (1998). Infection control guidelines: Hand washing, cleaning, disinfection and sterilization in health care. *Canada Communicable Disease Report 1998*, 24S8, 1–55.

9

General Survey, Vital Signs, and Pain

A complete physical assessment is initiated by performing general observations of the patient, obtaining the patient's vital signs, and assessing the patient for pain. Initial observations can provide data about the patient's general state of health. Vital signs include the patient's respirations, pulse, temperature, blood pressure (BP), and level of pain. These measurements provide information about the patient's basic physiological status. The presence of pain can affect a patient's physical, emotional, and mental health.

EQUIPMENT
- Stethoscope
- Watch with a second hand
- Thermometer (gloves and lubricant if using a rectal thermometer)
- Sphygmomanometer

GENERAL SURVEY

Initial observations include collecting information about the patient's physical and psychological presence, and signs and symptoms of distress.

Physical Presence

Observe the patient's:

E
1. Stated age versus apparent age
2. General appearance
3. Body fat
4. Stature
5. Motor activity
6. Body and breath odours

Stated Age versus Apparent Age

N   The patient's stated chronological age should be congruent with the apparent age.

General Appearance

N   The patient should exhibit body symmetry, no obvious deformity, and a well appearance.

Body Fat

N   Body fat should be evenly distributed. Body fat composition is difficult to estimate accurately without the use of immersion tanks or calipers. Research has indicated that body fat content, rather than actual body weight, is most closely linked to pathology (e.g., a person can be within normal limits on height and weight charts but have a high proportion of body fat to lean body mass.)

Stature

N   Limbs and trunk should appear proportional to body height; posture should be erect.

Motor Activity

N   Gait as well as other body movements should be smooth and effortless. All body parts should have controlled, purposeful movement.

E **Examination**   N **Normal Findings**   A **Abnormal Findings**   P **Pathophysiology**

Body and Breath Odours

N Normally, there is no apparent odour from patients. It is normal for some people to have bad breath related to the types of foods ingested or due to individual digestive processes.

Psychological Presence

Observe the patient's:

E 1. Dress, grooming, and personal hygiene
2. Mood and manner
3. Speech
4. Facial expressions

Dress, Grooming, and Personal Hygiene

N Generally, patients should appear clean and neatly dressed. Clothing choice should be appropriate for the weather. Norms and standards for dress and cleanliness may vary among cultures, age groups, and fashion trends.

Mood and Manner

N Generally, a patient should be cooperative and pleasant.

Speech

N The patient should respond to questions and commands easily. Speech should be clear and understandable. Pitch, rate, and volume should be appropriate to the situation.

Facial Expressions

N The patient should appear awake and alert. Facial expressions should be appropriate for what is happening in the environment and should change naturally.

Distress

Observe for:

E 1. Laboured breathing, wheezing or coughing, or laboured speech.
2. Painful facial expression, sweating, or physical protection of painful area.

3. Serious or life-threatening occurrences, such as seizure activity, active and severe bleeding, gaping wounds, and open fractures.
4. Signs of emotional distress or anxiety that may include but are not limited to tearfulness; nervous tics or laughter; avoidance of eye contact; cold, clammy hands; excessive nail biting; inability to pay attention; autonomic responses such as diaphoresis; or changes in breathing patterns.

N Breathing should be effortless, without coughing or wheezing. Speech should not leave a patient breathless. Face should be relaxed and the patient should be willing to move all body parts freely. There should be no serious or life-threatening conditions. The patient should not perspire excessively or show signs of emotional distress such as nail biting or avoidance of eye contact.

VITAL SIGNS

Vital sign measurements include respiration, pulse, temperature, and blood pressure, and level of pain.

Respiration

Respiration is the act of breathing, which supplies oxygen to the body and occurs in response to changes in the concentration of oxygen (O_2), carbon dioxide (CO_2), and hydrogen (H^+) in arterial blood. Inhalation, or inspiration, occurs when air is taken into the lungs. The diaphragm and the intercostal muscles contract and can be observed by the movement of the abdomen outward, and movement of the chest upward and outward, resulting in the lungs filling with air. Exhalation, or expiration, refers to the airflow out of the lungs. The external intercostal muscles and the diaphragm relax; the abdomen and the chest return to a resting position.

Respiratory rate is measured in breaths per minute. One respiratory cycle consists of one inhalation and one expiration.

To assess respiratory rate:

| E Examination | N Normal Findings | A Abnormal Findings | P Pathophysiology |

E 1. Stand in front of or to the side of the patient.
   2. Discreetly observe the patient's breathing (rise and fall of the chest)—the breathing pattern may be altered if the patient is being "watched."
   3. Count the number of respiratory cycles that occur in one minute.

N Table 9-1 lists the normal respiratory rates for different ages. Respiratory rates decrease with age and can vary with excitement, anxiety, fever, exercise, medications, and altitude.

A Tachypnea, respiratory rate greater than 20 breaths per minute in an adult.

P Hypoxia and metabolic acidosis, stress and anxiety.

A Bradypnea is a respiratory rate less than 12 breaths per minute in an adult at rest.

P Head injury, medications or chemicals such as opioids, barbiturates, or alcohol, sleep.

A Apnea is the absence of spontaneous breathing for 10 or more seconds.

P Traumatic injury to the brain stem.

Pulse

As the heart contracts, blood is ejected from the left ventricle (stroke volume) into the aorta. A pressure wave is created as the blood is carried to the peripheral vasculature. This palpable pressure is the pulse. Pulse assessment can determine heart rate, rhythm, and the estimated volume of blood being pumped by the heart.

Rate

Pulse rate is the number of pulse beats counted in one minute. Several factors influence heart rate or pulse rate. These include:

- The sinoatrial (SA) node, which fires automatically at a rate of 60–100 times per minute and is the primary controller of pulse rate and heart rate.
- Parasympathetic or vagal stimulation of the autonomic nervous system, which can result in decreased heart rate.
- Sympathetic stimulation of the autonomic nervous system, which results in increased heart rate.

TABLE 9-1   Respiratory Rate

AGE	RESTING RESPIRATORY RATE (Breaths/Minute)	AVERAGE
Newborn	30–50	40
1 year	20–40	30
3 years	20–30	25
6 years	16–22	19
10 years	16–20	18
14 years	14–20	17
Adult	12–20	18

- Baroreceptor sensors, which can detect changes in BP and influence heart rate. Elevated BP can decrease heart rate, whereas decreased BP can increase heart rate.

Other factors influencing heart rate include:

- Age: Heart rate generally decreases with age.
- Gender: The average female's pulse is higher than a male's pulse.
- Activity: Heart rate increases with activity. Athletes will have a lower resting heart rate than the average person because of their increased cardiac strength and efficiency.
- Emotional status: Heart rate increases with anxiety.
- Pain: Heart rate increases.
- Environmental factors: Temperature and noise level can alter heart rate.
- Stimulants: Caffeinated beverages and tobacco elevate heart rate.
- Medications: Digoxin decreases heart rate; amphetamines increase heart rate.
- Disease state: Abnormal clinical conditions can affect the heart rate (e.g., increased heart rate in hyperthyroidism, fever).

Rhythm

Pulse rhythm refers to the pattern of pulses and the intervals between pulses. A regular pulse occurs at regular intervals with even intervals

| E **Examination**   N **Normal Findings**   A **Abnormal Findings**   P **Pathophysiology** |

between each beat. Normal sinus rhythm is an example of a regular pulse.

An irregular pulse can be regularly irregular or irregularly irregular. A regular irregular rhythm is one in which an abnormal conduction occurs in the heart, but at regular intervals. Ventricular bigeminy is an example of a regularly irregular rhythm. In ventricular bigeminy, the irregular conduction, called a premature ventricular complex (PVC), occurs prior to the expected QRS complex. This PVC will occur at a regular rhythm (every other beat). An irregularly irregular rhythm has no predictable pattern, such as in atrial fibrillation.

Volume

Pulse volume (also called pulse strength or amplitude) reflects the stroke volume and the peripheral vasculature resistance (afterload). It can range from absent to bounding. Table 9-2 displays the two most commonly used scales: a 3-point and a 4-point scale. When reporting pulse volume, 2+/4+ indicates a normal pulse (2+) on a 4-point scale, whereas 2+/3+ indicates a normal pulse (2+) on a 3-point scale. If a pulse is not palpable, then attempt to ascertain its presence with a Doppler ultrasonic stethoscope.

TABLE 9-2	Scales for Measuring Pulse Volume

3-POINT SCALE

Scale	Description of Pulse
0	Absent
1+	Thready/weak
2+	Normal
3+	Bounding

4-POINT SCALE

Scale	Description of Pulse
0	Absent
1+	Thready/weak
2+	Normal
3+	Increased
4+	Bounding

The letter "D" in a pulse chart or stick figure represents the pulse that was detected by using this stethoscope.

Site

Peripheral pulses can be palpated where the large arteries are close to the skin surface. There are nine common sites for assessment of pulse (Figure 9-1). When routine vital signs are assessed, the pulse is generally measured at one of two sites: radial or apical.

Radial Pulse

To palpate the radial pulse:

E
1. Place the pad of your first, second, or third finger on the site of the radial pulse, which is along the radial bone on the thumb side of the inner wrist.
2. Press your finger gently against the artery with enough pressure so that you can feel the pulse. Pressing too hard will obliterate the pulse.
3. Count the pulse rate using the second hand of a watch. If the pulse is regular, count for 30 seconds and multiply by 2 to obtain the pulse rate per minute. If the pulse is irregular, count for 60 seconds.
4. Identify the pulse rhythm (regular or irregular) as you palpate.
5. Identify the pulse volume as you palpate (use scales from Table 9-2).

Apical Pulse

To assess the apical pulse:

E
1. Place the diaphragm of the stethoscope on the apical pulse site.
2. Count the pulse rate for 30 seconds if regular, 60 seconds if irregular.
3. Identify the pulse rhythm and volume.
4. Identify a pulse deficit (apical pulse rate greater than the radial pulse rate) by listening to the apical pulse and palpating the radial pulse simultaneously.

E Examination	N Normal Findings	A Abnormal Findings	P Pathophysiology

Rate

N Normal pulse rates vary with age (Table 9-3). The heart rate normally increases during periods of exertion. Athletes commonly have resting heart rates below 60 because of the increased strength and efficiency of the cardiac muscle.

Rhythm

N Normal pulse rhythm is regular with equal intervals between each beat.

Volume

N The pulse volume is normally the same with each beat. A normal pulse volume can be felt with a moderate amount of pressure of the fingers and obliterated with greater pressure.

Temperature

The Celsius scale is the official Canadian scale for measuring temperature, but many patients, especially the elderly, will report temperature in Fahrenheit degrees. Medical facilities use the Celsius scale. Figure 9-2 summarizes the temperature conversion formula.

Variables Affecting Body Temperature

Core body temperature is established by the temperature of blood perfusing the area of the hypothalamus (the body's temperature control centre), which triggers the body's physiological response to temperature. In addition, there are physiological variables that affect body temperature:

- Circadian rhythm
- Hormones
- Age
- Exercise
- Stress
- Environmental extremes of hot or cold

Measurement Routes

There are four basic routes by which temperature can be measured: oral, rectal, axillary, and tympanic, each of which has advantages and disadvantages (Table 9-4).

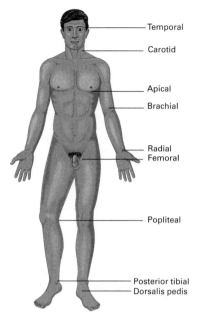

FIGURE 9-1 Peripheral Pulse Sites.

Temporal
Carotid
Apical
Brachial
Radial
Femoral
Popliteal
Posterior tibial
Dorsalis pedis

TABLE 9-3	Pulse Rate: Normal Range According to Age	
AGE	**RESTING PULSE RATE (Beats/Minute)**	**AVERAGE**
Newborn	100–170	140
1 year	80–160	120
3 years	80–120	110
6 years	70–115	100
10 years	70–110	90
14 years	60–110	85–90
Adult	60–100	72

Oral Method

E 1. Place the thermometer at the base of the tongue and to the right or left of the frenulum, and instruct the patient to close the lips around the

E **Examination**   N **Normal Findings**   A **Abnormal Findings**   P **Pathophysiology**

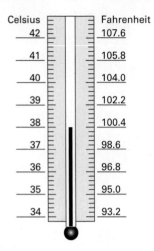

To convert:
(9/5 x temperature in Celsius) + 32 =
temperature in Fahrenheit

5/9 x (temperature in Fahrenheit − 32) =
temperature in Celsius

FIGURE 9-2 Correlation between Celsius and Fahrenheit Scales.

thermometer and to avoid biting the thermometer. Ensure that 15 minutes have passed if the patient has consumed a hot or cold beverage or food.
2. Leave the thermometer in the mouth for the time recommended by your agency or institution (usually 3–10 minutes).
3. Read the thermometer and record the temperature.

Rectal Method

E 1. Position patient with the buttocks exposed. Adults may be more comfortable lying on the side (with the knees slightly flexed), facing away from you, or prone.
2. Put on clean gloves.
3. Lubricate the tip of the thermometer with a water-soluble lubricant.
4. Ask the patient to take a deep breath; insert the thermometer into

the anus 1.25 to 3.50 cm, depending on the patient's age.
5. Do not force the insertion of the thermometer or insert into feces.
6. Hold the thermometer in place for 3–5 minutes or for the time recommended by your institution.

Axillary Method

E 1. Place the thermometer into the middle of the axilla and fold the patient's arm across the chest to keep the thermometer in place.
2. Leave the thermometer in place 5–10 minutes, depending on your institution's protocol.

Electronic Thermometer

E 1. Remove electronic thermometer from the charging unit.
2. Attach a disposable cover to the probe.
3. Using a method described (oral, rectal, or axillary), measure the temperature.
4. Listen for the sound or look for the symbol that indicates maximum body temperature has been reached.
5. Observe and record the reading.
6. Remove and discard the probe cover.
7. Return the electronic thermometer to the charging unit.

Tympanic Thermometer

E 1. Attach the probe cover to the nose of the thermometer.
2. Gently place the probe of the thermometer over the entrance to the ear canal. If the patient is under 3 years old, pull the pinna down, aiming the probe toward the opposite eye. If the patient is over 3 years old, grasp the pinna and pull gently up and back, aiming the probe toward the opposite ear. Make sure there is a tight seal.
3. Press the start button on the thermometer handle.
4. Wait for the beep, remove the probe from the ear, and read and record the temperature.

E Examination	N Normal Findings	A Abnormal Findings	P Pathophysiology

TABLE 9-4 Advantages and Disadvantages of Four Routes for Body Temperature Measurement

ROUTE	NORMAL RANGE	ADVANTAGES	DISADVANTAGES
Oral			
Average 37.0°C (slightly lower in the morning; slightly higher in late afternoon)	36.0°–38.0°C	Convenient; accessible	**Safety:** Glass thermometers are not recommended by the Canadian Paediatric Society.
			Physical abilities: Patients need to be able to breathe through the nose and be without oral pathology or recent oral surgery; route not applicable for comatose or confused patients.
			Accuracy: Oxygen therapy by mask, as well as ingestion of hot or cold drinks immediately before oral temperature measurement, affects accuracy of the reading.
Rectal			
Average 0.4°C higher than oral	36.7°–38.0°C	Considered most accurate	**Safety:** Contraindicated following rectal surgery. Risk of rectal perforation in children less than 2 years of age. Risk of stimulating Valsalva maneuver in cardiac patients. Possible source of infection in patients with mucositis or who are neutropenic.
			Physical aspects: Invasive and uncomfortable.
Axillary			
Average 0.6°C lower than oral	35.4°–37.4°C	Safe; noninvasive	**Accuracy:** Thermometer must be left in place for at least 5 minutes to obtain accurate measurement.
Tympanic			
Calibrated to oral or rectal scales	See oral or rectal	Convenient; fast; safe; noninvasive; does not require contact with any mucous membrane	**Accuracy:** Research is inconclusive as to accuracy of readings and correlations with other body temperature measurements. Technique affects reading. Tympanic membrane is thought to reflect the core body temperature.

5. Discard the probe cover.
6. Return the thermometer to the charger unit.

N Normal body temperatures are described in Table 9-4.

A Hyperthermia, pyrexia, or fever are conditions in which body temperatures exceed 38.5°C. Clinical signs of hyperthermia include increased respiratory rate and pulse, shivering, pallor, and thirst.

P There can be many causes of hyperthermia (including infection), which results from an increased basal metabolic rate.

A Hypothermia occurs when the body temperature is below 34°C.

P Clinical signs of hypothermia include decreased body temperature and initial shivering that ceases as drowsiness and coma ensue. Hypotension, decreased urinary output, lack of muscle coordination, and disorientation also occur as hypothermia progresses.

P Hypothermia can be caused by prolonged exposure to cold, such as immersion in cold water or administration of large volumes of unwarmed blood products.

P Hypothermia can be induced to decrease the tissues' need for oxygen, such as during cardiac surgery.

Blood Pressure

Blood pressure (BP) measures (in millimeters of mercury [mm Hg]) the force exerted by the flow of blood pumped into the large arteries. Arterial BP is determined by blood flow and the resistance to blood flow as indicated in the following formula:

$$MAP = CO \times TPR$$

mean arterial pressure (MAP) = cardiac output (CO) × total peripheral resistance (TPR)

Changes in BP can be used to monitor changes in cardiac output. Ineffective pumping, decreased circulating volume, as well as changes in the characteristics of the blood vessels can affect BP. There is a diurnal variation in BP as characterized by a high point in the early evening and a low point during the early deep stage of sleep.

It is important to assess BP at every opportunity, in particular as a means of screening for hypertension–known as the "silent killer"–which, even if severe, has no symptoms.

Korotkoff Sounds

Korotkoff sounds are generated when blood flow through the artery is altered by inflating the BP cuff that is wrapped around the extremity. Korotkoff sounds may be heard by listening over a pulse site that is distal to the BP cuff. As the air is released from the bladder of the cuff, the pressure on the artery changes from that which completely occludes blood flow to that which allows free flow. As the pressure against the artery wall decreases, five distinct sounds occur:

Phase I: The first audible sound heard as the cuff pressure is released. Sounds like clear tapping and correlates to systolic pressure (the force needed to pump the blood out of the heart).

Phase II: Sounds like swishing or a murmur. Created as the blood flows through blood vessels narrowed by the inflation of the BP cuff.

Phase III: Sounds like clear intense tapping. Created as blood flows through the artery but cuff pressure is still great enough to occlude flow during diastole.

Phase IV: Sounds are muffled and are heard when cuff pressure is low enough to allow some blood flow during diastole. The change from the tap of Phase III to the muffled sound of Phase IV is referred to as the first diastolic reading.

Phase V: No sounds are heard. Occurs when cuff pressure is released enough to allow normal blood flow. This is referred to as the second diastolic reading.

Measuring Blood Pressure

Systolic pressure represents the pressure exerted on the arterial wall during systole, when the ventricles are contracting. Diastolic pressure represents the pressure in the arteries when the ventricles are relaxed and filling. BP is recorded as a fraction with the top number representing the systole and the bottom number(s) repre-

---

| E Examination | N Normal Findings | A Abnormal Findings | P Pathophysiology |

senting the diastole. If first and second diastolic sounds are recorded, the first diastolic sound is written over the second. For example, 120/90/80 indicates that 120 mm Hg is the systolic pressure, 90 mm Hg is the first diastolic sound, and 80 mm Hg is the second diastolic sound. Pulse pressure is the difference between the diastolic and systolic blood pressures.

Measurement Sites

There are several potential sites for BP measurement. The preferred site is the brachial artery, which runs across the antecubital fossa. The posterior thigh, where the popliteal artery runs behind the knee joint, can also be used. A site should not be used if there is pain or injury around or near the site; for instance, a postmastectomy patient should have BP assessed on the unaffected side. Surgical incisions, intravenous, central venous, or arterial lines, or areas with poor perfusion should be avoided. Patients with arteriovenous (AV) fistulas or AV shunts should not have their BP measured in those extremities.

For the initial readings, it is recommended to take the BP in both arms (and legs if these are being used) with subsequent measures in the arm (or leg) with the highest reading.

Equipment

BP is measured indirectly with a stethoscope or Doppler and a sphygmomanometer, which consists of the BP cuff, connecting tubes and air pump, and manometer. The size of the BP cuff bladder should be 80% of the circumference of the limb being assessed.[1] The cuff should completely encircle the limb.

E
1. Ensure that the patient has not had any caffeine in the preceding hour, nor nicotine products in the 15–30 minutes prior to testing. The patient should not be experiencing any acute anxiety, stress, or pain. Bladder and bowel should be comfortable.
2. Measurements should be taken with a sphygmomanometer known to be accurate. A recently calibrated aneroid or a validated and recently calibrated electronic device can be used. Aneroid devices or mercury columns need to be clearly visible at eye level.
3. Choose a cuff with an appropriate bladder width matched to the size of the arm (Figure 9-3). For measurements taken by auscultation, bladder width should be close to 40% of arm

Cuff size

Arm circumference (cm)	Size of Cuff (cm)
From 18 to 26	9 x 18 (child)
From 26 to 33	12 x 23 (standard adult model)
From 33 to 41	15 x 33 (large, obese)
More than 41	18 x 36 (extra large, obese)

FIGURE 9-3 Cuff Size.

Source: *Reprinted from www.hypertension.ca with permission of the Canadian Hypertension Education Program.*

E Examination	**N Normal Findings**	**A Abnormal Findings**	**P Pathophysiology**

circumference and bladder length should cover 80%–100% of arm circumference. When using an automated device, select the cuff size as recommended by its manufacturer.

4. Place the cuff so that the lower edge is 3 cm above the elbow crease and the bladder is centered over the brachial artery. The patient should be resting comfortably for 5 minutes in the seated position with back support. The arm should be bare and supported with the antecubital fossa at heart level, as a lower position will result in erroneously higher SBP and DBP. There should be no talking and patients' legs should not be crossed (Figure 9-4). At least two measurements should be taken in the same arm with the patient in the same position. Blood pressure also should be assessed after 2 minutes of standing (with arm supported) and at times when patients report symptoms suggestive of postural hypotension. Supine BP measurements may also be helpful in the assessment of elderly and diabetic patients.

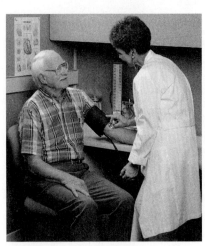

FIGURE 9-4 Position During Blood Pressure Measurement. © *Royalty-Free/Corbis.*

5. Increase the pressure rapidly to 30 mm Hg above the level at which the radial pulse is extinguished (to exclude the possibility of a systolic auscultatory gap).

6. Place the bell or diaphragm of the stethoscope gently and steadily over the brachial artery.

7. Open the control valve so that the rate of deflation of the cuff is approximately 2 mm Hg per heart beat. A cuff deflation rate of 2 mm Hg per beat is necessary for accurate systolic and diastolic estimation.

8. Read the systolic level—the first appearance of a clear tapping sound (phase I Korotkoff)—and the diastolic level (the point at which the sounds disappear (phase V Korotkoff). Continue to auscultate at least 10 mm Hg below phase V to exclude a diastolic auscultatory gap. Record the blood pressure to the closest 2 mm Hg on the manometer (or 1 mm Hg on electronic devices) as well as the arm used and whether the patient was supine, sitting or standing. Avoid digit preference by not rounding up or down. Record the heart rate. The seated blood pressure is used to determine and monitor treatment decisions. The standing blood pressure is used to examine for postural hypotension, which if present, may modify the treatment.

9. If Korotkoff sounds persist as the level approaches 0 mm Hg, then the point of muffling of the sound is used (phase IV) to indicate the diastolic pressure.

10. In the case of arrhythmia, additional readings may be required to estimate the average systolic and diastolic pressure. Isolated extra beats should be ignored. Note the rhythm and pulse rate.

11. Leaving the cuff partially inflated for too long will fill the venous system and make the sounds difficult to

---

E **Examination**   N **Normal Findings**   A **Abnormal Findings**   P **Pathophysiology**

Nursing Tip

Documenting Blood Pressure

The position of the patient during the BP measurement should be recorded. Use the following symbols to depict the patient's position:

○— supine   ○̦ sitting   ○̦ standing

Also, record where the BP was taken, using the following abbreviations:

RA = right arm   LA = left arm
RL = right leg   LL = left leg

Examples of BP readings are:

○—   160/122   LL   (supine)

○̦   98/52   RA   (sitting)

○̦   118/85   LA   (standing)

---

hear. To avoid venous congestion, it is recommended that at least 1 min should elapse between readings.

12. Blood pressure should be taken at least once in both arms and if an arm has a consistently higher pressure, that arm should be clearly noted and subsequently used for blood pressure measurement and interpretation.

N   Normal BP varies with age; it generally increases as a person ages (see Table 9-5). Normally, baroreceptors (located in the walls of most of the great arteries that sense hypotension and initiate reflex vasoconstriction and tachycardia to bring the BP back to normal) help a patient to maintain normal BP when changing from a supine to a sitting or a standing position. Processes increasing cardiac output, such as exercise, will usually increase BP. Pulse pressure is normally 30 to 40 mm Hg.

A   Hypertension, or high BP, is usually confirmed when an adult patient has sequential elevated BP readings. The CHEP recommends that the diagnosis of hypertension should be expedited with the goal of optimizing the diagnosis of hyperten-sion. Compared to previous algorithms that took up to six office visits or six months to diagnose hypertension, it is now diagnosed in as few as 1–5 visits (see Table 9-7).

P   The cause of hypertension in 90% of cases is unknown. It is thought that the mechanisms that maintain the therapeutic fluid volume in the body (e.g., the heart, kidneys, nervous system, renin-angiotensin-aldosterone system) may be abnormal. The other 10% of the population who have high BP have secondary hypertension. All of the following pathophysiologies of hypertension are secondary in nature.

P   Arteriosclerosis reduces arterial compliance. Elastic and muscular tissues of arteries are replaced with fibrous tissue as part of the normal aging process, making the vessels less able to contract and relax in response to systolic and diastolic pressures. When the systolic pressure alone is elevated in the elderly, it is called isolated systolic hypertension.

P   Processes decreasing the size of arterial lumen cause hypertension. Hypercholesterolemia results in deposits of plaque along the inner walls of the vessels, reducing the size of the lumen and increasing BP.

E   **Examination**   N   **Normal Findings**   A   **Abnormal Findings**   P   **Pathophysiology**

TABLE 9-5	Blood Pressure: Normal Range According to Age and Gender*	

AGE (FEMALE)	SYSTOLIC (mm Hg)	DIASTOLIC (mm Hg)
1	97–103	52–56
5	103–109	66–70
10	112–118	73–76
15	120–127	78–81
≥18	<120	<80
AGE (MALE)	**SYSTOLIC (mm Hg)**	**DIASTOLIC (mm Hg)**
1	94–103	49–54
5	104–112	65–70
10	111–119	73–78
15	122–131	76–81
≥18	<120	<80

*The National Heart, Lung, and Blood Institute of the National Institutes of Health developed pediatric BP guidelines based on gender, age, and height percentiles. The measurements listed for pediatric patients are consolidated for ease in reporting. Normal BP is defined as the systolic (SBP) and diastolic (DBP) blood pressures that are below the 90th percentile for age and gender. High-normal BP is defined as the SBP or DBP being at the 90th percentile and above, but not including, the 95th percentile. Hypertension is defined as a SBP or DBP greater than or equal to the 95th percentile on three different occasions.

P   Processes that increase the viscosity of the blood, such as sickle cell crisis, cause greater friction between molecules of the blood and, thus, higher BP.

P   Chronic steroid use, Cushing's syndrome, thyroid disease, and parathyroid dysfunction can all cause hypertension.

P   High BP may result from diseases affecting other regulatory BP processes. For example, kidney disease, which affects the production of antidiuretic hormone (helps control body fluid balance), can cause hypertension. An adrenal gland tumour, or pheochromocytoma, can increase BP because of epinephrine and norepinephrine secretion.

P   Overloads of fluids from poor renal function or indiscriminant IV fluid administration (particularly in children) can result in hypertension.

P   Stress can increase BP. Stimulation of the sympathetic nervous system increases cardiac output and vasoconstriction, thus increasing BP.

P   A patient's stress level can increase when in the presence of a health care provider. Patients who have elevated BP in a clinic or hospital environment only are said to have "white coat syndrome." When these patients have their BP taken in the community, it is frequently within an acceptable range.

A   BP falling below normal range is considered to be hypotension, or low BP, which results in inadequate tissue perfusion and oxygenation. If the standing SBP is more than 30 mm Hg below the supine systolic pressure, it may indicate that the person has orthostatic hypotension (see Chapter 16). Slow response by baroreceptors when an

E Examination	**N** Normal Findings	**A** Abnormal Findings	**P** Pathophysiology

individual transitions from a lying to a standing position can result in transitory orthostatic hypotension. When this occurs, the individual may feel dizzy and is at risk for falls.

P   Processes drastically reducing circulatory blood volume, such as hypovolemic shock, cause hypotension.

P   Medications such as nitroglycerin or anti-hypertensives lower BP.

P   Anaphylactic shock, resulting from massive histamine release, and circulatory collapse cause severe hypotension.

A   A difference of greater than 10–15 mm Hg between the BP in both arms is abnormal.

P   This can be caused by coarctation of the aorta, aortic aneurysm, atherosclerotic obstruction, and subclavian steal syndrome. These conditions all result in an increased pressure proximal to the narrowing and a decreased pressure distal to the narrowing of the aorta or whatever is causing the obstruction.

A   A SBP that is greater in the arms than in the legs is abnormal.

P   This is caused by constriction or obstruction of the aorta, which can result from an increase in stroke volume ejection velocity, increased cardiac output, peripheral vasodilation, and decreased distensibility of the aorta or major arteries.

A   A decreased pulse pressure is abnormal.

P   A decreased pulse pressure can result from a decreased stroke volume (cardiac tamponade, shock, and tachycardia) or increased peripheral resistance (aortic stenosis, coarctation of the aorta, mitral stenosis or mitral regurgitation, and cardiac tamponade).

P   An increased pulse pressure is abnormal.

P   An increased pulse pressure can result from increased stroke volume (aortic regurgitation) or increased peripheral vasodilatation (fever, anemia, heat, exercise, hyperthyroidism, and arteriovenous fistula).

PAIN

Pain is "an unpleasant sensory or emotional experience associated with actual or potential tissue damage, or described in terms of such damage."[2] It is a complex sensory experience that has received a lot of clinical attention in the past 35 years. Pain has become the focus of many clinical research projects as a single clinical phenomenon, not just a symptom of clinical pathology. Evidence about the prevalence and clinical significance of the pain experience has led to pain being classified as the "fifth vital sign."

Nociceptive Pain

Nociceptive pain arises from somatic or visceral stimulation. Nociception, or pain perception, is a multistep process that involves the nervous system as well as other body systems. A noxious stimulus (e.g., trauma, burn, chemical exposure, internal body inflammation, internal body growth of tissue) occurs that stimulates the nociceptors (receptive neurons of pain sensation that are located in the skin and various viscera). Transduction of the noxious stimulus travels to the spinal cord via the nociceptors, causing the conversion of one energy (travelling stimulus) from another (noxious stimulus). Cell damage from the noxious stimulus causes the release of certain chemicals or sensitizing nociceptors.

Neuropathic Pain

Neuropathic pain can result from lesions in the central nervous system (CNS) or peripheral nervous system (PNS). It is often characterized as a severe burning or tingling, such as that experienced with herpes zoster. Neuropathic pain may be difficult to treat clinically.

Types of Pain

Pain can be grouped by its origin as well as its duration. Cutaneous, somatic, visceral, and referred pain are the types grouped by origin. Cutaneous pain arises from the stimulation of cutaneous nerves and usually has a burning quality. Somatic pain originates from bone, tendons, ligaments, muscles, and nerves and is frequently caused by musculoskeletal injury. Visceral pain arises from the organs; diseased organs can change size, usually resulting in stretching of the organ, leading to pain. Acute appendicitis is an example of visceral pain. Referred pain is perceived in a location other

| E   **Examination** | N   **Normal Findings** | A   **Abnormal Findings** | P   **Pathophysiology** |

TABLE 9-7   Canadian Recommendations for the Management of Hypertension

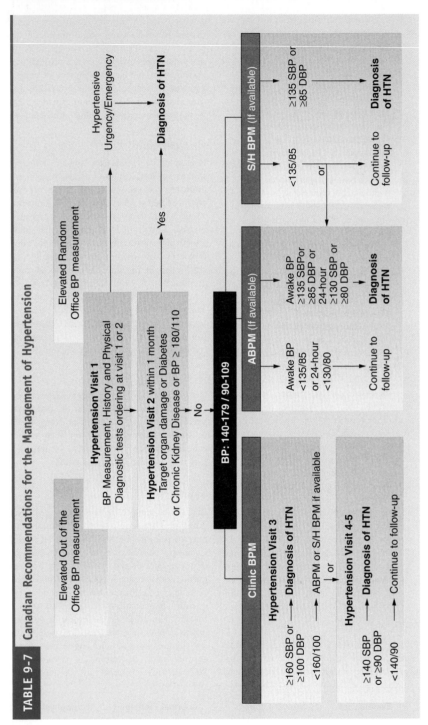

TABLE 9-7 Canadian Recommendations for the Management of Hypertension *continued*

Source: Reprinted from www.hypertension.ca with permission of the Canadian Hypertension Education Program.

The CHEP offers health care practitioners three validated technologies to diagnose hypertension: office or clinic BP monitoring; self/home blood pressure measurement (S/H BMP) that involves BP measurement morning and evening for an initial seven-day period using approved monitoring devices; ambulatory blood pressure monitoring (ABPM) by health professionals in the patient's home (especially for those suspected of office-induced hypertension).

Hypertension is diagnosed in the following scenarios:

On **Visit 1** to a health care professional if a hypertensive urgency or emergency is present. Examples include: asymptomatic DBP ≥130 mm Hg, hypertensive encephalopathy, acute aortic dissection, acute left ventricular failure, acute myocardial ischemia

After **Visit 2** to a health care professional if there is a sustained BP ≥180/110 mm Hg or sustained BP ≥140/90 mm Hg in the presence of diabetes, chronic kidney disease, or target organ damage.

After **3 Visits to a health care professional if there is** sustained BP between 160–179 mm Hg or DBP between 100–109 mm Hg (and not already diagnosed using the above criteria).

After **5 Visits to a health care professional if there is** sustained SBP ≥140 mm Hg or DBP ≥90 mm Hg.

When S/H BPM yields **duplicate home readings** in the morning and evening for **one week** (excluding day 1) ≥135/85 mm Hg.

When **ambulatory blood pressure** monitoring (ABPM) yields **average daytime** BP ≥135/85 mm Hg or **24-hour average** BP ≥130/80 mm Hg.

Nursing Tip

Assessing for Acuity Level of Pain

The Canadian Emergency Department Triage and Acuity Scale differentiates between pain presentations to determine level of acuity.[14]

- Central pain originating within a body cavity (e.g., head, chest, abdomen) or organ (e.g., eye, testicle) is more likely to predict life- or limb-threatening conditions than peripheral pain that originates within the skin, soft tissues, and axial skeleton.
- Acute central and peripheral pains are rated at higher acuity levels than central and peripheral chronic pains.

than where the pathology is occurring. The location of the referred pain is in the dermatome of the spinal cord that is innervating the affected viscera and where the organ was located in its embryonic stage. An example of referred pain is the pain of pancreatitis felt on the left shoulder.

Acute, chronic malignant, and chronic non-malignant pain are examples of pain grouped by their duration. Acute pain has a sudden onset, is of short duration, and is self-limiting. It ranges in intensity from mild to severe and usually has an identifiable cause, such as surgery or trauma. Chronic malignant pain is pain of more than six months' duration; for example, in a patient with cancer. This persistent pain can be due to a tumour, inflammation, blocked ducts, pressure on other body parts, and necrosis. Chronic nonmalignant pain also lasts more than six months and can occur with or without an identifiable cause. The pain can remain even after an initial injury is healed, such as in back pain and fibromyalgia.

Variables Affecting Pain

A patient's sex, age, previous experience with pain, and cultural expectations can affect an individual's response to pain. Studies have shown that females have a lower pain tolerance or threshold than males and report pain more frequently. Females tend to focus on the psychological aspects of pain, whereas males emphasize its physiological aspects.[3,4] Typically, young

children become sensitized to pain and may be greatly affected by the pain experience. As they reach adolescence, children may become more stoic about pain. Older adults, especially those who have chronic pain, may also not complain about their pain until it becomes debilitating. Lastly, cultural norms can determine what the patient's pain experience will be.

Effects of Pain on the Body

Pain affects everyone in different ways. Acute pain usually manifests itself differently from chronic pain, though there are some common elements. Physiological responses to pain include tachycardia, tachypnea, hypertension, diaphoresis, dilated pupils, and an altered immune response. Additional responses to pain include complaints of pain, crying, moaning, frowning, anger, fear, anxiety, depression, suicidal ideation, decreased appetite, sleep deprivation, altered concentration, pacing, and rubbing, protecting, or splinting the affected body part. Pain can affect every system in the human body, and unrelieved pain can take its toll on the health of the patient over time. Just as pain is a unique experience for the person in pain, so is the patient's response to pain.

Assessing Pain

Many patients present with a principal health issue or concern of pain. As with the experience of other symptoms, a thorough assessment includes asking questions about the following aspects of the pain experience:

- Location: Where is the pain located?
- Radiation: Does the pain move to another part of the body?
- Quality: How does the pain feel?
- Quantity: How severe is the pain?
- Associated manifestations: What other signs and symptoms are occurring with the pain?
- Aggravating factors: What makes the pain worse?
- Alleviating factors: What makes the pain better?
- Setting: Where were you (physically or emotionally or both) when the pain started?
- Timing: When did the pain start? How long does it last? How frequently does it occur?
- Meaning and impact: Does this pain have any special significance to you? How has it affected your life?

OUCHER!™

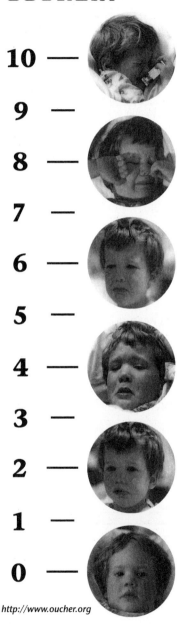

http://www.oucher.org

FIGURE 9-5 Oucher Pain Assessment Tool

Source: The Caucasian Version of the Oucher, developed and copyrighted by Judith E. Beyer, RN, PhD, 1983.

Pain intensity rating scales are available to assess the severity of a patient's pain experience. Examples of rating scales include the Oucher Pain Assessment Tool[5] (Figure 9-5), which is used with children 3–12 years old (Caucasian, Hispanic, and African American versions of this tool are available); the Wong-Baker FACES Pain Rating Scale[6] (Figure 9-6) which is recommended for children over the age of 3; and the Pain Intensity Scale[7] (Figure 9-7) which can be used with adults. Flow sheets can identify trends in the patient's pain, e.g., is the pain being alleviated or is it worsening; are treatment methods being effective?

REFERENCES

[1]Canadian Hypertension Education Program (CHEP) Recommendations (2006). Retrieved May 26, 2006, from http://www.hypertension.ca/CHEP2006/CHEP_2006_complete.pdf

[2]International Association for the Study of Pain (1979). *IASP pain terminology*. Retrieved May 26, 2006, from http://www.iasp-pain.org/terms-p.html

[3]Fillingim, R. B., & Maixner, W. (1995). Gender differences in response to noxious stimuli. *Pain Forum, 4*, 209–11.

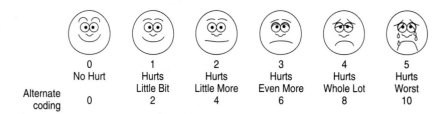

	0	1	2	3	4	5
	No Hurt	Hurts Little Bit	Hurts Little More	Hurts Even More	Hurts Whole Lot	Hurts Worst
Alternate coding	0	2	4	6	8	10

FIGURE 9-6 Wong-Baker FACES Pain Rating Scale.

Note. From Hockenberry, M., Wilson, D., & Winkelstein, M. (2005). *Wong's essentials of pediatric nursing* (7th ed.), St. Louis, MO: Mosby, Inc., p. 663. Reprinted with permission.

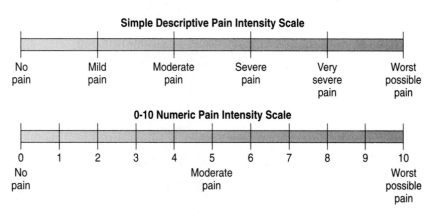

FIGURE 9-7 Pain Intensity Scale.

Note. From Acute Pain Management Guideline Panel. (1992). Acute pain management: Operative or medical procedures and trauma. Clinical Practice Guideline (AHCPR Publication No. 92-0032), Rockville, MD: Agency for Health Care Policy and Research.

[4]Berkeley, K. J., & Holdcroft, A. (1999). Sex and gender differences in pain. In P. D. Wall & R. Melzack (Eds.), *Textbook of pain* (4th ed.). Edinburgh: Churchill Livingstone.

[5]Beyer, J. (1983). *The Caucasian version of the Oucher.* Developed and copyrighted by Judith E. Beyer, RN, PhD, 1983.

[6]Hockenberry, M., Wilson, D., Winkelstein, M., & Kline, N. (2003). *Wong's nursing care of infants and children* (7th ed.). St. Louis, MO: Mosby.

[7]Acute Pain Management Guideline Panel. (1992). *Acute pain management: Operative or medical procedures and trauma. Clinical practice guideline* (AHCPR Publication No. 92-0032). Rockville, MD: Agency for Health Care Policy and Research.

BIBLIOGRAPHY

Abbott C., Schiffrin, E. L., Grover, S., Honos, G., Lebel, M., Mann, K., Wilson, T., Penner, B., Tremblay, G., Tobe, S. W., & Feldman, R. D. (2005). Canadian hypertension education program. The 2005 Canadian hypertension education program recommendations for the management of hypertension: Part 1— Blood pressure measurement, diagnosis and assessment of risk. *Canadian Journal of Cardiology. 21*(8), 645–56, Jun.

10

Skin, Hair, and Nails

ANATOMY AND PHYSIOLOGY

Skin

The surface area of the skin covers approximately 1.86 square metres (20 square feet) in the average adult, with a thickness varying from 0.2 mm to 1.5 mm, depending on the region of the body and the patient's age. Morphologically speaking, the skin is composed of three main layers: the epidermis, the dermis, and the subcutaneous tissue, or hypodermis (Figure 10-1).

Glands of the Skin

There are two main groups of glands in the skin: sebaceous glands and sweat glands.

The sebaceous glands are sebum-producing glands that are found almost everywhere in the dermis except for the palmar and plantar surfaces. They are part of the apparatus that contains the hair follicle and the arrector pili muscle, which contracts the skin and hair, resulting in "goose bumps." The ducts of the sebaceous glands open into the upper part of the hair follicle and produce sebum, an oily secretion that is thought to stop evaporation and water loss from the epidermal cells. Sebaceous glands are most prevalent in the scalp, forehead, nose, and chin.

The two main types of sweat glands are apocrine glands, which are associated with hair follicles, and eccrine glands, which are not

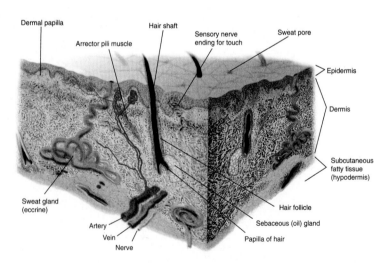

Dermal papilla

Hair shaft

Arrector pili muscle

Sensory nerve ending for touch

Sweat pore

Epidermis

Dermis

Subcutaneous fatty tissue (hypodermis)

Sweat gland (eccrine)

Artery

Vein

Nerve

Hair follicle

Sebaceous (oil) gland

Papilla of hair

FIGURE 10-1 Structures of the skin

associated with hair follicles. The secretory apparatus of both types of sweat glands is located in the subcutaneous tissue. Eccrine glands open directly onto the skin's surface and are widely distributed throughout the body. Apocrine glands are found primarily in the axillae, genital and rectal areas, nipples, and navel. These glands become functional during puberty, and secretion occurs during emotional stress or sexual stimulation. After puberty, apocrine glands are responsible for the characteristic body odour when sweat mixes with the natural bacterial flora normally present on the skin surface.

Hair

With few exceptions (the palmar and plantar surfaces, lips, nipples, and the glans penis), hair is distributed over the entire body surface. Its abundance and texture are dependent on an individual's age, sex, race, and heredity. Vellus hair, or fine, faint hair, covers most of the body. In general, terminal hair is the coarser, darker hair of the scalp, eyebrows, and eyelashes. In the axillary and pubic areas, terminal hair becomes increasingly evident in both males and females with the onset of puberty. Males also tend to develop coarser, thicker chest and facial hair.

Specialized epidermal cells are located in depressions at the base of each hair follicle and form each individual hair shaft. Blood vessels in the dermis nourish the cells so that they grow and divide, pushing the older cells toward the surface of the skin. Most hair shafts are composed of three layers: the cuticle, or outer layer; the cortex, or middle layer; and the medulla, or innermost layer. Hair colour is determined by the melanocytes produced in the cells at the base of each follicle; larger amounts of pigment produce darker hair colour and smaller amounts produce a lighter colour.

Nails

Nails are composed of keratinized, or horny, layers of cells that arise from undifferentiated epithelial tissue called the matrix. The nail plate, tissue that covers the distal portion of the digits and provides protection, is approximately 0.5–0.75 mm thick. The nails consists of the nail root, which lies posterior to the cuticle and is attached to the matrix; the nailbed, which is the vascular bed located beneath the nail plate; and the periungual tissues, which surround the nail plate and the free edge of the nail (Figure 10-2). At the proximal end of each nail is a white, crescent-shaped area known as the lunula, which is obscured by the cuticle in some individuals.

The normally translucent nail plate is given a pinkish cast by the underlying vascular bed in light-skinned individuals and a brownish cast in dark-skinned individuals. In many disease

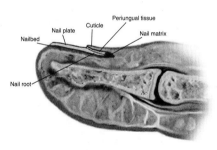

FIGURE 10-2 Structures of the nail.

HEALTH HISTORY

Skin Specific	Allergies, eczema, atopic dermatitis, melanoma, albinism, vitiligo, psoriasis, skin cancer, athlete's foot, birthmarks, body piercing, tattoos, urticaria
Hair Specific	Allergies, alopecia, lice, bacterial or fungal infections of the scalp, brittle hair, rapid hair loss, trichotillomania, trauma, congenital anomalies
Nail Specific	Allergies, psoriasis, bacterial or fungal infections, trauma, brittle nails, nail biting, congenital anomalies
Surgical History	Keloid and scar formation, plastic surgery for birthmarks, skin grafts, reconstructive surgery, excision biopsy

◀ NURSING CHECKLIST ▶

Specific Health History Questions Regarding the Skin, Hair, and Nails

Skin Care Habits

- Do you use lotions, perfumes, cologne, cosmetics, soaps, oils, shaving cream, after-shave lotion, or an electric or standard razor?
- What type of home remedies do you use for skin lesions and rashes?
- How often do you bathe or shower?
- Do you use a tanning bed or salon?
- What type of sun protection do you use?
- Have you ever had a reaction to jewelry that you wore?
- Do you wear hats, visors, gloves, long sleeves or pants, or sunscreen when in the sun?
- How much time do you spend in the sun?

Hair Care Habits

- Do you use shampoo, conditioner, hair spray, setting products?
- Do you colour, dye, bleach, frost, or use relaxants on your hair?
- What products do you use?
- Do you wear a wig or hairpiece?
- Do you have greying hair or hair loss?
- Do you use a hair dryer, heated curlers, or curling iron?
- Do you tightly braid your hair?

Nail Care Habits

- Do you get manicures or pedicures?
- What type of nail care do you practise (trimming, clipping, use of polish, nail tips, acrylics)?
- Do you bite your nails?
- Do you suffer from nail splitting or discoloration?

Nursing Alert

The A, B, C, D, E's of Screening

Patients should check nevi (moles) and other lesions in front of a mirror once a month. If a lesion is on a posterior surface, the patient should ask a partner to check it on a monthly basis. A photo can be taken for future comparisons. A skin lesion should be assessed further if any of the following are noted:

- **A**symmetry (Is the lesion asymmetrical?)
- **B**order irregularities (Are the borders of the lesion irregular?)
- **C**olour variegation (Is the colour of the lesion uneven, irregular, or multicoloured?)
- **D**iameter greater than 6 mm (Is the lesion greater than 6 mm?)
- **E**nlargement or evolution of colour change, shape, or symptoms (Is the lesion getting bigger or changing in shape, size or sensation?)

Nursing Tip

Reducing Exposure to Integumentary Irritants

- In the workplace, always follow health and safety guidelines. Review any Material Safety Data Sheet (MSDS) sources for precautionary measures on working with dangerous products.
- Follow the directions on the labels of all products; pay special attention to warning labels.
- If using a personal care product for the first time, perform a patch test to evaluate for sensitivity.
- Use rubber gloves when handling toxins or caustic substances.
- Contact a poison control centre for treatment guidelines if exposed to toxic or caustic substances.
- Notify appropriate officials if a dangerous chemical or toxin exposure occurs.

processes, the colour of the nailbed may vary. For instance, a decrease in oxygen content of the blood will cause the nailbeds to appear cyanotic, or blue.

EQUIPMENT

- Magnifying glass
- Good source of natural light
- Penlight
- Clean gloves
- Microscope slide
- Small centimeter ruler

For Special Techniques

- Wood's lamp
- #15 scalpel blade
- Microscope slide with cover slips
- Mineral oil
- Microscope

ASSESSMENT OF THE SKIN, HAIR, AND NAILS

Inspection of the Skin

In each area, observe for: colour, bleeding, ecchymosis, vascularity, lesions, moisture, temperature, texture, turgor, and edema.

E 1. Facing the patient, inspect the skin colour of the face, eyelids, ears, nose, lips, and mucous membranes.

2. Inspect the anterior and lateral aspects of the neck, then inspect behind the ears.

3. Inspect arms and dorsal and palmar surfaces of the hands. Pay special attention to the finger webs.

4. Have the patient move to a supine position, with arms placed over the head.

5. Lower gown to uncover chest and breasts.

6. Inspect intramammary folds and ridges. Pendulous breasts may need to be raised to complete this inspection.

7. Assess axillae, and cover chest and breasts with gown.

8. Raise gown to uncover abdomen and anterior aspect of the lower extremities; place a sheet over the genital area.

9. Inspect abdomen, anterior aspect of the lower extremities, dorsal and plantar surfaces of the feet, and toe webs.

10. Don gloves and uncover genital area.

11. Inspect inguinal folds and genitalia.

12. Remove gloves.

13. Have the patient turn to a side-lying position on the examination table so the patient's back is facing you.

14. Inspect back and posterior neck and scalp. Specifically look for nevi or other lesions.

15. Inspect posterior aspect of the lower extremities.

E Examination   N Normal Findings   A Abnormal Findings   P Pathophysiology

◀ NURSING CHECKLIST ▶

General Approach to Skin, Hair, and Nail Assessment

1. Ensure that the room is well lit. Daylight is the best source of light, especially when determining skin colour. However, if access to daylight is not possible, overhead fluorescent lights should be added.
2. Use a handheld magnifying glass to aid in inspection when simple visual inspection is not adequate.
3. Explain to the patient each step of the assessment process prior to initiating the assessment.
4. Ensure patient privacy by providing drapes.
5. Ensure the comfort of the patient by keeping the room at an appropriate temperature.
6. Warm hands by washing them in warm water before the assessment.
7. Gather equipment on a table prior to initiating the assessment.
8. Ask the patient to undress completely and to put on a patient gown, leaving the back untied.
9. Perform assessment in a cephalocaudal fashion.
10. For episodic illness, the skin examination is incorporated into the regional physical exam.

Nursing Alert

Frostbite

Damage to tissues from freezing results because of the formation of ice crystals within cells, which leads to rupture of the cells and, ultimately, cell death.

Frostnip

Initially cold, burning pain; the affected area becomes blanched (usually hands, feet, face, or other exposed areas). With rewarming, the area becomes reddened. Frostnip generally does not lead to permanent damage because only the top layers of skin are involved. However, it can lead to long-term sensitivity to heat and cold.

Frostbite

If freezing continues, frostbite develops. Symptoms include cold burning pain that progresses to tingling, and later, numbness or a heavy sensation. The area becomes pale or white and rewarming causes pain.

If further freezing continues, deep frostbite occurs; all of the muscles, tendons, blood vessels, and nerves freeze. The extremity is hard, feels woody, and use is lost temporarily, and in severe cases, permanently. The involved area appears deep purple or red with blisters that are usually filled with blood. This type of severe frostbite may result in the loss of fingers and toes.

Nursing Tip

Body Piercing and Tattoos

It is important to inspect the skin and note the presence and location of tattoos and body piercing. Some patients react to the ink in the tattoo and develop various skin disorders. Health Canada has deemed the use of the ingredient para-phenylenediamine (PPD) in "black henna" (temporary tattoo ink) as unsafe. Body piercing sites should be assessed for signs of infection (e.g., erythema, purulent discharge, increased skin temperature). Remember to assess all body areas and document the location of all tattoos and body piercing, such as the ears, umbilicus, eyebrows, lips, nares, tongue, labia, vagina, and scrotum. Health Canada warns that getting a tattoo or body piercing from an operator who does not use sterilized equipment or techniques places people at risk for blood-borne pathogens. Therefore, the nurse should screen patients with tattoos and body piercing for diseases such as hepatitis and HIV, among others.

---

16. Don clean gloves and raise the gluteal cleft and inspect the gluteal folds and perianal area; then remove and discard the gloves.
17. Cover the patient and assist to a sitting position.
18. Wash hands.

Colour

E Assess for coloration.

N Normally, the skin is a uniform whitish pink or brown colour, depending on the patient's race. Exposure to sunlight results in increased pigmentation of sun-exposed areas. Dark-skinned persons may have a freckling of the gums, tongue borders, and lining of the cheeks; the gingiva may appear blue or variegated in colour.

A The appearance of cyanosis (blue discoloration) of fingers, nailbeds, lips, or mucous membranes is abnormal in both light- and dark-skinned individuals. In light-skinned individuals, the skin has a bluish tint. The earlobes, lower eyelids, lips, oral mucosa, nailbeds, and palmar and plantar surfaces may be especially cyanotic. Dark-skinned individuals have an ashen- grey to pale tint, and the lips and tongue are good indicators of cyanosis.

P Cyanosis occurs when there is greater than 50 g/L of deoxygenated hemoglobin in the blood and does not usually appear until arterial oxygen saturation falls to 75% (severe respiratory failure occurs when oxygen saturation falls to 85–90%). In order for cyanosis to be an accurate indicator of arterial oxygen (PaO_2), two conditions must be met. The patient must have normal hemoglobin and hematocrit as well as normal perfusion. For example, a patient with polycythemia (elevated number of red blood cells) can be cyanotic but have adequate oxygenation. The problem is that the patient has too many red blood cells rather than too little oxygen. Conversely, a patient with anemia (reduced number of red blood cells) can be hypoxemic but not cyanotic. In this case, the patient has too little hemoglobin. Central cyanosis is secondary to marked heart and lung disease; peripheral cyanosis can be secondary to systemic disease or vasoconstriction stimulated by cold temperatures or anxiety.

A The appearance of jaundice (yellow-green to orange cast) of skin, sclera, mucous membranes, fingernails, and palmar or plantar surfaces in the light-skinned individual is abnormal. Jaundice in dark-skinned individuals may appear as yellow staining in the sclera, hard palate, and palmar or plantar surfaces.

P Jaundice is caused by an increased serum bilirubin level associated with liver disease

---

E Examination   N Normal Findings   A Abnormal Findings   P Pathophysiology

Nursing Alert

Signs of Abuse

Areas of ecchymosis at varying stages of healing (see Table 10-1) are often signs of trauma that could be the result of physical abuse. Ecchymotic areas at the base of the skull, or on the face, buttocks, breasts, or abdomen should warrant a high index of suspicion for abuse, especially if found in children or pregnant women, as should burns (e.g., cigarettes, iron) and ecchymoses that follow recognizable patterns (i.e., belt marks, fingerprints, bite marks). Any signs of abuse should be investigated further and referred as necessary.

or hemolytic disease and is only detected when the serum bilirubin is greater than 34μmol/L (twice the normal upper limit). Severe burns and sepsis also can produce jaundice.

A A yellow discoloration of the palmar and digital creases.

P Xanthoma striata palmaris is caused by hyperlipidemia.

A Orange-yellow coloration of palmar and plantar surfaces and forehead but no involvement of the mucous membranes.

P Carotenemia, elevated levels of serum carotene, results from the excessive ingestion of carotene-rich foods such as carrots.

TABLE 10-1	Estimating Age of Healing Bruises

COLOUR OF BRUISE	DAYS SINCE INJURY
Red	0–1
Bluish purple	1–4
Greenish yellow	5–7
Yellowish brown	8

Source: *Rudolph's Fundamentals of Pediatrics* (Rudolph and Kamei, 1998).

A A greyish cast to the skin.

P A greyish cast is seen in renal patients and is associated with chronic anemia along with retained urochrome pigments. Slight jaundice may also be found in the renal patient.

A A combination of pallor and ecchymosis with a jaundiced appearance.

P Uremia secondary to renal failure results in serum urochrome pigment retention.

A Sustained bright red or pink coloration in light-skinned individuals is abnormal. Dark-skinned individuals may have no underlying change in coloration. Palpation may be used to ascertain signs of warmth, swelling, or induration.

P Hyperemia occurs because of dilated superficial blood vessels, increased blood flow, febrile states, local inflammatory condition, or excessive alcohol intake.

A A bright red to ruddy sustained appearance that is evident on the integument, mucous membranes, and palmar or plantar surfaces is abnormal in both light- and dark-skinned individuals.

P Polycythemia, as noted earlier, is an increased number of red blood cells and results in this ruddy appearance.

A A dusky rubor of the extremities when in a dependent position, which can be associated with tissue necrosis.

P Venous stasis results from venule engorgement and diminished blood flow, which occurs in congestive heart failure and atherosclerosis.

A A pale cast to the skin that may be most evident in the face, mucous membranes, lips, and nailbeds is abnormal in light-skinned individuals. A yellow-brown to ashen-grey cast to the skin, along with pale or grey lips, mucous membranes, and nailbeds, is abnormal in dark-skinned individuals.

P Pallor (lack of colour) is due to decreased visibility of the normal oxyhemoglobin. This can occur when the patient has decreased blood flow in the superficial vessels, as in shock or syncope, or when there is a decreased amount of serum oxyhemoglobin, as in anemia. Localized pallor may be secondary to arterial insufficiency.

E Examination	N Normal Findings	A Abnormal Findings	P Pathophysiology

A   A brown cast to the skin can be generalized or discrete.

P   A brown coloration occurs when there is a deposition of melanin that can be caused by genetic predisposition, pregnancy, Addison's disease (deficiency in cortisol leads to enhanced melanin production), café au lait spots, and sunlight.

P   Acanthosis nigricans is a condition in which the skin becomes brownish and thicker, almost leathery in appearance. This usually occurs in the axillae, on the flexoral surfaces of the groin and neck, and around the umbilicus. Acanthosis nigricans occurs in obesity, diabetes mellitus, and with medications such as steroids.

A   A white cast to the skin as evidenced by generalized whiteness, including of the hair and eyebrows.

P   This lack of coloration is caused by albinism, a congenital inability to form melanin.

A   Vitiligo is a condition marked by patchy symmetrical areas of white on the skin.

P   This condition can be caused by an acquired loss of melanin. Trauma can also lead to hypopigmentation, especially in dark-skinned individuals.

A   An erythematous, confluent eruption in a butterfly-like distribution over the face.

P   Systemic lupus erythematosus, a connective tissue disorder, is the most likely etiology.

Bleeding, Ecchymosis, and Vascularity

E   Inspect the skin for evidence of bleeding, ecchymosis, or increased vascularity.

N   Normally, there are no areas of increased vascularity, ecchymosis, or bleeding.

A   Bleeding from the mucous membranes, previous venipuncture sites, or lesions.

P   Spontaneous bleeding can be indicative of clotting disorders, trauma, or use of antithrombolytic agents such as warfarin or heparin.

A   Petechiae are violaceous (red-purple) discolorations of less than 0.5 cm in diameter. Petechiae do not blanch. In dark-skinned individuals, evaluate for petechiae in the mucous membranes and axillae.

P   Increased bleeding tendency or embolism; causes include intravascular defects or infections.

A   Purpura is a condition characterized by the presence of confluent petechiae or confluent ecchymosis over any part of the body.

P   Purpura or peliosis is characterized by hemorrhage into the skin and can be caused by decreased platelet formation. Lesions vary based on the type of purpura; pigmentation changes may become permanent.

A   Ecchymosis is a violaceous discoloration of varying size, also called a black-and-blue mark. In dark-skinned patients, these discolorations are deeper in colour.

P   Extravasation of blood into the skin as a result of trauma and can also occur with heparin or warfarin use or liver dysfunction.

A   An erythematous dilation of small blood vessels is abnormal.

P   This describes telangiectasias. They tend to appear on the face and thighs and occur more frequently in women.

Nursing Tip

Enhancement Techniques

Magnification: Use of a magnifying glass may be beneficial in the evaluation of lesions and discolorations for morphology.

Wood's Lamp: Also known as a UV light, it is valuable in the diagnosis of certain skin and hair diseases. Dermatophytosis and erythrasma are easily diagnosed by the fluorescent changes that occur under UV exposure. Dermatophytosis in the hair shaft will appear green to yellow, and erythrasma will appear coral red.

E   **Examination**   N   **Normal Findings**   A   **Abnormal Findings**   P   **Pathophysiology**

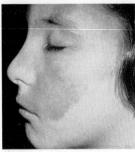

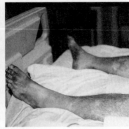

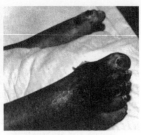

B. Necrosis. *Courtesy of Dr. Mark Dougherty, Lexington, KY.*

C. Gas gangrene

A. Nevus Flammeus. *Courtesy of Robert A. Silverman, M.D., Clinical Associate Professor, Department of Pediatrics, Georgetown University.*

FIGURE 10-3

A Spider angiomas are bright red and star-shaped. There is often a central pulsation noted with pressure and this results in blanching in the extensions. Most often, these lesions are noted on the face, neck, and chest. They are a type of telangiectasia.

P Causes include pregnancy, liver disease, and hormone therapy.

A Venous stars are linear or irregularly shaped blue vascular patterns that do not blanch with pressure.

P Increased venous pressure in the superficial veins.

A Cherry angiomas are bright-red circumscribed areas that may darken with age.

P Unknown etiology and are pathologically insignificant except for cosmetic appearance.

A A bright-red, raised area that has well-defined borders and does not blanch with pressure.

P Strawberry hemangiomas, or strawberry marks, are congenital malformations of closely packed immature capillaries.

A A burgundy, red, or violaceous macular vascular patch that is located along the course of a peripheral nerve.

P This is a nevus flammeus, or port-wine stain. Indicative of underlying disorders, such as Sturge-Weber syndrome (Figure 10-3A).

A In light-skinned individuals, a purple to black discoloration. In dark-skinned individuals, very dark to black discoloration.

P These findings can indicate different stages of necrosis, or tissue death. Conditions that starve the affected body part of oxygen, whether in acute or chronic situations, such as in diabetes mellitus, disseminated intravascular coagulation, acute hypovolemia, and severe electric charge, can cause necrosis (Figure 10-3B).

A Dark-brown or blackened areas of skin that are edematous and painful.

P Clostridial myonecrosis, more commonly referred to as gas gangrene, is a gram-positive infection that affects skeletal muscles that have decreased oxygenation (Figure 10-3C).

Lesions

E 1. Inspect the skin for lesions, noting the anatomic location. Lesions can be localized, regionalized, or generalized. They can involve exposed areas or skin folds.

  2. Note the grouping or arrangement of the lesions: discrete, grouped, confluent, linear, annular, polycyclic, generalized, or zosteriform (Figure 10-4).

E Examination	**N** Normal Findings	**A** Abnormal Findings	**P** Pathophysiology

3. Inspect the lesions for elevation (flat or raised).
4. Using a ruler, measure the lesions.
5. Describe the colour of the lesions.
6. Note any exudate for colour or odour.
7. Note the morphology of the skin lesions. Skin lesions can be primary (see Figure 10-5), originating from previously normal skin, or secondary (Figure 10-6), originating from primary lesions.

N   No skin lesions should be present except for freckles, birthmarks, or nevi (moles), which may be flat or elevated.

A/P   See Figures 10-4, 10-5, and 10-6.

PALPATION OF THE SKIN

Moisture

E   Palpate all nonmucous membrane skin surfaces for moisture using the dorsal surfaces of the hands and fingers.

N   Normally, the skin is dry with a minimum of perspiration. Moisture on the skin will vary from one body area to another, with perspiration normally present on the hands, axilla, face, and in between the skin folds. Moisture also varies with changes in environment, muscular activity, body temperature, stress, and activity levels. Body temperature is regulated by the skin's production of perspiration, which evaporates to cool the body.

A   Excessive dryness of the skin, xerosis, as evidenced by flaking of the stratum corneum and associated pruritus is abnormal.

P   Hypothyroidism and exposure to extreme cold and dry climates.

A   Very dry, large scales that are light coloured or brown.

P   Ichthyosis vulgaris is a skin abnormality originating from a keratin disorder. It can be associated with atopic dermatitis.

A   Diaphoresis is the profuse production of perspiration. Hyperhidrosis is abnormally increased axillary, plantar, facial and/or truncal perspiration, in excess of that required for regulation of body temperature.

> ### Nursing Tip
>
> **Use of Gloves**
>
> Use gloves for palpation of the skin only if there is any probability of contact with body fluids or if the patient is in isolation. Wearing gloves does not substitute for washing hands.

P   Hyperthyroidism, increased metabolic rate, sepsis, anxiety, or pain. Primary hyperhidrosis is idiopathic; secondary hyperhidrosis can be related to endocrine disorders, obesity, or menopause.

Temperature

E   Palpate all nonmucosal skin surfaces for temperature using the dorsal surfaces of the hands and fingers.

N   Skin surface temperature should be warm and equal bilaterally. Hands and feet may be slightly cooler than the rest of the body.

A   Hypothermia is a cooling of the skin and may be generalized or localized.

P   Generalized hypothermia is indicative of shock or some other type of central circulatory dysfunction. Localized hypothermia is indicative of arterial insufficiency in the affected area.

A   Generalized hyperthermia is the excessive warming of the skin and may be generalized or localized.

P   Generalized hyperthermia may be indicative of a febrile state, hyperthyroidism, or increased metabolic function caused by exercise. Localized hyperthermia may be caused by infection, trauma, sunburn, or windburn.

Tenderness

E   Palpate skin surfaces for tenderness using the dorsal surfaces of the hands and fingers.

N   Skin surfaces should be nontender.

A   Tenderness over the skin structures can be discrete and localized or generalized.

E **Examination**   N **Normal Findings**   A **Abnormal Findings**   P **Pathophysiology**

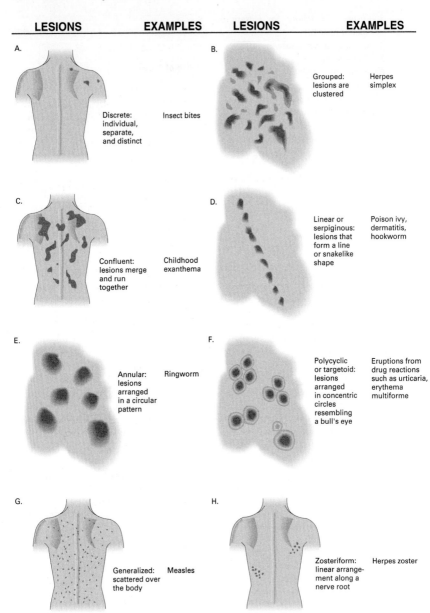

FIGURE 10-4 Arrangement of lesions.

NONPALPABLE

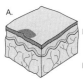

Macule:
  Localized changes in skin
  colour of less than 1 cm
  in diameter
Example:
  Freckle

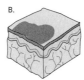

Patch:
  Localized changes in skin
  colour of greater than 1 cm
  in diameter
Example:
  Vitiligo, stage 1 of pressure
  ulcer

PALPABLE

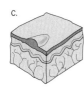

Papule:
  Solid, elevated lesion less
  than 0.5 cm in diameter
Example:
  Warts, elevated nevi,
  seborrheic keratosis

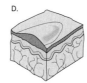

Plaque:
  Solid, elevated lesion
  greater than 0.5 cm
  in diameter
Example:
  Psoriasis, eczema,
  pityriasis rosea

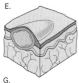

Nodules:
  Solid and elevated; however,
  they extend deeper than
  papules into the dermis or
  subcutaneous tissues,
  0.5-2.0 cm
Example:
  Lipoma, erythema nodosum,
  cyst, melanoma, hemangioma

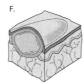

Tumour:
  The same as a nodule only
  greater than 2 cm
Example:
  Carcinoma (such as advanced
  breast carcinoma); **not** basal cell
  or squamous cell of the skin

Wheal:
  Localized edema in the
  epidermis causing irregular
  elevation that may be red
  or pale
Example:
  Insect bite, hive, angioedema

FLUID-FILLED CAVITIES WITHIN THE SKIN

Vesicle:
  Accumulation of fluid between
  the upper layers of the skin;
  elevated mass containing
  serous fluid; less than 0.5 cm
Example:
  Herpes simplex, herpes
  zoster, chickenpox, scabies

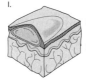

Bullae:
  Same as a vesicle only
  greater than 0.5 cm
Example:
  Contact dermatitis, large
  second-degree burns,
  bullous impetigo, pemphigus

Pustule:
  Vesicles or bullae that
  become filled with pus,
  usually described as less
  than 0.5 cm in diameter
Example:
  Acne, impetigo, furuncles,
  carbuncles, folliculitis

Cyst:
  Encapsulated fluid-filled or
  semi-solid mass in the
  subcutaneous tissue or
  dermis
Example:
  Sebaceous cyst, epidermoid
  cyst

FIGURE 10-5 Morphology of primary lesions.

ABOVE THE SKIN SURFACE

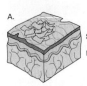

Scales:
Flaking of the skin's surface
Example:
Dandruff, psoriasis, xerosis

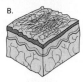

Lichenification:
Layers of skin become thickened and rough as a result of rubbing over a prolonged period of time
Example:
Chronic contact dermatitis

Crust:
Dried serum, blood, or pus on the surface of the skin
Example:
Impetigo, acute eczematous inflammation

Atrophy:
Thinning of the skin surface and loss of markings
Example:
Striae, aged skin

BELOW THE SKIN SURFACE

Erosion:
Loss of epidermis
Example:
Ruptured chickenpox vesicle

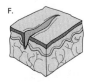

Fissure:
Linear crack in the epidermis that can extend into the dermis
Example:
Chapped hands or lips, athlete's foot

Ulcer:
A depressed lesion of the epidermis and upper papillary layer of the dermis
Example:
Stage 2 pressure ulcer

Scar:
Fibrous tissue that replaces dermal tissue after injury
Example:
Surgical incision

Keloid:
Enlarging of a scar past wound edges due to excess collagen formation (more prevalent in dark-skinned persons)
Example:
Burn scar

Excoriation:
Loss of epidermal layers exposing the dermis
Example:
Abrasion

FIGURE 10-6 Morphology of secondary lesions.

P Discrete tenderness may indicate a localized infection such as cellulitis; generalized tenderness can indicate systemic illness such as lymphoma or allergic reaction.

Texture

E 1. Evaluate the texture of the skin using the finger pads.

2. Evaluate surfaces such as the abdomen and medial surfaces of the arms first.
3. Compare these areas to areas that are covered with hair.

N Skin should normally feel smooth, even, and firm except where there is significant hair growth. A certain amount of roughness can be normal.

E **Examination**	**N** **Normal Findings**	**A** **Abnormal Findings**	**P** **Pathophysiology**

Nursing Alert

Stages of Pressure Ulcers

Defined by the National Pressure Ulcer Advisory Panel

Stage 1   An observable pressure-related alteration of intact skin whose indicators as compared to an adjacent or opposite area on the body may include changes in one or more of the following: skin temperature (warmth or coolness), tissue consistency (firm or boggy feel), and/or sensation (pain, itching). The ulcer appears as a defined area of persistent redness in lightly pigmented skin, whereas in darker skin tones, the ulcer may appear with persistent red, blue, or purple hues.

Stage 2   Partial-thickness skin loss involving epidermis, dermis, or both. The ulcer is superficial and presents clinically as an abrasion, blister, or shallow crater.

Stage 3   Full-thickness skin loss involving damage to, or necrosis of, subcutaneous tissue that may extend down to, but not through, underlying fascia.

Stage 4   Full-thickness skin loss with extensive destruction, tissue necrosis, or damage to muscle, bone, or supporting structures (e.g., tendon, joint, capsule).

Note: Wounds that are covered with debris and/or black discoloured tissuue cannot be staged accurately because the full extent of the wound is not visualized.

A   Roughness.

P   Wool clothing, cold weather, occupational exposures, or the use of soap. Generalized roughness can be associated with systemic diseases such as scleroderma, hypothyroidism, and amyloidosis. Localized thickening and roughness can be a result of chronic pruritus (lichenification) due to scratching, which causes a thickening of the epidermis.

A   Areas of hyperkeratosis and increased roughness that are found in the lower extremities are abnormal.

Nursing Alert

Evaluation of Edema

If the edema is severe enough, it can prohibit the evaluation of pathological conditions that are manifested by coloration changes. Plus two (+2) edema warrants referral if it is newly onset. Significant, severe edema (+3 to +4) warrants immediate evaluation.

P   Peripheral vascular disease, which causes abated circulation and diminished nourishment of cutaneous layers.

A   Very soft and silklike.

P   Hyperthyroidism secondary to elevated metabolism.

Turgor

Palpate the skin turgor, or elasticity, which reflects the skin's state of hydration.

E   1.   Pinch a small section of the patient's skin between your thumb and forefinger. The anterior chest, under the clavicle, and the abdomen are optimal areas to assess.

    2.   Slowly release the skin.

    3.   Observe the speed with which the skin returns to its original contour when released.

N   When the skin is released, it should return to its original contour rapidly.

A   Decreased skin turgor is present when the skin is released and it remains pinched, and slowly returns to its original contour.

P   Dehydration, or lack of fluid in the tissues, is the main cause of decreased skin turgor.

E   **Examination**   N   **Normal Findings**   A   **Abnormal Findings**   P   **Pathophysiology**

Nursing Tip

Wound Evaluation

Remove the dressing from the wound and assess the wound for location, colour, drainage, odour, size, and depth. Measure the borders of the wound with a centimetre ruler and draw a picture in your notes, if necessary, to depict necrotic areas, drains, and so on. Describe the nature of any wound exudate if there is any. Sanguinous exudate is bloody; serosanguineous exudate contains both serum and blood; serous exudate is straw-coloured serum; and mucopurulent drainage contains mucus and pus (a protein-rich liquid inflammation product made up of leukocytes, serum, and cellular debris).

The aging process and scleroderma can also decrease the turgor of the skin.

A   Increased turgor or tension causes the skin to return to its original contour too quickly.

P   Connective tissue disease.

Edema

Palpate the skin for edema, or accumulation of fluid in the intercellular spaces.

E   1. Firmly imprint your thumb against a dependent portion of the body (such as the arms, hands, legs, feet, ankle, or sacrum) for five seconds.
    2. Release pressure.
    3. Observe for an indentation on the skin.
    4. Rate the degree of edema. Pitting edema is rated on a 4-point scale:
       +0, no pitting
       +1, 1 cm pitting (mild)
       +2, 2 cm pitting (moderate)
       +3, 3 cm pitting (significant)
       +4, greater than 4 cm pitting (severe)
    5. Check for symmetry and measure circumference of affected extremities.

N   Edema is not normally present.

A   Edema is present if the skin feels puffy and tight. It can be localized or generalized (Table 10-3).

P   Localized edema may be due to dependency; however, generalized or bilateral edema is caused by increased hydrostatic pressure, decreased capillary osmotic pressure, increased capillary permeability, or obstruction to lymph flow. This occurs in congestive heart failure or kidney failure.

INSPECTION OF THE HAIR

Colour

E   Inspect scalp hair, eyebrows, eyelashes, and body hair for colour.

N   Hair varies from dark black to pale blonde based on the amount of melanin present. As melanin production diminishes, hair turns grey. Hair colour may also be chemically changed.

A   Patches of grey hair that are isolated or occur in conjunction with a scar.

P   Nerve damage, trauma.

Distribution

E   Evaluate the distribution of hair on the body, eyebrows, face, and scalp.

N   The body is covered in vellus hair. Terminal hair is found in the eyebrows, eyelashes, and scalp, and in the axilla and pubic areas after puberty. Males may experience a certain degree of normal balding and may also develop terminal facial and chest hair.

A   The absence of pubic hair, unless purposefully removed.

P   Endocrine disorders, such as anterior pituitary adenomas, or chemotherapy.

A   Male or female pattern baldness (alopecia); circumscribed bald area.

P   Androgenetic alopecia, progressive hair loss that is caused by a combination of genetic predisposition and androgenetic effects on the hair follicle; chemotherapy and radiation, infection, stress, drug reactions, lupus, and traction.

A   Total scalp baldness, or alopecia totalis.

P   Autoimmune diseases, emotional crisis, stress, or heredity.

E Examination	N Normal Findings	A Abnormal Findings	P Pathophysiology

Nursing Tip

The Braden Scale for Predicting Pressure Sore Risk (Table 10-2) enables nurses to identify patients at risk of pressure sores; accurate risk assessment helps to determine the nursing care plan to ensure the health of the patient.

Nursing Tip

Advise patients to follow the Canadian Cancer Society SunSense Guidelines to reduce the risk of skin cancer.

- Reduce sun exposure between 11 a.m. and 4 p.m. or any time of the day when the UV Index™ is 3 or more.
- Seek shade or create your own shade by using an umbrella.
- *SLIP!* on clothing to cover your arms and legs—loose fitting, tightly woven, and lightweight.
- *SLAP!* on a wide-brimmed hat that covers the head, face, ears, and neck.
- *SLOP!* on a broad spectrum (anti UVA and UVB) sunscreen with SPF (sun protection factor) 15 or higher and SPF 30 if working outdoors or if outside for most of the day. Apply sunscreen generously, 20 minutes before outdoor activities. Reapply at least every 2 hours and after swimming or exercise that causes perspiration.
- Avoid artificial tanning equipment, beds, and lamps.
- Use sunglasses with even shading, medium to dark lenses (grey, brown or green tint), with UVA and UVB protection.

Nursing Tip

Identifying Burns

A burn patient frequently has varying degrees of injury on the body. Parts of the body may have first-degree burns, and other parts may have second-, third-, or fourth-degree burns. The following descriptions will assist you in identifying burn injuries:

First-Degree Burn: the epidermis is injured or destroyed; there may be some damage to the dermis; hair follicles and sweat glands are intact; the skin is red and dry; painful.

Second-Degree Burn: also called partial-thickness burn; the epidermis and upper layers of the dermis are destroyed; the deeper dermis is injured; hair follicles, sweat glands, and nerve endings are intact; the skin is red and blistery with exudate; painful.

Third-Degree Burn: also called full-thickness burn; the epidermis and dermis are destroyed; subcutaneous tissue may be injured; hair follicles, sweat glands, and nerve endings are destroyed; the skin is white, red, black, tan, or brown with a leathery-looking appearance; painless because nerve endings are destroyed.

Fourth-Degree Burn: the epidermis and dermis are destroyed; subcutaneous tissue, muscle, and bone may be injured; hair follicles, sweat glands, and nerve endings are destroyed; the skin is white, red, black, tan, or brown with exposed and damaged subcutaneous tissue, muscle, or bone; painless.

TABLE 10-2 Braden Scale for Predicting Pressure Sore Risk

Patient's Name _____   Evaluator's Name _____   Date of Assessment _____

	1	2	3	4				
SENSORY PERCEPTION ability to respond meaningfully to pressure-related discomfort	**1. Completely Limited** Unresponsive (does not moan, flinch, or grasp) to painful stimuli, due to diminished level of consciousness or sedation. OR limited ability to feel pain over most of body.	**2. Very Limited** Responds only to painful stimuli. Cannot communicate discomfort except by moaning or restlessness OR has a sensory impairment which limits the ability to feel pain or discomfort over 1/2 of body.	**3. Slightly Limited** Responds to verbal commands, but cannot always communicate discomfort or the need to be turned OR has some sensory impairment which limits ability to feel pain or discomfort in 1 or 2 extremities.	**4. No Impairment** Responds to verbal commands. Has no sensory deficit which would limit ability to feel or voice pain or discomfort.				
MOISTURE degree to which skin is exposed to moisture	**1. Constantly Moist** Skin is kept moist almost constantly by perspiration, urine, etc. Dampness is detected every time patient is moved or turned.	**2. Very Moist** Skin is often, but not always moist. Linen must be changed at least once a shift.	**3. Occasionally Moist** Skin is occasionally moist, requiring an extra linen change approximately once a day.	**4. Rarely Moist** Skin is usually dry, linen only requires changing at routine intervals.				
ACTIVITY degree of physical activity	**1. Bedfast** Confined to bed.	**2. Chairfast** Ability to walk severely limited or nonexistent. Cannot bear own weight and/or must be assisted into chair or wheelchair.	**3. Walks Occasionally** Walks occasionally during day, but for very short distances, with or without assistance. Spends majority of each shift in bed or chair.	**4. Walks Frequently** Walks outside room at least twice a day and inside room at least once every two hours during waking hours.				
MOBILITY ability to change and control body position	**1. Completely Immobile** Does not make even slight changes in body or extremity position without assistance.	**2. Very Limited** Makes occasional slight changes in body or extremity position but unable to make frequent or significant changes independently.	**3. Slightly Limited** Makes frequent though slight changes in body or extremity position independently.	**4. No Limitation** Makes major and frequent changes in position without assistance.				

TABLE 10-2	Braden Scale for Predicting Pressure Sore Risk *continued*			

Patient's Name _____ Evaluator's Name _____ Date of Assessment _____

	1. Very Poor	2. Probably Inadequate	3. Adequate	4. Excellent
NUTRITION usual food intake pattern	Never eats a complete meal. Rarely eats more than 1/3 of any food offered. Eats 2 servings or less of protein (meat or dairy products) per day. Takes fluids poorly. Does not take a liquid dietary supplement OR is NPO and/or maintained on clear liquids or IVs for more than 5 days.	Rarely eats a complete meal and generally eats only about 1/2 of any food offered. Protein intake includes only 3 servings of meat or dairy products per day. Occasionally will take a dietary supplement OR receives less than optimum amount of liquid diet or tube feeding.	Eats over half of most meals. Eats a total of 4 servings of protein (meat, dairy products) per day. Occasionally will refuse a meal, but will usually take a supplement when offered OR is on a tube feeding or TPN regimen which probably meets most of nutritional needs.	Eats most of every meal. Never refuses a meal. Usually eats a total of 4 or more servings of meat and dairy products. Occasionally eats between meals. Does not require supplementation.
	1. Problem	**2. Potential Problem**	**3. No Apparent Problem**	
FRICTION & SHEAR	Requires moderate to maximum assistance in moving. Complete lifting without sliding against sheets is impossible. Frequently slides down in bed or chair, requiring frequent repositioning with maximum assistance. Spasticity, contractures or agitation leads to almost constant friction.	Moves feebly or requires minimum assistance. During a move skin probably slides to some extent against sheets, chair, restraints, or other devices. Maintains relatively good position in chair or bed most of the time but occasionally slides down.	Moves in bed and in chair independently and has sufficient muscle strength to lift up completely during move. Maintains good position in bed or chair.	

Total Score _____

Source: http://www.bradenscale.com/bradenscale.htm

TABLE 10-3	Types of Edema

TYPE	DESCRIPTION
Pitting	Edema that is present when an indentation remains on the skin after applying pressure
Nonpitting	Edema that is firm with discoloration or thickening of the skin; results when serum proteins coagulate in tissue spaces
Angioedema	Recurring episodes of noninflammatory swelling of skin, brain, viscera, and mucous membranes; onset may be rapid, with resolution requiring hours to days
Dependent	Localized increase of extracellular fluid volume in a dependent limb or area
Inflammatory	Swelling due to an extracellular fluid effusion into the tissue surrounding an area of inflammation
Noninflammatory	Swelling or effusion due to mechanical or other causes not related to congestion or inflammation
Lymphedema	Edema due to the obstruction of a lymphatic vessel

A Hair loss in linear formations.

P Traction alopecia caused by using curlers or wearing the hair in a tightly pulled ponytail common among individuals who wear cornrows.

A Excess facial and body hair.

P Hirsutism is indicative of endocrine disorders such as hypersecretion of adrenocortical androgens.

P Hirsutism can also result as a side effect of medications such as cyclosporin.

A Areas of broken-off hairs in irregular patterns with scaliness but no infection.

P Trichotillomania is the manipulation of the hair by twisting and pulling, leading to reduced hair mass.

A Broken-off hairs with scaliness and follicular inflammation.

P Tinea capitis (ringworm) is a fungal infection, frequently caused by dermatophytic trichomycosis.

A The scalp is covered with yellow-brown scales and crusts.

P Seborrheic dermatitis is caused by increased production of sebum by the scalp.

Lesions

E 1. Don gloves and lift the scalp hair by segments.
   2. Evaluate the scalp for lesions or signs of infestation.

N The scalp should be pale white to pink in light-skinned individuals and light brown in dark-skinned individuals. There should be no signs of infestation or lesions. Seborrhea, commonly known as dandruff, may be present.

A Head lice.

P Head lice (pediculosis capitis) are attached to the hair shaft and are difficult to remove.

PALPATION OF THE HAIR

Texture

E 1. Palpate the hair between your fingertips.
   2. Note the condition of the hair from the scalp to the end of the hair.

N Hair may feel thin, straight, coarse, thick, or curly. It should be shiny and resilient

E **Examination**   N **Normal Findings**   A **Abnormal Findings**   P **Pathophysiology**

when traction is applied and should not come out in clumps in your hands.

A Brittle hair that easily breaks off.

P Malnutrition, hyperthyroidism, use of chemicals such as permanents, or infections secondary to damage of the hair follicle.

INSPECTION OF THE NAILS

Colour

E 1. Inspect the fingernails and toenails, noting the colour of the nails.

2. Check capillary refill by depressing the nail until blanching occurs.

3. Release the nail and evaluate the time required for the nail to return to its previous colour.

4. Perform a capillary refill check on all four extremities.

N Normally, the nails have a pink cast in light-skinned individuals and are brown in dark-skinned individuals. Capillary refill is an indicator of peripheral circulation. Normal capillary refill may vary with age, but colour should return to normal within 2 or 3 seconds.

A White striations or dots in the nailbed.

P Leukonychia (Mees bands) may result from trauma, infections, vascular diseases, psoriasis, and arsenic poisoning.

A An entire nail plate that is white.

P Hypercalcemia, hypochromic anemia, leprosy, hepatic cirrhosis, and arsenic poisoning.

A A brown colour in the nail plate.

P Addison's disease and malaria.

A Bluish nails.

P Cyanosis, venous stasis, and sulfuric acid poisoning.

A Red or brown linear streaks in the nailbed.

P Splinter hemorrhages can result from subacute bacterial endocarditis, mitral stenosis, trichinosis, cirrhosis, and non-specific causes.

A Proximal end of the nailbed is white and the distal portion is pink.

P Lindsey's nails (half-and-half nails) can result from chronic renal failure and hypoalbuminemia.

Normal nail angle

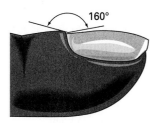

160°

Curved nail variant of normal

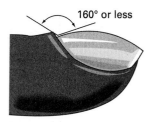

160° or less

Early clubbing

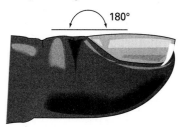

180°

FIGURE 10-7 Nail Angles.

A A yellow or white hue in a hyperkeratotic nailbed.

P Onychomycosis is a fungal infection of the nail.

Shape and Configuration

E 1. Assess the fingernails and toenails for shape, configuration, and consistency.

E Examination **N Normal Findings** **A Abnormal Findings** **P Pathophysiology**

2. View the profile of the middle finger and evaluate the angle of the nail base.

N   The nail surface should be smooth and slightly rounded or flat. Curved nails are a normal variant. Nail thickness should be uniform throughout, with no splintering or brittle edges. The angle of the nail base should be approximately 160° (Figure 10-7). Longitudinal ridging is a normal variant.

A   An angle of the nail base greater than 160°.

P   Clubbing can result from long-standing hypoxia and lung cancer.

PALPATION OF THE NAILS

Texture

E   1. Palpate the nail base between your thumb and index finger.
    2. Note the consistency.

N   The nail base should be firm on palpation.

A   A spongy nail base is an early indication of clubbing.

P   Impaired tissue oxygenation over a prolonged period of time, as in chronic bronchitis, emphysema, and heart disease.

E   **Examination**   N   **Normal Findings**   A   **Abnormal Findings**   P   **Pathophysiology**

11

Head, Neck, and Regional Lymphatics

ANATOMY AND PHYSIOLOGY

The skull is a complex bony structure that rests on the superior end of the vertebral column (Figure 11-1). The skull protects the brain from direct injury and provides a surface for the attachment of the muscles that assist with mastication and produce facial expressions.

Cranial bones of the skull are connected by immovable joints called sutures. The most prominent sutures are the coronal suture, the

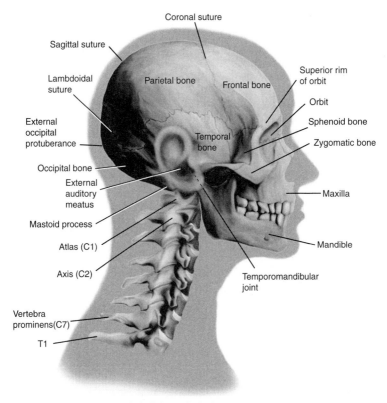

FIGURE 11-1 Bones of the Face and Skull (Lateral View).

sagittal suture, and the lambdoidal suture. The junction of the coronal and sagittal sutures is called the bregma.

The face of every individual has its own unique characteristics, which are influenced by race, state of health, emotions, and environment. Facial structures are symmetrical so that eyes, eyebrows, nose, mouth, nasolabial folds, and palpebral fissures look the same on both sides.

The neck is made up of seven flexible cervical vertebrae that support the head while allowing it maximum mobility.

The major muscles of the neck are the sternocleidomastoids and the trapezii. The anterior triangle is formed by the mandible, the trachea, and the sternocleidomastoid muscle and contains the anterior cervical lymph nodes, the trachea, and the thyroid gland. The posterior triangle, the area between the sternocleidomastoid and the trapezius muscles with the clavicle at the base, contains the posterior cervical lymph nodes (Figure 11-2).

The trapezii extend from the occipital bone down the neck to insert at the outer third of the clavicles, at the acromion process of the scapula, and along the spinal column to the level of T12.

The thyroid gland, the largest endocrine gland in the body, secretes thyroxine (T_4) and triiodothyronine (T_3), which regulate the rate of cellular metabolism. The gland, a flattened, butterfly-shaped structure with two lateral lobes connected by the isthmus, weighs about 25 to 30 grams and is slightly larger in females (Figure 11-3). The

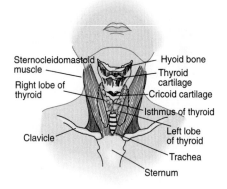

FIGURE 11-3 Structure of the Thyroid Gland.

isthmus rests on top of the trachea, inferior to the cricoid cartilage.

An extensive system of lymphatic vessels is an important part of the immune system (Figure 11-2). Lymphatic tissue in the nodes filter and sequester pathogens and other harmful substances. Lymph nodes are usually less than 1 cm, round or ovoid in shape, and smooth in consistency. If a tender or enlarged lymph node is found on the clinical examination, assess the entire lymph node area and note the direction in which each node drains.

Major arteries that carry blood to the head and neck include the common carotids (which bifurcate into the internal and external carotid

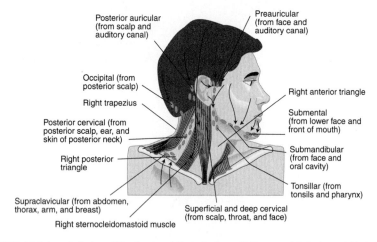

FIGURE 11-2 Lymph Nodes of the Head and Neck: Drainage Patterns and Anterior and Posterior Cervical Triangles.

HEALTH HISTORY

Medical History	(See also Table 11-1.)
Head and Neck Specific	Hypo- or hyperthyroidism, sinus infections, migraine headache, cancer, closed head injury or skull fracture
Surgical History	Thyroidectomy, facial reconstruction, cosmetic surgery, neurosurgery, and other surgery related to the head or neck

TABLE 11-1 Classification of Headaches

VASCULAR ETIOLOGIES
Migraine headaches
Cluster headaches
Subarachnoid hemorrhage
Subdural hematoma
Infarction
Cerebral aneurysm
Temporal arteritis
Vasculitis

MUSCLE CONTRACTION
Tension headache

INTRACRANIAL ETIOLOGIES
Brain tumours
Increased intracranial pressure from hydrocephalus, pseudotumor cerebri
Intracranial infection, e.g., meningitis, encephalitis, abscess
Ischemic cerebrovascular disease

SYSTEMIC ETIOLOGIES
Infection
Post-lumbar puncture
Hypertension
Exertion from coitus, cough, exercise
Postictal
Pheochromocytoma
Premenstrual syndrome

FOOD-RELATED ETIOLOGIES
Nitrites (e.g., hot dogs, bacon)
Tyramine (e.g., red wine, cheese, chocolate)
Monosodium glutamate (e.g., Chinese food)
Food allergy

FACIAL OR CERVICAL ETIOLOGIES
Sinusitis
Temporomandibular joint (TMJ) dysfunction
Dental lesions

Trigeminal neuralgia
Cervical spine radiculopathies

OCULAR-RELATED ETIOLOGIES
Narrow angle glaucoma
Uveitis
Extraocular muscle paralysis
Eye strain

METABOLIC ETIOLOGIES
Hypoxia
Hypercapnia
Hypoglycemia

DRUG ETIOLOGIES
Alcohol and alcohol withdrawal
Caffeine withdrawal
Nitrates
Oral contraceptives
Estrogen

ENVIRONMENTAL ETIOLOGIES
Change in barometric pressure (from weather or altitude)
Carbon monoxide poisoning
Tobacco smoke
Glaring or flickering lights
Odours

MISCELLANEOUS ETIOLOGIES
Fever
Influenza
Head trauma
Otitis media
Parotitis
Pregnancy
Fatigue and decreased sleep
Psychogenic disorders

Nursing Alert

Tell patients that they need to seek help for a headache when:

- They have a very sudden, severe, "thunderclap" headache that seems to come on instantly and is unlike any headache they have had before.
- It begins abruptly and they have no previous history of them, especially if the pain is sudden and severe.
- They experience any signs of a brain attack (stroke), such as sudden numbness, weakness, and inability to move one side of the entire body, or sudden problems speaking and understanding speech.
- A headache occurs with a stiff neck, fever, nausea, vomiting, lethargy, drowsiness, and confusion.
- A headache occurs with weakness, paralysis, numbness, visual disturbances, slurred speech, confusion, behaviour changes, or loss of consciousness.
- Headaches occur after a recent fall or blow to the head.
- Headaches develop gradually and occur with confusion, lethargy, problems with walking, or loss of bladder or bowel control.
- Headaches cause people to wake up at night.
- Headaches occur daily or become worse.
- Headaches occur after physical exercise, sexual activity, coughing, or sneezing.
- Life is being disrupted by the headaches (for example, missing work or school regularly).

◄ NURSING CHECKLIST ►

General Approach to Head and Neck Assessment

1. Greet the patient and explain the assessment techniques that you will be using.
2. Ensure that the room temperature is at a comfortable level for the patient.
3. Use a quiet room free from interruptions.
4. Ensure that the light in the room provides sufficient brightness to allow adequate observation of the patient.
5. Place the patient in an upright sitting position on the examination table, or
5a. Gain access to the head of the supine, bedridden patient by removing nonessential equipment or bedding (for patients who cannot tolerate the sitting position).
6. If the patient is wearing a wig or headpiece, ask the patient to remove it.
7. Visualize the underlying anatomic structures during the assessment process to permit an accurate description of the location of any pathology.
8. Always compare the right and left sides of the head, neck, and face to one another.
9. Use the same systematic approach every time an assessment is performed.

arteries), the brachiocephalic artery (the right common carotid artery branches from this), the subclavian arteries, and the temporal arteries. Deoxygenated blood from the head and neck is returned to the heart via the internal and external jugular veins, the brachiocephalic vein, and the subclavian veins.

EQUIPMENT
- Stethoscope
- Cup of water

ASSESSMENT OF THE HEAD AND NECK

Inspection of the Shape of the Head

E   1. Have the patient sit in a comfortable position.
    2. Face the patient, with your head at the same level as the patient's head.
    3. Inspect the head for shape and symmetry.

N   The head should be normocephalic and symmetrical.

A   Hydrocephalus is an enlargement of the head without enlargement of the facial structures.

P   Abnormal accumulation of cerebrospinal fluid within the skull.

A   Acromegaly is an abnormal enlargement of the skull and bony facial structures.

P   Excessive secretion of growth hormone from the pituitary gland.

A   Craniosynostosis is characterized by abnormal shape of the skull or bone growth at right angles to suture lines, exophthalmos, and drooping eyelids.

P   Premature closure of one or more sutures of the skull before brain growth is complete.

PALPATION OF THE HEAD

E   1. Place the finger pads on the scalp and palpate all of its surface, beginning in the frontal area and continuing over the parietal, temporal, and occipital areas.

    2. Assess for contour, masses, depressions, and tenderness.

    3. Palpate the superficial temporal artery, which is located anterior to the tragus of the ear.

N   The normal skull is smooth, nontender, and without masses or depressions. The temporal artery is usually a weaker peripheral pulse (1+/4+ or 1+/3+) than the other peripheral pulses of the body. The artery is nontender, smooth, and readily compressible.

A   Masses in the cranial bones that feel hard or soft.

P   Carcinomatous metastasis from other regions of the body or from lymphomas, multiple myeloma, or leukemia.

A   Palpation elicits localized edema over the bony frontal portion of the skull.

P   Osteomyelitis of the skull may develop following acute or chronic sinusitis if the infection extends out from the sinuses into the surrounding bone.

A   Softening of the outer bone layer.

P   Craniotabes is a softening of the skull caused by hydrocephalus or demineralization of the bone due to rickets, hypervitaminosis A, or syphilis.

A   A temporal artery that is hard in consistency and tender.

P   Temporal arteritis.

INSPECTION AND PALPATION OF THE SCALP

E   1. Part the hair repeatedly all over the scalp and inspect for lesions or masses.

    2. Place the finger pads on the scalp and palpate for lesions or masses.

N   The scalp should be shiny, intact, and without lesions or masses.

A   A laceration, or a laceration with bleeding.

P   Direct trauma.

A   A gaping laceration with profuse bleeding.

P   A deep wound that may involve a compound skull fracture as a result of some type of trauma.

A   Localized, easily movable accumulation of blood in the subcutaneous tissue.

E Examination	**N** Normal Findings	**A** Abnormal Findings	**P** Pathophysiology	

P Hematomas can result from direct trauma to the skull.

A Single or multiple masses that are easily movable. They are round, firm, nontender, and arise from either the skin or the subcutaneous tissue.

P Sebaceous cysts form as a result of a retention of secretions from sebaceous glands.

A Nonmobile, fatty masses with smooth, circular edges palpated deeper in the scalp.

P Benign fatty tumours known as lipomas.

INSPECTION OF THE FACE

Symmetry

E 1. Have the patient sit in a comfortable position facing you.
   2. Observe the patient's face for expression, shape, and symmetry of the eyebrows, eyes, nose, mouth, and ears.

N The facial features should be symmetrical. Both palpebral fissures should be equal and the nasolabial fold should present bilaterally. It is important to remember that slight variations in symmetry are common. Slanted eyes with inner epicanthal folds are normal findings in patients of Asian descent.

A Structures are absent or deformed. There is a definite asymmetry of expression, the palpebral fissures, the nasolabial folds, and the corners of the mouth.

P Damage to the nerves innervating facial muscles (cranial nerve VII), as in stroke or Bell's palsy (Figure 11-4).

Shape and Features

E 1. Face the patient.
   2. Observe the shape of the patient's face.
   3. Note any swelling, abnormal features, or unusual movement.

N The shape of the face can be oval, round, or slightly square. There should be no edema, disproportionate structures, or involuntary movements.

A Slanted eyes with inner epicanthal folds; a short, flat nose; and a thick, protruding tongue.

P Down syndrome (trisomy 21), a chromosomal aberration.

A An abnormally wide distance between the eyes is hypertelorism.

P Hypertelorism is a congenital anomaly.

A Facial skin is shiny, contracted, and hard. The face appears to have furrows around the mouth.

P Scleroderma is a collagen disease of unknown cause. Sclerosis of the skin, as well as visceral organs (esophagus, lungs, heart, muscles, and kidneys) occurs.

A The face is thin with sharply defined features and prominent eyes (exophthalmos) in Graves' disease.

P Graves' disease is an autoimmune disorder associated with increased circulating levels of T_3 and T_4.

A The patient's face is round and swollen with characteristic periorbital edema and dry, dull skin.

P Myxedema is associated with hypothyroidism.

A The eyes are sunken and cheeks are hollow in cachexia.

P A profound state of wasting of the vital tissues associated with cancer, malnutrition, and dehydration.

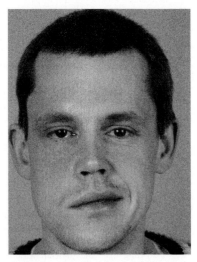

FIGURE 11-4 Bell's Palsy. © *NIH/Phototake.*

| E Examination | N Normal Findings | A Abnormal Findings | P Pathophysiology |

Reflective Thinking

Facial Piercing

Your patient has a history of acne, chronic sinusitis, and allergies. She informs you that she plans to get her eyebrows and nares pierced. How would you respond to her? How would you counsel this patient to have her body piercing done safely?

Reflective Thinking

Sensitivity to Patients with Severe Facial Burns

During your first day working in the burn unit, you are assigned to care for a patient who has multiple second-degree burns to his face and upper extremities. When you meet him for the first time, he says, "I look horrible; you won't be able to stand to look at me." How would you respond verbally and nonverbally to his comment and his disfigurement?

A   The patient's face is immobile and expressionless, with a staring gaze and raised eyebrows in Parkinson's disease.

P   Parkinson's disease is the degeneration of basal ganglia, resulting from a deficiency of the neurotransmitter dopamine.

A   The face of Caucasians shows a dusky blue discoloration beneath the eyes (allergic shiners), creases below the lower eyelids (Dennie's lines).

P   Chronic allergies.

A   The patient's face has a rounded "moon-face," red cheeks, and excess hair on the jaw and upper lip.

P   Cushing's syndrome, which is caused by increased production of adrenocorticotropic hormone (ACTH) or prolonged steroid ingestion.

PALPATION AND AUSCULTATION OF THE MANDIBLE

E   1. Use the fingertips of both index and middle fingers to locate the TMJ anterior to the tragus of the ear on both sides.

2. Hold the fingertips firmly in place over the joints and ask the patient to open and close the mouth.

3. As the patient opens and closes the mouth, observe the relative smoothness of the movement and whether or not the patient notices any discomfort.

4. Remove your hands.

5. Hold the bell of the stethoscope over the joint.

6. Listen for any sound while the patient opens and closes the mouth.

N   The patient should experience no discomfort with movement. The TMJ should articulate smoothly, without clicking or crepitus.

A   Tenderness when the mouth is opened or closed. Clicking or crepitus.

P   Inflammation of migratory arthritis.

A   Crepitus or clicking.

P   Osteoarthritis.

A   Mouth remains in an open and fixed position.

P   The temperomandibular joint   is dislocated and will not function. This condition requires reduction.

E   **Examination**   N   **Normal Findings**   A   **Abnormal Findings**   P   **Pathophysiology**

INSPECTION AND PALPATION OF THE NECK

Inspection of the Neck

E 1. Have the patient sit facing you, with the patient's head held in a central position.

    2. Inspect for symmetry of the sternocleidomastoid muscles anteriorly, and the trapezii posteriorly.

    3. Have the patient touch the chin to the chest, to each side, and to each shoulder.

    4. Assess for limitation of motion.

    5. Note the presence of a stoma or tracheostomy.

N The muscles of the neck are symmetrical with the head in a central position. The patient is able to move the head through a full range of motion without complaint of discomfort or noticeable limitation. The patient may be breathing through a stoma or tracheostomy.

A Pain with flexion or rotation of the head.

P Pain with flexion: muscle spasm caused by meningeal irritation of meningitis (see Chapter 19). Generalized discomfort: trauma, spasm, inflammation of muscles, or diseases of the vertebrae.

A Slight or prominent lateral deviation of the patient's neck. The sternocleidomastoid muscles, and to a lesser extent the trapezius and scalene muscles, may also be prominent on affected side.

P This condition is called torticollis. Causes can be:

    1. Congenital: resulting from a hematoma or partial rupture at birth of the sternocleidomastoid, causing a shortening of the muscle.

    2. Ocular: a head posture assumed to correct for ocular muscle palsy and resulting diplopia.

    3. Acute spasm: commonly associated with the inflammation of viral myositis or trauma such as sleeping with the head in an unusual position.

Nursing Alert

Neck Injury

If a neck injury is suspected, stabilize the neck and do not proceed with the assessment. Refer the patient immediately to a qualified specialist for further evaluation.

    4. Other: hysteria, phenothiazine therapy, and Parkinson's disease as the result of increased cholinergic activity in the brain.

A Range of motion of the neck is reduced.

P Degenerative changes of osteoarthritis, usually painless unless nerve root irritation has occurred.

Palpation of the Neck

E 1. Stand in front of the patient.

    2. Use your finger pads to palpate the sternocleidomastoids.

    3. Note the presence of masses or tenderness.

    4. Stand behind the patient.

    5. Palpate the trapezius with your finger pads.

    6. Note the presence of masses or tenderness.

N The muscles should be symmetrical without palpable masses or spasm.

A A mass is palpated in the musculature.

P Tumour, either primary or metastatic.

A A spasm may be felt in the muscles.

P Infections, trauma, chronic inflammatory processes, or neoplasms.

INSPECTION OF THE THYROID GLAND

E 1. Secure tangential lighting and shine it at an oblique angle on the patient's anterior neck.

    2. Face the patient.

| E **Examination** | N **Normal Findings** | A **Abnormal Findings** | P **Pathophysiology** |

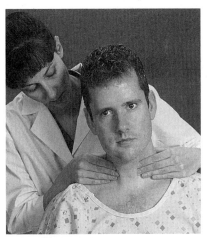

A. Posterior Approach.

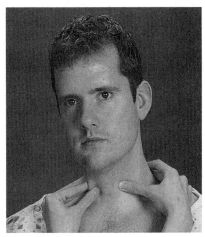

B. Anterior Approach.

FIGURE 11-5   Examination of the Thyroid Gland.

3. Ask the patient to look straight ahead with the head slightly extended.
4. Have the patient take a sip of water and swallow twice.
5. While the patient swallows, observe the front of the neck in the area of the thyroid and the isthmus for masses and symmetrical movement.

N   Thyroid tissue moves up with swallowing but often the movement is so small it is not visible on inspection. In males, the thyroid cartilage, or Adam's apple, is more prominent than in females.

A   A mass or enlargement of the thyroid that moves upward with swallowing.

P   Many goiters (enlarged thyroid glands) or thyroid nodules are visible and may indicate a variety of thyroid diseases.

PALPATION OF THE THYROID GLAND

Palpation of the thyroid gland may be done using both anterior and posterior approaches (Figure 11-5).

Posterior Approach

E   1. Have the patient sit comfortably. Stand behind the patient.

2. Have the patient lower the chin slightly in order to relax the neck muscles.
3. Place your thumbs on the back of the patient's neck and bring the other fingers around the neck anteriorly with their tips resting on the lower portion of the neck over the trachea.
4. Move the finger pads over the tracheal rings.
5. Instruct the patient to swallow. Palpate the isthmus for nodules or enlargement.
6. Have the patient incline the head slightly forward.
7. Press the fingers of the left hand against the left side of the thyroid cartilage to stabilize it while placing the fingers of the right hand gently against the right side.
8. Instruct the patient to swallow sips of water.
9. Note consistency, nodularity, or tenderness as the gland moves upward.
10. Repeat on the other side.

| E Examination | N Normal Findings | A Abnormal Findings | P Pathophysiology |

Anterior Approach

E   1. Stand in front of the patient.
    2. Ask the patient to flex the head slightly forward.
    3. Place the right thumb on the thyroid cartilage and displace the cartilage to the patient's right.
    4. Grasp the elevated and displaced right lobe of the thyroid gland with your thumb and index and middle fingers of the left hand.
    5. Palpate the surface of the gland for consistency, nodularity, and tenderness.
    6. Have the patient swallow, and palpate the surface again.
    7. Repeat the procedure on the opposite side.

N   No enlargement, masses, or tenderness should be noted on palpation.

A   Palpation reveals the gland to be smooth, soft, and slightly enlarged but less than twice the size of a normal thyroid gland.

P   Physiological hyperplasia can be seen premenstrually, during pregnancy, or from puberty to young adulthood in females. Symmetrical enlargement may also be noted in patients who live in areas of iodine deficiency. These are referred to as nontoxic diffuse goiters or endemic goiters.

A   Palpation reveals the gland to be two to three times larger than normal size.

P   Diffuse toxic hyperplasia of the thyroid, or Graves' disease.

A   Asymmetrical enlargement of the thyroid and the presence of two or more nodules.

P   Thyroid adenomas (benign epithelial tumours).

A   Solitary nodule in the thyroid tissue.

P   Suggestive of carcinoma.

A   Lateral deviation of the trachea, but no specific goiter.

P   This may be a retrosternal goiter.

A   Tenderness of the thyroid.

P   Suggests thyroiditis.

AUSCULTATION OF THE THYROID GLAND

If the thyroid is enlarged, auscultation should be done.

E   1. Stand in front of the patient.
    2. Place the bell of the stethoscope over the right thyroid lobe.
    3. Auscultate for bruits.
    4. Repeat on the left thyroid lobe.

N   Auscultation should not reveal bruits.

A/P Bruit over an enlarged thyroid gland.

P   Increased vascularization due to diffuse toxic goiter.

INSPECTION OF THE LYMPH NODES

    1. Stand in front of the patient.
    2. Expose the area of the head and neck to be assessed.
    3. Inspect the nodal areas of the head and neck for any enlargement or inflammation.

N   Lymph nodes should not be visible or inflamed.

A   Enlargement and inflammation in specific nodes.

P   Localized or generalized infection.

PALPATION OF THE LYMPH NODES

E   1. Have the patient sit comfortably.
    2. Face the patient and assess both sides of the neck simultaneously.
    3. Move the pads and tips of your middle three fingers in small circles of palpation using gentle pressure.
    4. Follow a systematic, routine sequence beginning with the preauricular, postauricular, occipital, submental, submandibular, and tonsillar nodes. Moving down to the neck, evaluate the anterior and the posterior cervical chains, and the supraclavicular nodes (Figure 11-6).
    5. Note size, shape, delimitation (discrete or matted together), mobility, consistency, and tenderness.

E Examination   N Normal Findings   A Abnormal Findings   P Pathophysiology

N   Lymph nodes should not be palpable in the healthy adult patient; however, small, discrete, movable nodes are sometimes present but are of no significance.

A   Palpable lymph nodes greater than 0.5 cm.

P   Palpable lymph nodes can result from a variety of other pathological processes, including blood dyscrasias, AIDS, tuberculosis, surgical procedures that traumatize the nodes, blood transfusions, or chronic illness.

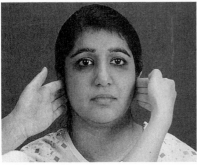

A. Preauricular

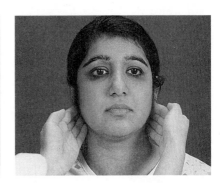

B. Postauricular

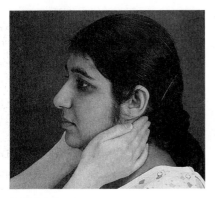

C. Occipital

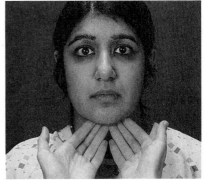

D. Submental

FIGURE 11-6 Palpation of Lymph Nodes.

| E **Examination** | N **Normal Findings** | A **Abnormal Findings** | P **Pathophysiology** |

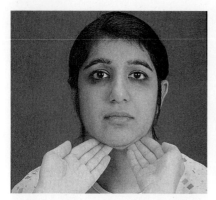

E. Submandibular

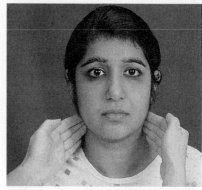

F. Tonsillar

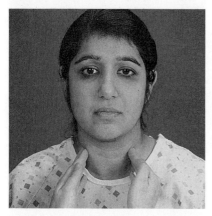

G. Anterior Cervical Chain

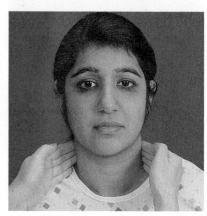

H. Posterior Cervical Chain

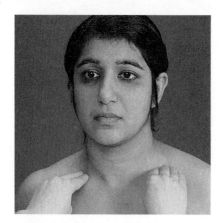

I. Supraclavicular

FIGURE 11-6 Palpation of Lymph Nodes. *continued*

12

Eyes

ANATOMY AND PHYSIOLOGY

External Structures

The external structures of the eyes comprise the eyelids or palpebra, the conjunctiva, the lacrimal glands, and the extraocular muscles. The eyelids consist of smooth muscle covered with a very thin layer of skin; they admit light to the eye while protecting and maintaining lubrication of the eye. The interior surface of the lid muscle is covered with a pink mucous membrane called the palpebral conjunctiva. Contiguous with the palpebral conjunctiva is the bulbar conjunctiva, which folds back over the anterior surface of the eyeball and merges with the cornea at the limbus, the junction of the sclera and the cornea (Figure 12-1). The conjunctiva contains blood vessels and pain receptors that respond quickly to outside insult. Eyelashes are evenly spaced along lid margins and curve outward to protect the eye by filtering particles of dirt and dust from the external environment.

The opening between the eyelids is called the palpebral fissure. Upper and lower eyelids meet at the inner canthus on the nasal side and at the outer canthus on the temporal side. Embedded

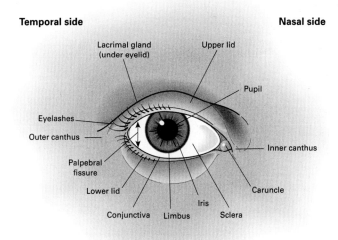

RIGHT EYE

FIGURE 12-1 External View of the Eye.

just beneath the lid margins are the meibomian glands, which secrete a lubricating substance onto the surface of the eye.

The lacrimal glands, located above and on the temporal side of each eye, are responsible for the production of tears, which lubricate the eye.

Six extraocular muscles (superior, inferior, medial, and lateral recti, and the superior and inferior obliques) extend from the scleral surface of each eye and attach to the bony orbit.

Internal Structures

The eye itself is approximately 2.5 cm in diameter and has three layers: a tough, outer, fibrous tunic (sclera); a middle, vascular tunic; and the innermost layer, which contains the retina (Figure 12-2).

The innermost layer of the eyeball, or the retina, is an extension of the optic nerve, which lines the inside of the globe and receives light impulses that are transmitted to the occipital lobe of the brain.

The optic disc is a round or oval area with distinct margins located on the nasal side of the retina.

The physiologic cup is a pale, central area in the optic disc occupying one-third to one-fourth of the disc. In the temporal area of the retina, the tiny, darker macula, with the fovea centralis at its centre, contains a high concentration of cones necessary for colour vision, reading ability, and other tasks requiring fine visual discrimination. The fovea is the area of sharpest vision. Other portions of the retina contain a high concentration of rods, which provide dark and light discrimination and peripheral vision.

EQUIPMENT

- Ophthalmoscope
- Penlight
- Clean gloves
- Snellen chart, Snellen E chart, Rosenbaum near-vision pocket screening card
- Vision occluder
- Cotton-tipped applicator

ASSESSMENT OF THE EYE

Visual Acuity

The assessment of visual acuity (cranial nerve II, or CN II) is a simple, noninvasive procedure

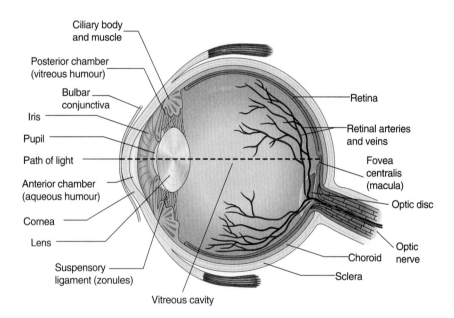

FIGURE 12-2 Lateral Cross Section of the Interior Eye.

HEALTH HISTORY

Medical History	Myopia, hyperopia, strabismus, astigmatism, glaucoma, cataracts, conjunctivitis, hordeolum, pterygium, blepharitis, chalazion, trachoma, macular degeneration
Surgical History	Cataract extraction, lens implant, LASIK (laser-assisted in situ-keratomileusis) [laser vision correction], repair of detached retina, neurosurgery, enucleation of eye, optic nerve decompression

Nursing Alert

Glaucoma

Although there is no cure for glaucoma, it can be managed through treatment. Early detection is important. Individuals should have an eye examination every three to five years until the age of 40 and then every two to four years until the age of 65. As so many eye diseases tend to occur in the elderly, those over 65 should have an eye examination every two years—annually if they have any risk factors.

◀ NURSING CHECKLIST ▶

General Approach to Eye Assessment

1. Greet the patient and explain the assessment techniques that you will be using.
2. Use a quiet room free from interruptions.
3. Ensure that the light in the room provides sufficient brightness to allow adequate observation of the patient.
4. Place the patient in an upright sitting position on the examination table.
5. Visualize the underlying structures during the assessment process to allow adequate description of findings.
6. Always compare right and left eyes.
7. Use a systematic approach that is followed consistently each time the assessment is performed.

that uses a Snellen chart and also an occluder to cover the patient's eye.

Distance Vision

E   1. Ask the patient to stand or sit facing the Snellen chart at a distance of 20 feet.

2. If the patient normally wears glasses, ask that they be removed. Contact lenses may be left in the eyes.
3. Instruct the patient to cover the left eye with the occluder and to read as many lines on the chart as possible.

E	**Examination**	N	**Normal Findings**	A	**Abnormal Findings**	P	**Pathophysiology**

4. Note the number at the end of the last line the patient was able to read.
5. If the patient is unable to read the letters at the top of the chart, move the patient closer to the chart. Note the distance at which the patient is able to read the top line.
6. Repeat the test, occluding the right eye.
7. If the patient normally wears glasses, the test should be repeated with the patient wearing the glasses, and it should be so noted (corrected or uncorrected).

N   The patient who has a visual acuity of 20/20 is considered to have normal visual acuity.

A   The patient is unable to read the chart with an uncorrected visual acuity of 20/30 in one eye, vision in both eyes is different by two lines or more, or acuity is absent.

P   Myopia (nearsightedness); corneal opacities that are congenital, from lesions that have scarred the cornea (e.g., herpes simplex), from trauma, or from degeneration and dystrophies; opacities of the lens caused by senile or traumatic cataracts; inflammation of the iris (iritis); inflammation of the retina caused by toxoplasmosis or by the presence of blood in the vitreous humour following hemorrhage; hypertension; diabetes mellitus; trauma.

Near Vision

E   1. Use a pocket Snellen chart, Rosenbaum card, or any printed material written at an appropriate reading level.
    2. If the pocket vision card is available, have the patient sit comfortably and hold the card 35 cm (14 inches) from the face without moving it.
    3. Ask the patient to read the smallest line possible. If other printed material is used, you will be able to gain only a general understanding of the patient's near vision.

N   Until a patient is in the late 30s to the late 40s, reading is generally possible at a distance of 35 cm.

A   Presbyopic (farsightedness).

P   The normal aging process causes the lens to harden (nuclear sclerosis), decreasing its ability to change shape and therefore focus on near objects.

Colour Vision

E   For routine testing of colour vision, test the patient's ability to identify primary colours found on the Snellen chart or in the examining room. For more specific testing, ask the patient to view Ishihara plates and identify the numerals on them.

E **Examination**   N **Normal Findings**   A **Abnormal Findings**   P **Pathophysiology**

N   The patient who is able to identify all six screening Ishihara plates correctly has normal colour vision.

A   The colour vision defect is designated as red/green, blue/yellow, or complete when the patient sees only shades of grey.

P   Diseases of the optic nerve, macular degeneration, pathology of the fovea centralis, nutritional deficiency, or heredity.

Visual Fields

The confrontation technique is used to test visual fields of each eye (CN II). The visual field of each eye is divided into quadrants, and a stimulus is presented in each quadrant.

E   1.   Sit or stand approximately 60–90 cm (2–3 feet) opposite the patient, with your eyes at the same level as the patient's.
     2.   Have the patient cover the right eye with the right hand or an occluder.
     3.   Cover your left eye in the same manner.
     4.   Have the patient look at your uncovered eye with his or her uncovered eye.
     5.   Hold your free hand at arm's length equidistant from you and the patient, and move your hand, or a held object such as a pen, into your and the patient's field of vision from nasal, temporal, superior, inferior, and oblique angles.
     6.   Ask the patient to say "now" when your hand is seen moving into the field of vision. Use your own visual fields as the control for comparison to the patient's.
     7.   Repeat the procedure for the other eye.

N   The patient is able to see the stimulus at about 90° temporally, 60° nasally, 50° superiorly, and 70° inferiorly.

A   If the patient is unable to identify movement that you perceive, a defect in the visual field is presumed.

P   Tumours or strokes, or neurological diseases such as glaucoma or retinal detachment.

External Eye and Lacrimal Apparatus

Eyelids

E   1.   Ask the patient to sit facing you.
     2.   Observe the patient's eyelids for drooping, infection, tumours, or other abnormalities.
     3.   Note the distribution of the eyelashes and eyebrows.
     4.   Instruct the patient to focus on an object or a finger held about 25–30 cm (10–12 inches) away and slightly above eye level.
     5.   Move the object or finger slowly downward and observe for a white space of sclera between the upper lid and the limbus.
     6.   Observe the blinking of the eyes.
     7.   Ask the patient to elevate the eyelids.

N   The eyelids should appear symmetrical with no drooping, infections, or tumours of the lids. Eyelids of people of Asian descent normally slant upward. When the eyes are focused in a normal frontal gaze, the lids should cover the upper portion of the iris. The patient can raise both eyelids symmetrically (CN III). Slight ptosis, or drooping of the lid, can be normal. When the eye is closed, no portion of the cornea should be exposed. Normal lid margins are smooth with the lashes evenly distributed and sweeping upward from the upper lids and downward from the lower lids. Eyebrows are present bilaterally and are symmetrical and without lesions or scaling.

A   The patient has either unilateral or bilateral, constant or intermittent ptosis of the lid.

P   In congenital ptosis there is failure of the levator muscle to develop. If the ptosis is acquired, it is related to one of three factors:
     1.   Mechanical: heavy lids from lesions, adipose tissue, swelling, or edema.
     2.   Myogenic: muscular diseases such as myasthenia gravis or multiple sclerosis.

E   **Examination**   N   **Normal Findings**   A   **Abnormal Findings**   P   **Pathophysiology**

3. Neurogenic: paralysis from damage or interruption of the neural pathways.

A An area of white sclera between the upper lid and the limbus, widening as the eye looks downward.

P Thyrotoxicosis.

A The patient is unable to bring about complete lid closure. This is generally a unilateral condition.

P Lagophthalmos and can be associated with Bell's palsy, stroke, trauma, or ectropion (everted eyelid).

A Disparity of the palpebral fissure with apparent lid retraction, indicating a protrusion of the globe.

A Exophthalmos (or proptosis) can be present unilaterally in orbital tumours, thyroid disease, trauma, or inflammation. Bilateral exophthalmos is related to thyroid disease.

A Turning inward, or inversion, of the lower lid—referred to as entropion.

P Spasms or advancing age (senile).

A Turning outward, or eversion, of the lower lid—referred to as ectropion.

P Normal aging process, Bell's palsy.

A Excessive blinking that may or may not be accompanied by increased tearing and pain.

P Voluntary: irritation to the cornea or the conjunctiva, or stress and anxiety; Involuntary: tonic spasms of the orbicularis oculi muscle, called blepharospasm; often seen in elderly individuals and in patients with CN VII lesions, irritation of the eye, fatigue, and stress.

A Lids are black and blue, bluish, yellow, or red, depending on race and skin colour.

P 1. Redness: generalized redness is nonspecific; redness in the nasal half of the lid; frontal sinusitis. Redness adjacent to the lower lid; disease of the lacrimal sac or nasolacrimal duct, such as dacryocystitis; redness in the temporal portion of the lid; dacryoadenitis, an inflammation of the lacrimal gland.

2. Bluish: orbital vein thrombosis, orbital tumours, or aneurysms in the orbit.

3. Black and blue: bleeding into the surrounding tissues following trauma (black eye).

A Swelling or edema in the eyelid.

P Allergies, systemic diseases, medications that contribute to swelling from fluid overload, trichinosis, early myxedema, thyrotoxicosis, or contact dermatitis.

A Acute localized inflammation, tenderness, and redness, with pain in the infected area. This is called a hordeolum (sty).

P *Staphylococcus.*

A Chronic inflammation of the meibomian gland in either the upper or the lower lid. There is no redness or tenderness.

P Chalazion, cause is unknown.

A Lids are inflamed bilaterally and are red rimmed, with scales clinging to both the upper and the lower lids.

P Blepharitis, which may be either staphylococcal or seborrheic.

A Raised, yellow, nonpainful plaques on upper and lower lids near the inner canthus.

P Xanthelasma, a form of xanthoma frequently associated with hypercholesterolemia.

Lacrimal Apparatus

Inspection

E 1. Have the patient sit facing you.

2. Identify the area of the lacrimal gland. Note any swelling or enlargement of the gland or elevation of the eyelid. Note any enlargement, swelling, redness, increased tearing, or exudate in the area of the lacrimal sac at the inner canthus.

3. Compare this eye to the other eye in order to determine whether there is unilateral or bilateral involvement.

N There should be no enlargement, swelling, or redness, no large amount of exudate, and minimal tearing.

A Inflammation and swelling in the upper lateral aspect of one or both eyes, and pain in the affected area.

P Acute inflammation of the lacrimal gland is called dacryoadenitis; it does not occur commonly and may result from trauma or

---

E **Examination**   N **Normal Findings**   A **Abnormal Findings**   P **Pathophysiology**

may be found in association with measles, mumps, and mononucleosis.

A Inflammation and painful swelling beside the nose and near the inner canthus and possibly extending to the eyelid.

P Dacryocystitis is caused by inflammatory or neoplastic obstruction of the lacrimal duct.

Palpation

E 1. To assess the lacrimal sac for obstruction, don gloves.
   2. Gently press the index finger near the inner canthus, just inside the rim of the bony orbit of the eye.
   3. Note any discharge from the punctum.

N There should not be excessive tearing or discharge from the punctum.

A Mucopurulent discharge.

P Obstruction anywhere along the lacrimal apparatus.

A Overflowing of tears from the eye.

P Epiphora, which is caused by obstruction of the lacrimal duct.

Extraocular Muscle Function

Six extraocular muscles control the movement of each eye in relation to three axes: vertical, horizontal, and oblique (Figure 12-3). Assessing extraocular function is carried out by observing corneal light reflex or alignment, using the cover/uncover test, and by testing the six cardinal fields of gaze (CN III, IV, and VI).

Corneal Light Reflex (Hirschberg Test)

E 1. Instruct the patient to look straight ahead.
   2. Focus a penlight on the corneas from a distance of 30–38 cm away at the midline.
   3. Observe the location of reflected light on the cornea.

N The reflected light (light reflex) should be seen symmetrically in the centre of each cornea.

A A discrepancy in the placement of one of the light reflections.

P The condition of one eye constantly being deviated is called strabismus, or tropia: esotropia is an inward turning of the eye; exotropia is an outward turning of the eye (Figure 12-4).

Cover/Uncover Test

E 1. Ask the patient to look straight ahead and to focus on an object in the distance.
   2. Place an occluder over the patient's left eye for several seconds and observe for movement in the uncovered right eye.
   3. As the occluder is removed, observe the covered eye for movement.

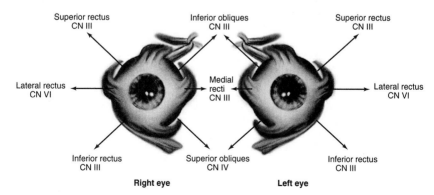

FIGURE 12-3 Direction of Movement of Extraocular Muscles.

E **Examination** N **Normal Findings** A **Abnormal Findings** P **Pathophysiology**

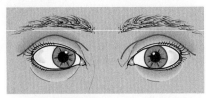

A. Right Esotropia

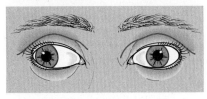

B. Right Exotropia

FIGURE 12-4 Strabismus.

4. Repeat the procedure with the same eye, having the patient focus on an object held close to the eye.
5. Repeat on the other side.

N If the eyes are in alignment, there will be no movement of either eye.

A If the uncovered eye shifts position as the other eye is covered, or if the covered eye shifts position as it is uncovered, a phoria, or latent misalignment of an eye, exists.

P Mild weakness has two forms: esophoria, nasal or inward drift, and exophoria, a temporal or outward drift.

Cardinal Fields of Gaze (Extraocular Muscle Movements)

E 1. Place the patient in a sitting position facing you.
2. Place your nondominant hand just under the patient's chin or on top of the patient's head as a reminder to hold the head still.
3. Ask the patient to follow an object (finger, pencil, or penlight) with the eyes.
4. Move the object through the six fields of gaze in a smooth and steady manner, pausing at each extreme position to detect any nystagmus, or involuntary movement, and

returning to the centre after each field is tested.

5. Note the patient's ability to move the eyes in each direction.
6. Move the object forward to about 12 cm (5 inches) in front of the patient's nose at the midline.
7. Observe for convergence of gaze.

N Both eyes should move smoothly and symmetrically in each of the six fields of gaze and converge on the held object as it moves toward the nose. A few beats of nystagmus with extreme lateral gaze can be normal.

A Lack of symmetrical eye movement in a particular direction.

P Weakness in the muscle that moves the eye in that direction.

A Failure of an eye to move outward (CN VI), inability of the eye to move downward when deviated inward (CN IV), or other defects in movement (CN III).

P Traumatic ophthalmoplegia may be caused by fracture of the orbit near the foramen magnum, causing damage to the extraocular muscles or CN II, III, IV, and VI; basilar skull fractures; vitamin deficiency, especially thiamine; Herpes zoster; syphilis; scarlet fever; whooping cough; botulism.

A Ophthalmoplegia is paralysis of one or more of the optic muscles.

P Increased intracranial pressure; parasellar meningiomas or tumours in the sphenoid sinus.

A Vertical gaze is a paralysis of upward gaze.

P Destruction at the area of the midbrain–diencephalic junction or the medial longitudinal fasciculus, or tumours of the pineal gland.

A Paralysis of horizontal gaze.

P Damage to the motor areas of the cerebral cortex so the eyes tend to deviate toward the side of the lesion.

A If one eye deviates down and the other eye deviates up, it is called skew deviation.

P Cerebellar disease or a lesion in the pons on the same side as the eye that is deviated down.

| E Examination | N Normal Findings | A Abnormal Findings | P Pathophysiology |

A Rhythmic, beating, involuntary oscillation of the eyes as the object is held at points away from the midline.

P Nystagmus may be caused by a lesion in the brain stem, cerebellum, vestibular system, or along the visual pathways in the cerebral hemispheres.

Anterior Segment Structures

Conjunctiva

To assess the bulbar conjunctiva:

E
1. Separate the patient's lid margins with your fingers.
2. Have the patient look up, down, and to the right and left.
3. Inspect the surface of the bulbar conjunctiva for colour, redness, swelling, exudate, or foreign bodies. Note whether injection or redness is around the cornea, foreign bodies, or toward the periphery.
4. With your thumb, gently pull the lower lid toward the cheek and inspect the surface of the bulbar conjunctiva for colour, inflammation, edema, lesions, or foreign bodies.

N The bulbar conjunctiva is transparent with small blood vessels visible in it. It should appear white except for a few small blood vessels, which are normal. No swelling, injection, exudate, foreign bodies, or lesions are noted.

The palpebral conjunctiva is examined only when there is a concern about its condition. To examine the palpebral conjunctiva of the upper lid:

E
1. Explain the procedure to the patient to alleviate the fear of pain or damage to the eye.
2. Don gloves, and have the patient look down to relax the levator muscle.
3. Gently pull the eyelashes downward and place a sterile, cotton-tipped applicator about 1 cm above the lid margin.
4. Gently exert downward pressure on the applicator while pulling the eye-lashes upward to evert the lid (Figure 12-5).
5. Inspect the palpebral conjunctiva for injection, swelling or chemosis, exudate, and foreign bodies.
6. Return the lid to its normal position by instructing the patient to look up and then pulling the eyelid outward and removing the cotton-tipped applicator. Ask the patient to blink.

N The palpebral conjunctiva should appear pink and moist. It is without swelling, lesions, injection, exudate, or foreign bodies.

A Bilateral injected conjunctiva with purulent, sticky discharge and lid edema.

P Bacterial conjunctivitis.

A Unilateral injection with moderate pain and without purulent discharge.

P Viral conjunctivitis most commonly due to adenovirus.

A Mild inflammation and injection and follicles of palpebral conjunctiva are present with scant discharge.

P Allergic conjunctivitis.

A A yellow nodule on the nasal side of the bulbar conjunctiva adjacent to the cornea.

P Pinguecula is a nodular degeneration of the conjunctiva due to increased exposure to UV light.

A Unilateral or bilateral triangle-shaped encroachment onto the conjunctiva.

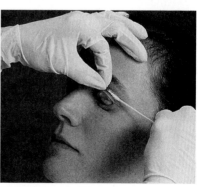

B. Everting the Eyelid

FIGURE 12-5 Assessing Palpebral Conjunctiva.

P Pterygium is caused by excessive UV light exposure.

A Sudden onset of a painless, bright-red appearance on the bulbar conjunctiva.

P Subconjunctival hemorrhage from the pressure exerted during coughing, sneezing, or a Valsalva maneuver; also attributed to anticoagulant medications or uncontrolled hypertension.

Sclera

E While assessing the conjunctiva, inspect the sclera for colour, exudate, lesions, and foreign bodies.

N In light-skinned individuals, the sclera should be white with some small, superficial vessels and without exudate, lesions, or foreign bodies. In dark-skinned individuals, the sclera may have tiny brown patches of melanin or a greyish blue or "muddy" colour.

A The colour of the sclera is uniformly yellow.

P Jaundice or scleral icterus is due to colouring of the sclera with bilirubin (an early manifestation of systemic conditions such as hepatitis, sickle cell disease, gallstones, and physiological jaundice of the newborn).

A The sclera is blue.

P Osteogenesis imperfecta due to thinning of the sclera.

Cornea

E 1. Stand in front of the patient.
   2. Shine a penlight directly on the cornea.

3. Move the light laterally and view the cornea from that angle, noting colour, discharge, and lesions.

N The corneal surface should be moist and shiny, with no discharge, cloudiness, opacities, or irregularities.

A A greyish, well-circumscribed ulcerated area on the cornea.

P Bacterial invasion.

A A treelike configuration on the corneal surface. The patient complains of mild discomfort, photophobia, and in some cases blurred vision.

P This type of ulceration is caused by the herpes simplex virus.

A A hazy grey ring about 2 mm in width just inside the limbus.

P Arcus senilis, a bilateral, benign degeneration of the peripheral cornea.

A A steamy or cloudy cornea.

P Glaucoma is caused by increased intraocular pressure.

Iris

E With the penlight, inspect the iris for colour, nodules, and vascularity.

N Normally, the colour is evenly distributed over the iris, although there can be a mosaic variant. It is normally smooth and without apparent vascularity.

A Heavily pigmented, slightly elevated area visible in the iris.

P This lesion can be a benign iris nevus or a malignant melanoma.

A The inferior portion of the iris is obscured by blood.

Nursing Alert

Screening for Retinopathy in People with Diabetes Mellitus

- Initiate screening five years after diagnosis of type 1 diabetes mellitus (DM) in all individuals 15 years of age and older. In the absence of retinopathy, rescreen annually.
- Screen all individuals at diagnosis of type 2 DM. In the absence of retinopathy, rescreen every one to two years.
- For all people with DM, review the ABC's (A1C, blood pressure, and cholesterol).

E **Examination**   N **Normal Findings**   A **Abnormal Findings**   P **Pathophysiology**

P   Hyphema is caused by bleeding from vessels in the iris as a result of direct trauma to the globe; eye surgery.

A   Absent wedge portion of the iris.

P   Surgical removal of a cataract.

Pupil

E   1. Stand in front of the patient in a darkened room.

2. Note the shape and size of the pupils in millimetres.

3. Move a penlight from the side to the front of one eye without allowing the light to shine on the other eye.

4. Observe the pupillary reaction in that eye. This is the direct light reflex. Note the size of the pupil receiving light stimulus and the speed of pupillary response to light.

5. Repeat in the other eye.

6. Move the penlight in front of one eye and observe the other eye for pupillary constriction. This is the consensual light reflex.

7. Repeat the procedure on the other eye.

8. Instruct the patient to shift the gaze to a distant object for 30 seconds.

9. Instruct the patient to then look at your finger or an object held in your hand about 10 cm from the patient.

10. Note the reaction and size of the pupils. Accommodation occurs when pupils constrict and converge to focus on objects at close range.

N   The pupils should be deep black, round, and of equal diameter, ranging from 2–6 mm. Pupils should constrict briskly to direct and consensual light and to accommodation (CN III). Small differences in pupil size (anisocoria) may be normal in some people.

A   The pupil that constricts to less than 2 mm in diameter is termed miotic. The pupil that dilates to more than 6 mm in diameter is termed mydriatic.

P   Medications such as sympathomimetics or parasympathomimetics, iritis, or disorders such as CN III paralysis, which can occur as a result of a carotid artery aneurysm (see Table 12-1 for further pathologies).

A   The pupil has an irregular shape.

P   Surgical removal of cataracts and iridectomy.

A   When the direct light reflex is defective, the pupil dilates in response to light, but consensual reaction is appropriate. This is called a Marcus Gunn pupil.

P   Optic nerve damage in the optic chiasm, such as in trauma.

A   The hippus phenomenon occurs after the pupil has been stimulated by direct light. Light causes the pupil to constrict, but then the pupil appears to rhythmically vacillate in size from a larger to a smaller diameter.

P   Lesion in the midbrain.

Lens

E   1. Stand in front of the patient.

2. Shine a penlight directly on the pupil. The lens is behind the pupil.

3. Note the colour.

N   The lens is transparent in colour.

A   One or more of the pupils are not deep black; a pearly grey appearance of one or both pupils may indicate an opacity (cloudiness) in the lens (cataract).

P   Senile cataract; unilateral cataract; bilateral cataracts found in infants or young children are congenital cataracts.

Posterior Segment Structures

The funduscopic assessment (CN II) requires the use of a direct ophthalmoscope to assess the structures in the posterior segment of the eye.

E   1. Instruct the patient to look at a distant object across the room. This will help to dilate the eyes.

2. Set the ophthalmoscope on the 0 lens and hold it in front of your right eye with your index finger on the lens selector.

3. From a distance of 20–30 cm (8–12 inches) from the patient and about 15° to the lateral side, shine the light

| E | Examination | N | Normal Findings | A | Abnormal Findings | P | Pathophysiology |

TABLE 12-1   Pupil Abnormalities

A.

A: The size of pupils is unequal but both pupils react to light and accommodation.
P: Inequality of pupillary size is called **anisocoria** and may be congenital or due to inflammation of ocular tissue or disturbances of neurophthalmic pathways.

B.

A: A fixed and dilated pupil is observed on one side. The abnormal pupil does not react to direct or consensual light stimulation and does not accommodate. Ptosis and lateral downward deviation may also be noted.
P: This abnormality is caused by **oculomotor nerve damage** due to head trauma and increased intracranial pressure. Atropine-like agents applied topically may cause an even more widely fixed and dilated pupil.

C.

A: A unilateral, small, regularly shaped pupil is observed. Both pupils react directly and consensually and accommodate. Ptosis and diminished or absent sweating on the affected side may also be noted.
P: This finding is **Horner's syndrome**, which is caused by a lesion of the sympathetic nerve pathway.

D.

A: Pupils are bilaterally small and irregularly shaped. They react to accommodation but sluggishly or not at all to light.
P: These abnormalities are **Argyll Robertson** pupils and are usually caused by central lesions of neurosyphilis. Other causes include encephalitis, drugs, diabetes, brain tumors, and alcoholism.

E.

A: A unilateral, large, regularly shaped pupil is noted. The affected pupil's reaction to light and accommodation is sluggish or absent. The patient may report blurred vision because of the slow accommodation. You may observe diminished ankle and knee deep-tendon reflexes.
P: This abnormality, a tonic or **Adie's** pupil, is due to impaired sympathetic nerve supply.

F.

A: Both pupils are **small, fixed,** regularly shaped, and do not react to light or accommodation.
P: This abnormality may be caused by opiate ingestion, topical application of miotic drops, or lesions in the brain.

A: Pupils are small, equal, and reactive.
P: Diencephalic injury or metabolic coma may cause these findings.

G.

A: Both pupils are **dilated** and **fixed**, and do not react to light or accomodation.
P: Severe head trauma, brain stem infarction, cardiopulmonary arrest (after 4 to 6 min).

H.

Blind eye

Light

A: Light shone into a blind eye (amaurotic pupil) will cause no reaction (direct or consensual) in either pupil. If light is shone in the other eye, and CN III is intact, both pupils should constrict.
P: Due to a lesion in the retina or the optic nerve, the light stimulus shown in the amaurotic pupil is unable to pass along the sensory pathway; therefore, the oculomotor response in both eyes is absent.

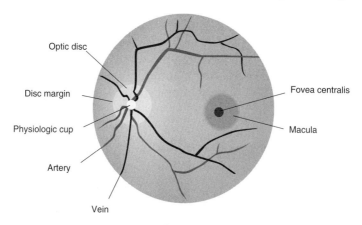

LEFT EYE

FIGURE 12-7 Optic Disc.

into the patient's right pupil, eliciting a light reflection from the retina; this is called the red reflex.

4. While maintaining the red reflex in view, move closer to the patient and move the lens selector from 0 to the + or black numbers in order to focus on the anterior ocular structures.

5. For optimum visualization, keep the ophthalmoscope within an inch of the patient's eye (Figure 12-6).

6. At this point, move the lens selector from the + or black numbers, through 0, and into the × or red numbers in order to focus on structures progressively more posterior.

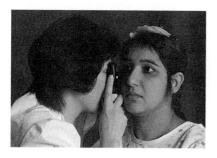

FIGURE 12-6 Examining Retinal Structures.

7. Focus on the optic disc at the nasal side of the retina by following any retinal vessels centrally (Figure 12-7).

8. You may need to reverse direction along the vessel if the disc does not appear.

9. Observe the retina for colour and lesions; the retinal vessels for configuration and characteristics of their crossing; and the optic disc for colour, shape, size, margins, and comparison of cup-to-disc ratio.

10. Describe the size, position, and location of any abnormality. Use the diameter of the disc (DD) as a guide to describe the distance of the abnormality from the optic disc. Use the optic disc as a clock face as a reference point to describe the location of the abnormality. Describe the size of the abnormality in relation to the size of the optic disc.

11. Repeat on the left eye.

N Refer to Table 12-2. The red reflex is present. The optic disc is pinkish orange in colour, with a yellow-white excavated centre known as the physiologic cup (Figure 12-7). The ratio of the cup diameter to that of the entire disc is 1:3. The border of the disc may range from a

| E Examination | N Normal Findings | A Abnormal Findings | P Pathophysiology |

TABLE 12-2   Retinal Colour Variations

FINDINGS	CHARACTERISTICS
Fair-skinned individual	• Retina appears a lighter red-orange colour
	• Tessellated appearance of the fundi (pigment does not obscure the choroid vessels)
Dark-skinned individual	• Fundi appear darker in colour; greyish purple to brownish (from increased pigment in the choroid and retina)
	• No tessellated appearance
	• Choroidal vessels usually obscured
Aging individual	• Vessels are straighter and narrower
	• Choroidal vessels are easily visualized
	• Retinal pigment epithelium atrophies and causes the retinal colour to become paler

sharp, round demarcation from the surrounding retina to a more blended border, but should be on the same plane as the retina. In general, there are four main vascular branches emanating from the disc, each branch consisting of an arteriole and a venule. The venules are approximately four times the size of the accompanying arterioles and are darker in colour. Light often produces a glistening "light reflex" from the arteriolar vessel. Normal arterial-to-venous width is a ratio of 2:3 or 4:5.

A   The red reflex is absent.

P   Cataracts.

A   The red reflex is absent and the pupil appears white.

P   Leukocoria, or white reflex, is found in retinoblastoma, congenital cataracts, and retinal detachment.

P   Optic atrophy caused by increased intracranial pressure or from congenital syphilis.

A   The physiologic cup exceeds the normal 1:3 ratio. The disc appears elevated above the plane of the surrounding retina.

P   Papillitis resulting from optic neuritis; without loss of vision: increased intracranial pressure.

A   Superficial retinal hemorrhages found in the fundi, or red hemorrhages with white centres called Roth's spots.

P   Severe hypertension, occlusion of the central retinal vein, and papilledema. Roth's spots are sometimes associated with infective endocarditis.

A   Deep retinal hemorrhages, or dot hemorrhages, appear as small red dots or irregular spots in the deep layer of the retina.

P   Diabetes mellitus.

A   Diffuse preretinal hemorrhages occur in the small space between the vitreous and the retina.

P   Sudden increase in intracranial pressure.

A   Microaneurysms are tiny, round, red dots that can be seen in peripheral and macular areas of the retina.

P   Diabetic retinopathy.

A   Neovascularization is the formation of new vessels that are very narrow and disorderly in appearance and may extend into the vitreous.

P   Diabetic retinopathy.

A   Fluffy white or grey slightly irregular areas that appear on the retina and are ovoid in shape are abnormal.

E   Examination   N   Normal Findings   A   Abnormal Findings   P   Pathophysiology

P Cotton wool spots represent microscopic infarcts of the nerve fibre layer and are due to diabetic or hypertensive retinopathy.

P Drusen are small white dots in the fundus that are arranged in an irregular pattern.

P Normal aging process.

A The red-orange retinal reflex is absent in the area of a retinal detachment. The area appears pearly grey and is elevated and wrinkled.

P Severe myopia, cataract surgery, diabetic retinopathy, trauma.

Macula

When the retinal structures and the optic disc have been assessed:

E 1. Move the ophthalmoscope approximately two disc diameters temporally to view the macula, or ask the patient to look at the light. The red-free filter lens of the ophthalmoscope may be helpful in assessing the macula, which is not clearly demarcated and is very light sensitive. The patient tends to turn away when the light strikes the fovea, making it difficult to assess details of the macular area.

2. Note the fovea centralis and observe for colour, shape, and lesions.

3. Repeat with the other eye.

N The macula is a darker, avascular area with a pinpoint reflective centre known as the fovea centralis.

A The retina is pale with the macular region appearing as a cherry-red spot.

P Retinal artery occlusion, an indication of Tay-Sachs disease.

A An enlarged macula.

P Diabetes mellitus, hypertension, ARMD, retinal blood vessel obstruction.

A Sharply defined, small red spots found in and around the macula.

P Diabetes mellitus.

A Macular borders are blurred, with a few spots of pigment near the macula; a hole may appear to be present in the centre of the region, or a hemorrhage may have occurred.

P ARMD (Age-Related Macular Degeneration).

E **Examination** N **Normal Findings** A **Abnormal Findings** P **Pathophysiology**

13

Ears, Nose, Mouth, and Throat

ANATOMY AND PHYSIOLOGY

Ear

External Ear

The external ear, also called the auricle or pinna, extends through the auditory canal to the tympanic membrane (TM). The auricle is composed of cartilage and receives sound waves and funnels them through the auditory canal to produce vibrations on the TM (Figure 13.1).

The external auditory canal (EAC) is lined with tiny hairs and modified sweat glands that secrete a thick, waxlike substance called cerumen, which can vary in consistency from dry and flaky to wet and waxy. Cerumen ranges from a pale, honey colour in light-skinned individuals to dark-brown or black in dark-skinned people.

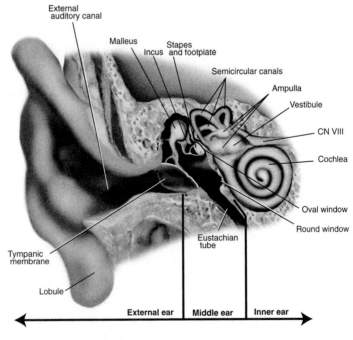

External auditory canal

Malleus

Incus Stapes and footplate

Semicircular canals

Ampulla

Vestibule

CN VIII

Cochlea

Oval window

Round window

Eustachian tube

Tympanic membrane

Lobule

External ear | Middle ear | Inner ear

FIGURE 13-1 Cross Section of the Ear.

Middle Ear

The middle ear is composed of the TM, the ossicles, and the tympanic cavity. The cavity is an air-filled compartment that separates the external ear from the internal ear. The TM is circular or oval and is about 2.5 cm in diameter (Figure 13-2).

Vibrations set up in the TM by sound waves reaching it through the EAC are transmitted to the inner ear by rapid movement of the ossicles.

The middle ear is connected to the nasopharynx by the auditory or eustachian tube (ET).

Inner Ear

The inner ear is a complex, closed, fluid-filled system of interconnecting tubes called the labyrinth, which is essential for hearing and equilibrium. The labyrinth has bony and membranous portions. The bony labyrinth is composed of the cochlea, the semicircular canals, and the vestibule. The human ear is capable of hearing within a frequency range of 20 to 20,000 Hz, and a decibel (dB) range of 0 to 140.

Nose

The nose consists of the external or outer nose, and the nasal fossae or internal nose (Figure 13-3). The outer nose is made up of bone and cartilage and is divided internally into two nasal fossae by

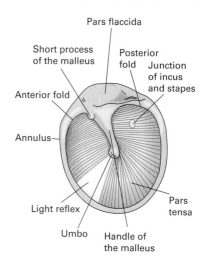

FIGURE 13-2 Landmarks of the Left Tympanic Membrane.

the nasal septum. Anterior openings into the nasal fossae are nostrils, or nares.

Air enters the anterior nares, passes through the vestibule, which contains nasal hairs and sebaceous glands, and enters the fossa.

Olfactory receptor cells are located in the upper parts of the nasal cavity, the superior nasal conchae, and on parts of the nasal septum

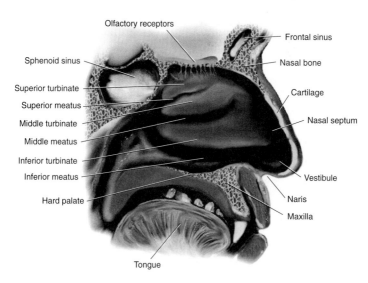

FIGURE 13-3 Lateral Cross Section of the Nose.

and are covered by cilia that project into the cavity. The chemical component of odours binds with the receptors, causing nerve impulses to be transmitted to the olfactory cortex, located in the base of the frontal lobe.

Sinuses

Air-filled cavities lined with mucous membranes are present in some of the cranial bones and are referred to as paranasal sinuses (Figure 13-4). The frontal, maxillary, ethmoid, and sphenoid paranasal sinuses open into the nose. Only the frontal and maxillary sinuses can be assessed in the physical examination.

Mouth and Throat

The lips are sensory structures at the opening of the mouth (Figure 13-5). The area where the lips meet the facial skin is called the vermilion border. The median groove superior to the upper lip is called the philtrum.

The roof of the mouth consists of the hard palate anteriorly and the soft palate posteriorly (Figure 13-6). The linear raphe is a linear ridge in the middle of the hard palate.

Situated in the floor of the mouth, the tongue is a muscular organ connected to the hyoid bone posteriorly and to the floor of the mouth anteriorly by the frenulum. The tongue assists with mastication, swallowing, speech, and mechanical cleansing of the teeth.

The mucous membrane covering the upper surface of the tongue has numerous projections called papillae that assist in handling food and contain taste buds. Four qualities of

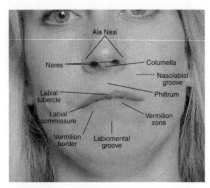

FIGURE 13-5 Landmarks of the Area around the Mouth.

taste are found in taste buds distributed over the surface of the tongue: bitter is located at the base, sour along the sides, and salty and sweet near the tip. The sulcus terminalis is the midline depression that separates the anterior two-thirds of the tongue from the posterior one-third.

Gums, or gingivae, hold the teeth in place and appear pink or coral in light-skinned individuals, and brown with a darker melanotic line along the edges in dark-skinned individuals. Adults have 32 permanent teeth: four incisors, two canines, four premolars, and six molars in each half of the mouth (Figure 13-7). The three parts of the tooth are the top, or the crown, the root, which is embedded in the gum, and the neck, which connects the root and the crown. The uvula is a fingerlike projection of tissue that hangs down from the centre of the soft palate.

EQUIPMENT

- Otoscope with earpieces of different sizes and pneumatic attachment
- Nasal speculum
- Penlight
- Tuning fork, 512 Hz
- Tongue blade
- Watch
- Gauze square
- Clean gloves
- Transilluminator
- Cotton-tipped applicator

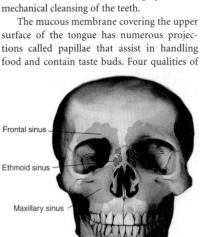

FIGURE 13-4 Location of the Sinuses (Sphenoid sinuses are directly behind ethmoid sinuses.)

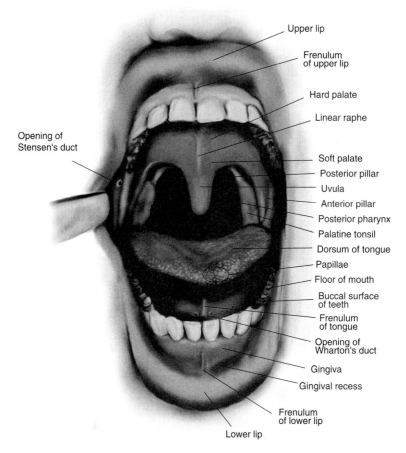

FIGURE 13-6 Structures of the Mouth.

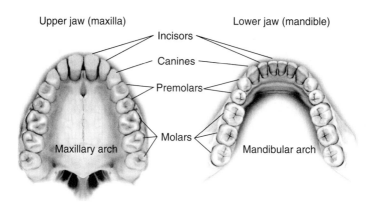

FIGURE 13-7 Permanent Teeth.

HEALTH HISTORY

Medical History

Ear Specific — Acute otitis media (AOM), acute otitis externa (AOE), serous otitis media, hearing difficulties

Nose Specific — Polyps, septal deviation, sinus infection, allergic rhinitis, anosmia

Mouth and Throat Specific — Tonsillitis, caries, herpes simplex virus, *Candida* infections, strep throat, frequent URIs, tonsillar abscess

Surgical History — Neurosurgery, tonsillectomy, adenoidectomy, tumour removal, cosmetic surgery of head or neck, repair of septal deviation, oral surgery, tympanostomy tube placement

Allergies — Pollen: sneezing, nasal congestion, watery or itchy eyes, cough
Insect stings: swelling of the throat, around the eyes
Animal dander: sneezing, nasal congestion, watery or itchy eyes, cough

Special Needs — Deafness, speech disorders

Childhood Illnesses — Frequent tonsillitis, frequent ear infections

Social History

Drug Use — Snorting cocaine may cause perforation of the nasal septum

Tobacco Use — Snuff or chewing tobacco predisposes the patient to mouth, lip, or throat cancer

◄ NURSING CHECKLIST ►

General Approach to Ears, Nose, Mouth, and Throat Assessment

1. Greet the patient and explain the assessment techniques that you will be using.
2. Use a quiet room free from interruptions.
3. Ensure that the light in the room provides sufficient brightness to allow adequate observation of the patient.
4. Place the patient in an upright sitting position on the examination table, or
4a. For patients who cannot tolerate the sitting position, gain access to the patient's head so that it can be rotated from side to side for assessment.
5. Visualize the underlying structures during the assessment process to allow adequate description of findings.
6. Always compare right and left ears, as well as right and left sides of the nose, sinuses, mouth, and throat.
7. Use a systematic approach that is followed consistently at each assessment.

ASSESSMENT OF THE EAR

Physical assessment of the ear consists of three parts:

1. Auditory screening (CN VIII)
2. Inspection and palpation of the external ear
3. Otoscopic assessment

Auditory Screening

Voice-Whisper Test

E
1. Instruct the patient to occlude one ear with a finger.
2. Stand 0.6 metres behind the patient's other ear and whisper a two-syllable word or phrase that is evenly accented.
3. Ask the patient to repeat the word or phrase.
4. Repeat the test with the other ear.

N The patient should be able to repeat words whispered from a distance of 0.6 metres.

A The patient is unable to repeat the words correctly or states that he or she was unable to hear anything.

P Hearing loss in the high-frequency range that may be caused by excessive exposure to loud noises.

Tuning Fork Tests

Weber and Rinne tests help to determine whether the type of hearing loss the patient is experiencing is conductive or sensorineural. Air conduction refers to the transmission of sound through the ear canal, TM, and ossicular chain to the cochlea and auditory nerve. Bone conduction refers to the transmission of sound through the bones of the skull to the cochlea and auditory nerve.

Weber Test

E
1. Hold the handle of a 512 Hz tuning fork and strike the tines on the ulnar border of the palm to activate it.
2. Place the stem of the fork firmly against the middle of the patient's forehead, on the top of the head at the midline, or on the front teeth (Figure 13-8).
3. Ask the patient if the sound is heard centrally or toward one side.

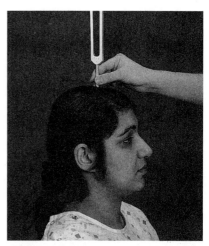

FIGURE 13-8 Weber Test.

N The patient should perceive the sound equally in both ears or "in the middle." No lateralization of sound is known as a negative Weber test.

A The sound lateralizes to the affected ear.

P Conductive hearing loss occurs when there are external or middle ear disorders such as impacted cerumen, perforation of the TM, serum or pus in the middle ear, or a fusion of the ossicles.

A The sound lateralizes to the unaffected ear.

P Sensorineural hearing loss occurs when there is a disorder in the inner ear, the auditory nerve, or the brain; disorders include congenital defects, effects of ototoxic drugs, and repeated or prolonged exposure to loud noise.

Rinne Test

E
1. Stand behind or to the side of the patient and strike the tuning fork.
2. Place the stem of the tuning fork against the patient's right mastoid process to test bone conduction (Figure 13-9A).
3. Instruct the patient to indicate if the sound is heard.
4. Ask the patient to tell you when the sound stops.

E Examination	N Normal Findings	A Abnormal Findings	P Pathophysiology

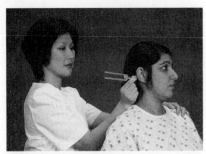

A. Assessing Bone Conduction

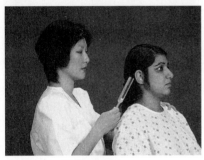

B. Assessing Air Conduction

FIGURE 13-9 Rinne Test.

5. When the patient says that the sound has stopped, move the tuning fork, with the tines facing forward, in front of the right auditory meatus, and ask the patient if the sound is still heard. Note the length of time the patient hears the sound (testing air conduction) (Figure 13-9B).
6. Repeat the test on the left ear.

N   Air conduction is heard twice as long as bone conduction when the patient hears the sound through the external auditory canal (air) after it is no longer heard at the mastoid process (bone). This is denoted as AC>BC.

A   The patient reports hearing the sound longer through bone conduction.

P   Conductive hearing loss resulting from disease, obstruction, or damage to the outer or middle ear.

External Ear

Inspection

E   1. Inspect the ears and note their position, colour, size, and shape.
    2. Note any deformities, nodules, inflammation, or lesions.
    3. Note colour, consistency, and amount of cerumen.

N   The ear should match the flesh colour of the patient's skin and should be positioned centrally and in proportion to the head. The top of the ear should cross an imaginary line drawn from the outer canthus of the eye to the occiput. Cerumen should be moist and not obscure the TM. There should be no foreign bodies, redness, drainage, deformities, nodules, or lesions.

A   The ears are pale, red, or cyanotic.

P   Vasomotor disorders, fevers, hypoxemia, and cold weather.

A   Purulent drainage.

P   Infection.

A   Clear or bloody drainage.

P   Cerebrospinal fluid leaking as a result of head trauma or surgery.

A   A hematoma behind an ear over the mastoid bone.

P   This is called Battle's sign and indicates head trauma to the temporal bone of the skull.

A   A hard, painless, irregular-shaped nodule on the pinna.

P   Tophi are uric acid nodules and may indicate the presence of gout or benign fibromas.

A   Sebaceous cysts.

P   Blockage of the ducts to the sebaceous gland.

A   Lymph nodes anterior to the tragus or overlying the mastoid. Malignancy or an infection.

Palpation

E   1. Palpate the auricle between your thumb and the index finger, noting any tenderness or lesions. If the patient has ear pain, assess the unaffected ear first, then cautiously assess the affected ear.

E   **Examination**   N   **Normal Findings**   A   **Abnormal Findings**   P   **Pathophysiology**

2. Using the tips of the index and middle fingers, palpate the mastoid tip, noting any tenderness.

3. Using the tips of the index and middle fingers, press inward on the tragus, noting any tenderness.

4. Hold the auricle between the thumb and the index finger and gently pull up and down, noting any tenderness.

N The patient should not complain of pain or tenderness during palpation.

P Acute otitis externa (AOE).

A Auricular pain or tenderness.

A Tenderness over the mastoid process.

P Middle-ear inflammation or mastoiditis.

A The tragus is edematous or sensitive.

P Inflammation of the external or middle ear.

Otoscopic Assessment

E 1. Ask the patient to tip his or her head away from the ear being assessed.

2. Select the largest speculum that will comfortably fit the patient.

3. Hold the otoscope securely in your dominant hand, with the patient's head held downward, and the handle held like a pencil between your thumb and forefinger.

4. Rest the back of your dominant hand on the right side of the patient's head (Figure 13-10).

5. Use the ulnar aspect of your free hand to pull the right ear in a manner that will straighten the canal. In adults, and in children over 3 years old, pull the ear up and back. See Chapter 24 for the assessment of children.

6. If hair obstructs visualization, moisten the speculum with water or a water-soluble lubricant.

7. If wax obstructs visualization, it should be removed only by a skilled practitioner, either by curettement (if the cerumen is soft or the TM is ruptured) or by irrigation (if the cerumen is dry and hard and the TM is intact).

8. Slowly insert the speculum into the canal, looking at the canal as the speculum passes.

9. Assess the canal for inflammation, exudates, lesions, and foreign bodies.

10. Continue to insert the speculum into the canal, following the path of the canal until the TM is seen.

11. If the TM is not visible, gently pull the pinna slightly farther in order to straighten the canal to allow an adequate view.

12. Identify the colour, light reflex, umbo, the short process, and the long handle of the malleus. Note the presence of perforations, lesions, bulging or retraction of the TM, dilatation of blood vessels, bubbles, or fluid.

13. Ask the patient to close the mouth, pinch the nose closed, and blow gently while you observe for movement of the TM. A pneumatic attachment may be used to create this movement if one is available.

14. Gently withdraw the speculum and repeat the process with the left ear.

N The ear canal should have no redness, swelling, tenderness, lesions, drainage, foreign bodies, or scaly surface areas. Cerumen varies in amount, consistency, and colour. The TM should be pearly grey with clearly defined landmarks and a distinct cone-shaped light reflex extending from the umbo toward the anteroinferior aspect of the membrane.

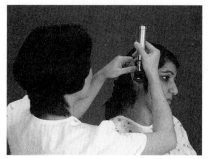

FIGURE 13-10 Position for Otoscopic Examination.

E **Examination** N **Normal Findings** A **Abnormal Findings** P **Pathophysiology**

Nursing Alert

Risk Factors for Otitis Media

- Less than 2 years of age
- Frequent upper respiratory tract infections
- Males
- Family history (parents, siblings)
- Pacifier use after 6 months of age
- Passive smoking
- Day care attendance
- Bottle fed
- Down syndrome
- Craniofacial disorders

This light reflex is seen at 5 o'clock in the right ear and at 7 o'clock in the left ear. Blood vessels should be visible only on the periphery, and the membrane should not bulge, be retracted, or have any evidence of fluid behind it. The TM should move when the patient blows against resistance.

A   A painful, boil-like pustule in the EAC.
P   Furunculosis.
A   There is redness, swelling, narrowing, and pain of the external ear.

P   Acute otitis externa (AOE) is caused by infectious organisms or allergic reactions. Predisposing factors include excessive moisture in the ear related to swimming, trauma from cleansing the ears with a sharp instrument, or allergies to substances such as hairspray.
A   Hard, dry, and very dark yellow-brown cerumen.
P   Old cerumen is harder and drier, and may become impacted if not removed.
A   The TM is red, with decreased mobility and possible bulging.
P   Acute otitis media (AOM), or an inflammation of the middle ear.
A   Amber-yellow fluid on the TM is abnormal and may be accompanied by a fluid line or bubbles behind the membrane. Bulging may be present and mobility of the eardrum may be decreased.
P   OME or serous otitis media can be caused by allergies, infections, and a blocked ET. Table 13-1 compares AOM, OME, and otitis externa.
A   The TM is pearly grey and has dark patches.
P   Old perforations in the TM.
A   The TM is pearly grey and has dense white plaques.
P   Calcific deposits of scarring of the TM from frequent past episodes of otitis media.

TABLE 13-1   Comparison of Acute Otitis Media (AOM), Otitis Media with Effusion (OME), and Otitis Externa (AOE)

	AOM	OME	AOE
TM colour	Diffuse red, dilated peripheral vessels	Yellowish	WNL
TM appearance	Bulging	Bubbles, fluid line	WNL
TM landmarks	Decreased	Retracted with prominent malleus	WNL
Movement of tragus	Painless	Painless	Painful
Hearing	WNL/decreased	WNL/decreased	WNL
EAC	WNL	WNL	Erythematous, edematous

E **Examination**   N **Normal Findings**   A **Abnormal Findings**   P **Pathophysiology**

ASSESSMENT OF THE NOSE

External Inspection

E Inspect the nose, noting any trauma, bleeding, lesions, masses, swelling, and asymmetry.

N The shape of the external nose can vary greatly among individuals. Normally, it is located symmetrically in the midline of the face and is without swelling, bleeding, lesions, or masses.

A The nose is misshapen, broken, or swollen.

P Genetics, trauma, cosmetic surgery.

Patency

E 1. Have the patient occlude one nostril with a finger.
   2. Ask the patient to breathe in and out through the nose as you observe and listen for air movement in and out of the nostril.
   3. Repeat on the other side.

N Each nostril is patent.

A You observe or the patient states that air cannot be moved through the nostril(s).

P Deviated septum, foreign body, URI, allergies, or nasal polyps.

Internal Inspection

E 1. Position the patient's head in an extended position.
   2. Place your nondominant hand firmly on top of the patient's head.
   3. Using the thumb of the same hand, lift the tip of the patient's nose.
   4. Gently insert a nasal speculum or an otoscope with a short, wide nasal speculum. If using a nasal speculum, use a penlight to view the nostrils.
   5. Assess each nostril separately.
   6. Inspect the mucous membranes for colour and discharge.
   7. Inspect the middle and inferior turbinates and the middle meatus for colour, swelling, drainage, lesions, and polyps.
   8. Observe the nasal septum for deviation, perforation, lesions, and bleeding.

N The nasal mucosa should be pink or dull red without swelling or polyps. The septum is at the midline and without perforation, lesions, or bleeding. A small amount of clear, watery discharge is normal.

A The nasal mucosa is red and swollen with copious, clear, watery discharge. This is called rhinitis, an inflammation of the nasal mucosa.

P Common cold (coryza) when there is an acute onset of symptoms. Discharge may become purulent if a secondary bacterial infection develops.

A Nasal mucosa is pale and edematous with clear, watery discharge.

P Allergies or hay fever.

A Following trauma to the head, there is a clear, watery nasal discharge with normal-appearing mucosa. This discharge tests positive for glucose.

P Presence of cerebrospinal fluid. This may occur following head injury or complications of nose or sinus surgery or dental work.

A Nasal mucosa is red and swollen with purulent nasal discharge.

P Bacterial sinusitis.

A Smooth, round masses that are pale and shiny are noted protruding from the middle meatus.

P Nasal polyps.

A Bleeding is noted from an area of the lower portion of the nasal septum.

P Kiesselbach's plexus is the site of most nosebleeds.

A Unilateral purulent discharge; however, the patient does not experience other symptoms of an URI.

P Local infection. A common cause of localized infection is the presence of a foreign body.

A Nasal mucosa is inflamed and friable with possible septal perforation.

P Nasal inhalation of cocaine or amphetamines or the overuse of nasal spray.

E **Examination**   N **Normal Findings**   A **Abnormal Findings**   P **Pathophysiology**

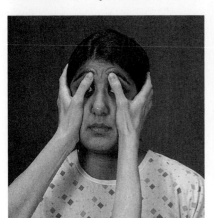

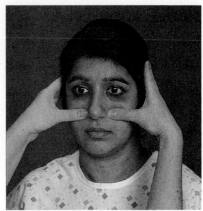

A. Palpation of Frontal Sinuses

B. Palpation of Maxillary Sinuses

FIGURE 13-11 Palpation of Sinuses.

ASSESSMENT OF THE SINUSES
Inspection

E   Observe the patient's face for any swelling around the nose and eyes.

N   There is no evidence of swelling around the nose and eyes.

A   Swelling is noted above or below the eyes.

P   Acute sinusitis.

Palpation and Percussion

To palpate and percuss the frontal sinuses:

E   1. Stand facing the patient.
    2. Gently press your thumbs under the bony ridge of the upper orbits (Figure 13-11A). Avoid applying pressure on the globes themselves.
    3. Observe for the presence of pain.
    4. Percuss the areas using the middle or index finger of your dominant hand (immediate percussion).
    5. Note the sound.

To palpate and percuss the maxillary sinuses:

E   1. Stand in front of the patient.
    2. Apply gentle pressure in the area under the infraorbital ridge using your thumb or middle finger (Figure 13-11B).
    3. Observe for the presence of pain.
    4. Percuss the area using your dominant middle or index finger.
    5. Note the sound.

N   The patient should experience no discomfort during palpation or percussion. The sinuses should be air filled and therefore resonant to percussion.

A   The patient complains of pain or tenderness at the site of palpation or percussion.

P   Sinusitis can be due to viral, bacterial, or allergic processes.

A   Percussion of the sinuses elicits a dull sound.

P   Fluid or cells present in the sinus cavity from an infectious or allergic process, or congenital absence of a sinus.

ASSESSMENT OF THE MOUTH AND THROAT
Assessment of the Mouth
Breath

E   1. Stand facing the patient and about 30 cm away.
    2. Smell the patient's breath.

N   The breath should smell fresh.

A   The breath smells foul.

E **Examination**   N **Normal Findings**   A **Abnormal Findings**   P **Pathophysiology**

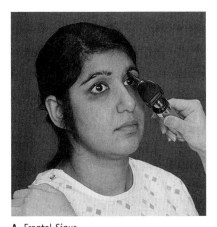

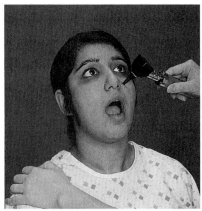

A. Frontal Sinus

B. Maxillary Sinus

FIGURE 13-12 Transillumination of Sinuses.

P   Halitosis can be a symptom of tooth decay, poor oral hygiene, or diseases of the gums, tonsils, or sinuses.

A   The breath smells of acetone.

P   Acetone or "fruity" breath is common in patients who are malnourished or who have diabetic ketoacidosis.

A   The breath smells musty.

P   Fetor hepaticas is the musty smell of the breath of a patient in liver failure.

A   The breath smells of ammonia.

P   End-stage renal failure (uremia).

ADVANCED TECHNIQUES

Transillumination of the Sinuses

If palpation and percussion of the sinuses suggest sinusitis, transillumination of the frontal and maxillary sinuses should be performed.

To evaluate the frontal sinuses:

E   1. Place the patient in a sitting position facing you in a dark room.

    2. Place a strong light source, such as a transilluminator, penlight, or the tip of an otoscope with the speculum, under the bony ridge of the upper orbits (Figure 13-12A).

    3. Observe the red glow over the sinuses and compare the symmetry of the two sides.

To evaluate the maxillary sinuses:

E   1. Place the patient in a sitting position facing you in a dark room.

    2. Place the light source firmly under each eye and just above the infraorbital ridge (Figure 13-12B).

    3. Ask the patient to open his or her mouth; observe the red glow on the hard palate, and compare the two sides.

N   The glow on each side is equal, indicating air-filled frontal and maxillary sinuses.

A   Absence of glow is abnormal.

P   Absence of glow suggests sinus congestion or the congenital absence of a sinus.

E   **Examination**   N   **Normal Findings**   A   **Abnormal Findings**   P   **Pathophysiology**

◀ NURSING CHECKLIST ▶

Preparing for the Assessment of the Mouth and Throat

1. Physical assessment of the oral cavity should include the following: breath, lips, tongue, buccal mucosa, gums and teeth, hard and soft palates, throat (oropharynx), and temporomandibular joint.
2. If the patient is wearing dentures or removable orthodontia, ask that they be removed before the examination begins.
3. Use gloves and a light source for optimum visualization of the oral cavity and pharynx.

Lips

Inspection

E   1. Observe the lips for colour, moisture, swelling, lesions, or other signs of inflammation.
   2. Instruct the patient to open his or her mouth.
   3. Use a tongue blade to inspect the membranes that connect the upper and lower lips to the gums for colour, inflammation, lesions, and hydration.

N   The lips and membranes should be pink and moist with no evidence of lesions or inflammation.

A   The lips are pale or cyanotic.
P   Refer to Chapter 16.
A   Swelling of the lips.
P   Allergic reactions.
A   The skin at the outer corners of the mouth is atrophic, irritated, and cracked.
P   Angular cheilosis occurs in nutritional deficiencies (such as riboflavin), poorly fitting dentures, and deficiencies of the immune system. *Candida* infections may also be present.
A   Vesicles on erythematous bases with serous fluid are found on the lips, gums, or hard palate, either singly or in clusters.
P   These are herpes simplex lesions, which are also called cold sores or fever blisters.
A   A round, painless lesion with central ulceration.

P   Chancre, the primary lesion of syphilis.
A   A plaque, wart, nodule, or ulcer, usually on the lower lip.
P   Squamous cell carcinoma, the most common form of oral cancer; basal cell carcinoma lesions can have pearly borders, crusting, and central ulcerations.
A   Persistent, painless, white, painted-looking patches on the lips.
P   These patches are called leukoplakia and are considered premalignant lesions.

Palpation

E   1. Don clean gloves.
   2. Gently pull down the patient's lower lip with the thumb and index finger of one hand and pull up the patient's upper lip with the thumb and index finger of the other hand.
   3. Note the tone of the lips as they are manipulated.
   4. If lesions are present, palpate them for consistency and tenderness.

N   Lips should not be flaccid and lesions should not be present.
A/P   See inspection of the lips for pathologies.

Tongue

E   1. Ask the patient to stick out his or her tongue (CN XII assesses tongue movement).
   2. Observe the dorsal surface for colour, hydration, texture, symmetry, fasci-

---

| E | **Examination** | N | **Normal Findings** | A | **Abnormal Findings** | P | **Pathophysiology** |

culations, atrophy, position in the mouth, and the presence of lesions.

3. Ask the patient to move the tongue from side to side and up and down.

4. With the patient's tongue back in the mouth, ask the patient to press it against the cheek. Provide resistance with your finger pads held on the outside of the cheek. Note the strength of the tongue and compare bilaterally.

5. Ask the patient to touch the tip of the tongue to the roof of the mouth. You may also grasp the tip of the tongue with a gauze square held between the thumb and the index finger of the gloved hand (Figure 13-13).

6. Inspect the ventral surface of the tongue, the frenulum, and Wharton's ducts for colour, hydration, lesions, inflammation, and vasculature.

7. With the gauze square, pull the tongue to the left and inspect and palpate the tongue using your finger pads.

8. Repeat with the tongue held to the right side.

N The tongue is in the midline of the mouth. The dorsum of the tongue should be pink, moist, rough (from the taste buds), and without lesions. The tongue is symmetrical and moves freely. The strength of the tongue is symmetrical and strong. The ventral surface of the tongue has prominent blood vessels and should be moist and without lesions. Wharton's ducts are patent and without inflammation or lesions. The lateral aspects of the tongue should be pink, smooth, and lesion free.

A The tongue is enlarged.

P Myxedema, acromegaly, Down syndrome, amyloidosis. Transient enlargement may be associated with glossitis, stomatitis, cellulitis of the neck, angioneurotic edema, hematoma, or abscess.

A The tongue is red and smooth with absent papillae.

P Vitamin B_{12}, iron, or niacin deficiency. May also be a side effect of chemotherapy.

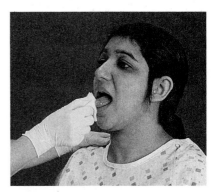

FIGURE 13-13 Tongue Assessment.

A There is a thick, white, curdlike coating on the tongue that leaves a raw, red surface when it is scraped off.

P Candidiasis, or thrush, due to chemotherapy, radiation therapy, disorders of the immune system such as AIDS, antibiotic therapy, or excessive use of alcohol, tobacco, or cocaine.

A Thin, pearly white lesions that coalesce and become thick and palpable on the sides of the tongue.

P This is leukoplakia. It is considered a premalignant lesion.

A A painful, small, round, white, ulcerated lesion with erythematous borders.

P Aphthous ulcer (canker sore), which can be associated with stress, extreme fatigue, food allergies, and oral trauma.

A A short lingual frenulum.

P Ankyloglossia is a congenital abnormality.

A The tongue has a hairy appearance and is yellow, black, or brown.

P Hairy leukoplakia, or hairy tongue, a benign condition that can result from antibiotic therapy.

A Lesions are noted on the ventral surface of the tongue.

P Malignancies, especially in patients who drink alcohol and smoke or use smokeless tobacco.

A Indurations, or ulcerations, on the lateral surfaces of the tongue.

P Lingual cancers.

E Examination   N Normal Findings   A Abnormal Findings   P Pathophysiology

Nursing Alert

Oral Cancer Risk Factors

- Male gender
- Age >50 years
- Tobacco use (snuff, chewing tobacco, pipes, cigars, cigarettes)
- Chewing betel nut
- Excessive alcohol use
- Excessive sun exposure to the lips
- History of leukoplakia or erythroplakia

A Engorged blood vessels of the tongue.

P Hemangioma of the tongue is a benign overgrowth of vascular tissue.

A Deviation of the tongue toward one side, atrophy, and asymmetrical shape of the tongue.

P Unilateral paralysis of the tongue muscles will cause the tongue to deviate toward the affected side.

Buccal Mucosa

E 1. Ask the patient to open his or her mouth as wide as possible.

 2. Use a tongue depressor and a penlight to assess the inner cheeks and the openings of Stensen's ducts.

 3. Observe for colour, inflammation, hydration, and lesions.

N The colour of the oral mucosa on the inside of the cheek may vary according to race. Blacks have a bluish hue; Caucasians have pink mucosa. Freckle-like macules may appear on the inside of the buccal mucosa. The buccal mucosa should be moist, smooth, and free of inflammation and lesions. Some patients may have torus mandibularis, which are bony nodules in the mandibular region.

A Leathery, painless, white, painted-looking patches.

P Leukoplakia.

A The mucosa is pale.

P Anemia or vasoconstriction, such as shock.

A The mucosa is cyanotic.

P Systemic hypoxemia.

A The mucosa is erythematous.

P Stomatitis.

A There is excessive dryness of the mucosa.

P Xerostomia, which occurs when salivary gland activity is decreased or obstructed, or when the patient is hypovolemic, breathes through the mouth, or has Sjögren's syndrome.

A Flat-topped papules with thin, bluish white spider-web lines resembling leukoplakia.

P Wickham's striae are the lesions of lichen planus, which is an inflammatory and pruritic disease of the skin and mucous membranes.

Gums

E 1. Instruct the patient to open his or her mouth.

 2. Observe dentures or orthodontics for fit.

 3. Remove any dentures or removable orthodontia.

 4. Shine the penlight in the patient's mouth.

 5. Use the tongue depressor to move the tongue to visualize the gums.

 6. Observe for redness, swelling, bleeding, retraction from the teeth, or discoloration.

N In light-skinned individuals, the gums have a pale-red stippled surface. Patchy brown pigmentation may be present in dark-skinned patients. The gum margins should be well defined with no pockets existing between the gums and the teeth and no swelling or bleeding.

A The gingiva are red, tender, and swollen and bleed easily.

P Gingivitis, which may be caused by poor dental hygiene, improperly fitted dentures, and scurvy. Gingivitis can also occur with stomatitis that occurs in mouth infections and upper respiratory tract infections.

A Gingival borders are red and there is infection of the pockets formed between receding gums and teeth. Purulent drainage may be present.

P Periodontitis due to chronic gingivitis.

| E Examination | N Normal Findings | A Abnormal Findings | P Pathophysiology |

A   Blue lines are noted approximately 1 mm from the gingival margin.

P   Chronic exposure to lead or bismuth.

A   The gums are brownish.

P   Addison's disease.

A   Hypertrophy of gum.

P   Gingival hyperplasia occurs in pregnancy, in wearers of orthodontic braces, by dental plaque, or with the use of medications such as phenytoin.

Teeth

E   1. Instruct the patient to open his or her mouth.

   2. Count the upper and lower teeth.

   3. Observe the teeth for discoloration, loose or missing teeth, caries, mal-occlusion, and malformation.

N   The adult normally has 32 teeth, which should be white with smooth edges, in proper alignment, and without caries.

A   Teeth are absent.

P   Due to loss or failure of development.

A   White or black patches on the surface of a tooth.

P   Dental caries, or cavities, resulting from poor oral hygiene.

A   The teeth are worn at an angle.

P   Repetitive biting on hard substances or objects or grinding of teeth, called bruxism.

A   A tooth is dark in colour and the patient reports insensitivity to cold.

P   This is usually a dead tooth.

Palate

E   1. Ask the patient to tilt his or her head back and open the mouth as wide as possible.

   2. Shine the penlight in the patient's mouth.

   3. Observe both the hard and the soft palates.

   4. Note their shape and colour, and the presence of any lesions or mal-formations.

N   The hard and soft palates are concave and pink. The hard palate has many ridges; the soft palate is smooth. No lesions or malformations are noted.

A   The palates are red, swollen, tender, or with lesions.

P   Infection.

A   A fibrous, encapsulated tissue growth on the palate.

P   A fibroma may be idiopathic or neoplastic in origin.

A   A lesion that has become eroded on the palate.

P   Cancerous lesion in the epithelium of the hard palate.

A   The palate is highly arched.

P   Turner's syndrome, Marfan's syndrome.

A   There is a hole in the hard palate.

P   Palatine perforation is related to syphilis or radiation therapy.

Inspection of the Throat

E   1. Ask the patient to tilt his or her head back and to open the mouth widely. The patient can either stick out the tongue or leave it resting on the floor of the mouth.

   2. Use your right hand to place the tongue blade on the middle third of the tongue.

   3. With your left hand, shine a light at the back of the patient's throat.

   4. Ask the patient to say "ah."

   5. Observe the position, size, colour, and general appearance of the tonsils and uvula.

   6. Touch the posterior third of the tongue with the tongue blade.

   7. Note movement of the palate and the presence of the gag reflex.

   8. Assess the colour of the oropharynx. Note any swelling, exudate, or lesions.

N   When the patient says "ah," the soft palate and the uvula should rise symmetrically (CN IX and X). The uvula is midline. The throat is normally pink and vascular and without swelling, exudate, or lesions. The gag reflex should be present but is congenitally absent in some patients (CN IX and X).

A   The posterior pharynx is red with white patches. The tonsils are large and red with

---

E   **Examination**   N   **Normal Findings**   A   **Abnormal Findings**   P   **Pathophysiology**

white patches, and the uvula is red and swollen.

P   Viral pharyngitis and tonsillitis are common illnesses with these findings.

A   Tonsils, pillars, and uvula are very red and swollen, with patches of white or yellow exudate on the tonsils. The posterior pharynx is bright red. The patient reports soreness of the throat with swallowing.

P   Streptococcal pharyngitis; tonsillitis.

A   There is a greyish membrane covering the tonsils, uvula, and soft palate.

P   Diphtheria, acute tonsillitis, or infectious mononucleosis.

14

Breasts and Regional Nodes

ANATOMY AND PHYSIOLOGY

Breasts

The female breasts are a pair of mammary glands located on the anterior chest wall, extending vertically from the second to the sixth rib and laterally from the sternal border to the axilla. Anatomically, the breast can be divided into four quadrants: the upper inner quadrant, the lower inner quadrant, the upper outer quadrant, and the lower outer quadrant (Figure 14-1). The upper outer quadrant, which extends into the axilla, is known as the tail of Spence. The breasts are supported by a bed of muscles: the pectoralis major and minor, latissimus dorsi, serratus anterior, rectus abdominus, and external oblique muscles, which extend vertically from the deep fascia (Figure 14-2). Cooper's ligaments extend vertically from the deep fascia through the breast to the inner layer of the skin, providing support for the breast tissue (Figure 14-3).

In the centre of each breast is the nipple, a round, hairless, pigmented protrusion of erectile tissue approximately 0.5 to 1.5 cm in diameter. The 12 to 20 minute openings on the surface of the nipple consist of lactiferous ducts through which milk and colostrum are excreted.

Surrounding the nipple is the areola, a pigmented area approximately 2.5 to 10 cm in diameter, with hair follicles punctuating the border. Several sebaceous glands (Montgomery's

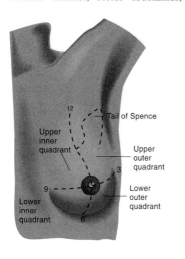

FIGURE 14-1 Quadrants of the Left Breast.

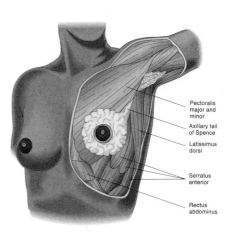

FIGURE 14-2 Muscles Supporting the Breast.

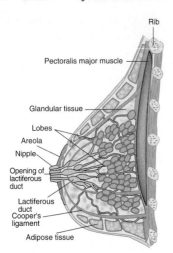

FIGURE 14-3 Cross Section of the Left Breast.

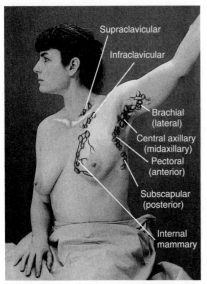

FIGURE 14-4 Regional Lymphatics and Drainage Patterns of the Left Breast.

tubercles) that are present on the surface of the areola lubricate the nipple, helping to keep it supple during lactation.

The breast is composed of glandular, connective (Cooper's ligaments), and adipose tissue. Glandular tissue is arranged radially in the form of 12 to 20 lobes. Each lobe is composed of 20 to 40 lobules that contain milk-producing glands called alveoli or acini.

The function of the female breast is to produce milk for the nourishment and protection of neonates and infants. In many cultures, breasts provide pleasure during sexual foreplay and breastfeeding, in addition to providing some protection to the anterior thoracic chest wall.

The male breast is composed of a well-developed areola and a small nipple that has immature tissue underneath.

Regional Nodes

The lymphatic drainage of the breast is via a complex network of lymph vessels and nodes (Figure 14-4). The axillary nodes are composed of four groups: central axillary nodes (midaxillary), pectoral nodes (anterior), subscapular nodes (posterior), and brachial nodes (lateral).

Because of their superficial location, axillary nodes can be easily palpated. The internal mammary nodes, however, are very deep in the chest wall and are inaccessible by palpation.

EQUIPMENT

- Towel
- Drape
- Centimetre ruler
- Teaching aid for BSE

ASSESSMENT OF THE FEMALE BREASTS AND REGIONAL NODES

Inspection of the Breasts

E 1. Position the patient uncovered to the waist, seated at the edge of the examination table, and facing you.
   2. Instruct the patient to let her arms relax by her sides (Figure 14-5).
   3. Inspect the breasts, axillae, areolar areas, and nipples for colour, vascularity, thickening, edema, size, symmetry, contour, lesions or masses, and exudates.
   4. Repeat the above inspection sequence with the patient's arms raised over her head (Figure 14-6). This will

| E Examination | N Normal Findings | A Abnormal Findings | P Pathophysiology |

HEALTH HISTORY

Medical History
Benign breast disease, cysts, fibroadenomas, intraductal papillomas, mammary duct ectasia, mastitis, areas of greater density, breast cancer, masses, breast abscess, Paget's disease

Surgical History
Breast biopsy, lumpectomy, quadrantectomy, partial mastectomy, radical mastectomy, breast reduction or augmentation

Medications
Oral contraceptives, chlorpromazine, alpha-methyldopa, diuretics, digitalis, steroids, and tricyclics may precipitate nipple discharge; use of hormone replacement therapy has been linked with increased incidences of breast cancer

Family Health History
8% to 20% of breast cancers are thought to have a familial link via a primary relative, for example, mother, sister, grandmother. The link is stronger if the family history includes bilateral breast cancer. *BRCA 1* or *BRCA 2* gene mutation (*BRCA 1* and *2* are defective genes associated with the development of familial breast cancer)

accentuate any retraction (tissue drawn back) if present.

5. Repeat inspection sequence with patient pressing hands into hips, which will contract the pectoral muscles (Figure 14-7). Once again, if retraction is present, it will be more pronounced with this maneuver.

6. Have the patient lean forward to allow the breasts to hang freely away from the chest wall (Figure 14-8), and repeat the inspection sequence.

Provide support to the patient as necessary.

Colour

E Inspect the breasts, areolar areas, nipples, and axillae for coloration.

N The breasts and axillae are flesh-coloured and the areolar areas and nipples are darker in pigmentation. This pigmentation is normally enhanced during pregnancy. Moles and nevi are normal variants, and terminal hair may be present on the areolar areas.

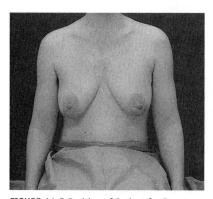

FIGURE 14-5 Position of Patient for Breast Inspection: Arms at Side.

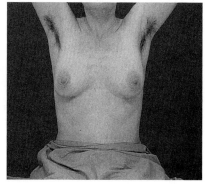

FIGURE 14-6 Position of Patient for Breast Inspection: Arms Overhead.

| E Examination | N Normal Findings | A Abnormal Findings | P Pathophysiology |

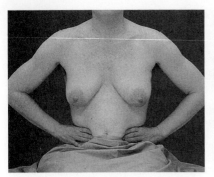

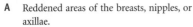

FIGURE 14-7 Position of Patient for Breast Inspection: Hands Pressed against Hips.

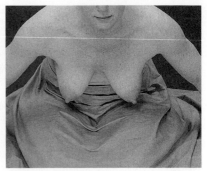

FIGURE 14-8 Position of Patient for Breast Inspection: Leaning Forward.

A Reddened areas of the breasts, nipples, or axillae.

P Inflammation, an infection such as mastitis, or inflammatory carcinoma.

A Striae are streaks over the breasts or axillae. In light-skinned individuals, new striae are red and become silver to white in coloration with age. In dark-skinned individuals, new striae are a ruddy, dark-brown colour, and older striae become lighter than the skin colour.

P Rapid stretching of the skin. Although normal in pregnancy, striae are often observed with obesity.

Vascularity

E Observe the entire surface of each breast for superficial vascular patterns.

N Normal superficial vascular patterns are diffuse and symmetrical.

A Abnormal patterns of vascularity are focal or unilateral.

P Increased blood supply may indicate tumour formation.

Thickening or Edema

E Observe the breasts, axillae, and nipples for thickening or edema.

N Normally, thickening or edema is not found in the breasts, axillae, or nipples.

A Enlarged skin pores give the appearance of an orange rind (peau d'orange).

P Obstructed lymphatic drainage due to a tumour.

Size and Symmetry

E Observe the breasts, axillae, areolar areas, and nipples for size and symmetry.

N It is not unusual for there to be some difference in the size of the breasts and areolar areas, with the breast on the side of the dominant arm being larger. Nipple inversion, which is present from puberty, is a normal variant. Nipples should point upward and laterally, or they may point outward and downward. Supernumerary nipples are a variant of normal.

A Asymmetry in the directions in which the nipples are pointed.

P Underlying invasive process.

A Significant differences in the size or symmetry of the breasts, axillae, areolar areas, or nipples.

P Tumour formation.

A Recent inversion, flattening, or depression of a nipple.

P Underlying cancer.

A Nipples that have been inverted since puberty and become broader or thicker.

P Tumour formation.

A Lack of breast tissue unilaterally.

P Trauma, mastectomy, or breast reduction.

Contour

E 1. Assess the breasts for contour.
     2. Compare the breasts to each other.

N The breast is normally convex, without flattening, retractions, or dimpling.

E **Examination**   **N** **Normal Findings**   **A** **Abnormal Findings**   **P** **Pathophysiology**

◀ NURSING CHECKLIST ▶

General Approach to Clinical Breast Examination

Prior to the assessment:

1. When possible, instruct the patient to neither use creams, lotions, or powders, nor shave her underarms 24 to 48 hours before the scheduled examination. These products may mask or alter the nature of the surface integument of the breasts, and shaving the underarms may cause folliculitis, which may result in pain upon palpation.
2. Encourage the patient to express any anxieties and concerns about the physical examination. Acknowledge anxieties and validate concerns. Many women avoid having their breasts assessed because they fear Abnormal Findings.
3. Inform the patient that the examination should not be painful but may be uncomfortable at times. This is especially true if the patient is currently experiencing menses, ovulation, or pregnancy.
4. Adopt a nonjudgmental and supportive attitude and remain sensitive to the patient's views of having her breasts touched by another person.
5. Be aware of the impact of the patient's culture on the breast examination. Women of certain cultures may not accept a male performing this assessment; even within the dominant Canadian culture, some women may feel uncomfortable with the clinical breast examination because of beliefs about the potential sexual nature of the procedure.
6. Instruct the patient to remove any jewelry that might interfere with the assessment.
7. Ensure that the room is warm enough to prevent chilling, and provide additional draping material as necessary.
8. Warm your hands with warm water or by rubbing them together prior to the assessment.
9. Ensure that privacy is maintained during the examination by providing screens, closing doors, and posting a door sign stating that an examination is in progress.

During the assessment:

1. Inform the patient of what you are going to do before you do it.
2. Use this time to educate the patient about her body.
3. Offer the patient the opportunity to ask questions about her body and sexuality.
4. Keep body areas not being assessed appropriately draped.
5. Always compare right and left breasts.
6. Wear gloves if the patient has any discharge from the breast.

After the assessment:

1. Assess whether the patient needs assistance in dressing.
2. After the patient is dressed, discuss the experience with her, invite questions and comments, listen carefully, and provide her with information regarding the examination.

A Dimpling, retractions, flattening, or other changes in breast contour.

P Suggestive of cancer; fat necrosis; and mammary duct ectasia.

E Examination   N Normal Findings   A Abnormal Findings   P Pathophysiology

TABLE 14-1	Characteristics of Common Breast Masses

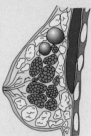 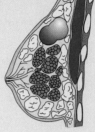 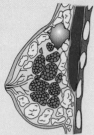

	Gross Cyst	Fibroadenoma	Carcinoma
Age	30–50; diminishes after menopause	puberty to menopause; peaks between ages 20–30	most common after 50 years
Shape	round	round, lobular, or ovoid	irregular, stellate, or crab-like
Consistency	soft to firm	usually firm	firm to hard
Discreteness	well defined	well defined	not clearly defined
Number	single or grouped	most often single	usually single
Mobility	mobile	very mobile	may be mobile or fixed to skin, underlying tissue, or chest wall
Tenderness	tender	nontender	usually nontender
Erythema	no erythema	no erythema	may be present
Retraction/ dimpling	not present	not present	often present

Lesions or Masses

E Inspect the breasts, axillae, areolar areas, and nipples for lesions or masses.

N The breasts, axillae, areolar areas, and nipples are free of masses, tumours, and primary or secondary lesions.

A Breast masses, tumours, nodules, or cysts.

P See Table 14-1 for common pathologies of breast masses.

A A scaly, eczema-like erosion of the nipple, or persistent dermatitis of the areola and nipple.

P Suggestive of Paget's disease.

Discharge

E Observe for spontaneous discharge from the nipples or other areas of the breast.

N In the nonpregnant, nonlactating female, there should be no discharge. During pregnancy and up through the first week after birth, there may be a yellow discharge known as colostrum. During lactation, there is a white discharge of breast milk.

A The presence of nipple discharge in the nonpregnant, nonlactating woman is abnormal.

P Nipple discharge may be caused by the use of medications such as tranquilizers and

E Examination	N Normal Findings	A Abnormal Findings	P Pathophysiology

Nursing Alert

Examining Nipple Discharge

If a patient is found to have abnormal nipple discharge:

1. Don gloves before proceeding with the assessment.
2. Note the colour, odour, consistency, and amount of discharge, and whether the discharge is unilateral or bilateral, and spontaneous or provoked.
3. With a sterile, cotton-tipped swab, obtain a sample of the discharge so that a culture, sensitivity, and gram stain can be obtained.
4. Consider checking the sample for occult blood.
5. Follow your institution's guidelines for sample preparation.

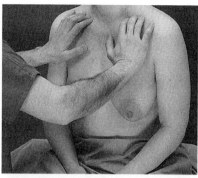

FIGURE 14-9 Palpation of Supraclavicular Nodes.

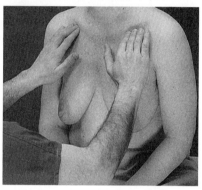

FIGURE 14-10 Palpation of Infraclavicular Nodes.

oral contraceptives, manual stimulation, pituitary tumour, or infection. It may also be indicative of malignant or benign breast disease.

Palpation

Palpation is performed in a sequential manner:

1. Supraclavicular and infraclavicular lymph node areas
2. Breasts, with the patient in sitting position
   a. Arms at sides
   b. Arms raised over head
3. Axillary lymph node regions
4. Breasts, with the patient in supine position

Supraclavicular and Infraclavicular Lymph Nodes

E   1. Have patient seated and uncovered to the waist.
   2. Encourage the patient to relax the muscles of her head and neck because this pulls the clavicles down and allows a thorough exploration of the supraclavicular area.

3. Flex the patient's head to relax the sternocleidomastoid muscle.
4. Standing in front of the patient, in a bilateral and simultaneous motion, place your finger pads over the patient's clavicles, lateral to the tendinous portion of the sternocleidomastoid muscles.
5. Using a rotary motion of the palmar surfaces of the fingers, probe deeply into the scalene triangles in order to palpate the supraclavicular lymph nodes (Figure 14-9).
6. Palpate the infraclavicular nodes using the same rotary motion of the palmar surfaces of the fingers (Figure 14-10).

N   Palpable lymph nodes less than 1 cm in diameter are usually considered normal

---

E   Examination   N   Normal Findings   A   Abnormal Findings   P   Pathophysiology

Nursing Alert

Risk factors for breast cancer in women

There is no single cause of breast cancer but some factors appear to increase the risk of developing it.[1,2]

Factors consistently found to increase risk

- Being overweight or obese (only after menopause), based on BMI
- Taking hormone replacement therapy (estrogen plus progestin for more than 5 years)
- Exposure of the breasts to high levels of ionization radiation (e.g., X-rays) or lower levels before age 2
- Having a first baby after age 30 or never having a baby
- Never breastfeeding
- Having a close relative(s) with breast cancer (especially in a mother, sister, or daughter diagnosed before menopause or if the *BRCA 1* or *BRCA 2* genes are present)
- Age (breast cancer can occur in women of any age but increases with age, especially after 50)
- Early menstruation (before the age of 12); late menopause (after age 55)
- Significant mammographic breast density (this indicates greater amount of glandular tissue)

Factors less consistently found to increase breast cancer risk

- Drinking alcohol
- Being physically inactive
- Smoking tobacco
- Taking birth control pills appears to slightly increase a woman's risk of breast cancer, though the risk of ovarian cancer is decreased.

and clinically insignificant provided that there are no additional enlarged lymph nodes found in other regions such as the axilla. Palpation should not elicit pain.

A Fixed, firm, immobile, irregular lymph nodes more than 1 cm in diameter.

P These nodes are considered suspicious for metastasis from a variety of sources or primary lymphoma.

A Enlarged, painful, or tender nodes that are matted together.

P Systemic infection or carcinoma.

Breasts: Patient in Sitting Position

E 1. Place the patient in a sitting position with arms at her sides.
2. Stand to the patient's right side, facing the patient.
3. Using the palmar surfaces of the fingers of your dominant hand, begin the palpation at the outer quadrant of the patient's right breast.

4. Use the other hand to support the inferior aspect of the breast.
5. In small-breasted patients, the dominant hand can palpate the tissue against the chest wall, but if the breasts are pendulous, use a bimanual technique of palpation (Figure 14-11).
6. Palpate in a downward fashion, sweeping from the outer quadrants to the sternal border of each breast.
7. Repeat this sequence on the other breast.
8. Repeat the entire assessment with the patient's arms raised over her head to enhance any potential retraction.

N The consistency of the breasts is widely variable, depending on age, time in menstrual cycle, and proportion of adipose tissue. The breasts may have a nodular or granular consistency that may be enhanced prior to the onset of menses. The inferior

E **Examination**   N **Normal Findings**   A **Abnormal Findings**   P **Pathophysiology**

aspect of the breast will be somewhat firmer due to a transverse inframammary ridge. Palpation should not elicit significant tenderness, though the breasts and especially the nipples may become full and slightly tender premenstrually. Breasts that feel fluid-filled or firm throughout with accompanying inferior suture-line scars are indicative of breast augmentation.

A   Any lump, mass, thickening, or unilateral granulation that is noticeably different from the rest of the breast tissue.

P   For a description of breast masses and their pathologies, see Table 14-1.

A   Significant breast tenderness.

P   Mammary duct ectasia: benign condition in which lactiferous ducts become inflamed.

A   Erythema and swelling.

P   Mastitis usually caused by *Staphylococcus aureus*.

Axillary Lymph Node Region

E   1. Stand at the patient's right side, facing the patient.

2. Tell the patient to take a deep breath and to relax her shoulders and arms (this relaxes the areas to be palpated).

3. Using your left hand, adduct the patient's right arm so that it is close to her chest wall. This maneuver relaxes the muscles.

4. Support the patient's right arm with your left hand.

5. Using the palmar surfaces of the finger pads of your right hand, place your fingers into the apex of the axilla so that they are positioned behind the pectoral muscles.

6. Gently roll the tissue against the chest wall and axillary muscles as you work downward.

7. Locate and palpate the four axillary lymph node groups:

   a. Brachial (lateral) at the inner aspect of the upper part of the humerus, close to the axillary vein.

   b. Central axillary (midaxillary) at the thoracic wall of the axilla.

   c. Pectoral (anterior) behind the lateral edge of the pectoralis major muscle.

   d. Subscapular (posterior) at the anterior edge of the latissimus dorsi muscle.

8. Repeat this method of palpation with the patient's arm abducted—instruct the patient to remain in the same position and lift the upper arm and elbow away from her body. Support the patient's abducted arm on your left shoulder (Figure 14-12).

9. Palpate the patient's left axilla using the same technique.

N   Palpable lymph nodes less than 1 cm in diameter are usually considered normal and clinically insignificant provided that

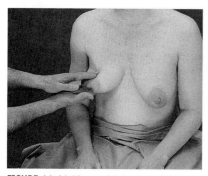

FIGURE 14-11 Bimanual Palpation of the Breasts while Patient Is Sitting.

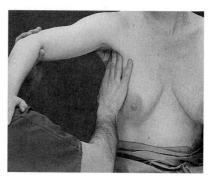

FIGURE 14-12 Palpatation of Axillary Nodes.

E **Examination**	N **Normal Findings**	A **Abnormal Findings**	P **Pathophysiology**

there are no additional enlarged lymph nodes found in other regions. Palpation should not elicit pain.

A   Fixed, firm, immobile, irregular lymph nodes more than 1 cm in diameter.

P   Suggestive of metastasis from a variety of sources or primary lymphoma.

A   Enlarged, painful, or tender nodes that are matted together.

P   Systemic infection or carcinoma.

Breasts: Patient in Supine Position

E   1. Keep the patient uncovered to the waist.

2. Instruct the patient to assume a supine position, which spreads the breast tissue thinly and evenly over the chest wall. Palpation is more accurate when there is the least amount of breast tissue between the skin and the chest wall.

3. If the breasts are large, place a small towel or folded sheet under the patient's right shoulder. This helps to flatten the breast more.

4. Stand at the patient's right side. Palpation can be performed with the patient's arms at her sides or with her right arm above her head.

5. Using the palmar surfaces of your fingers, palpate the right breast by compressing the mammary tissues gently against the chest wall. Do not press too hard; you may mistake a rib for a hard breast mass. Palpation may be performed from the periphery to the nipple, in either concentric circles, in wedge sections, or parallel lines.

6. Palpation must include the tail of Spence, periphery (Figure 14-13A), and areola (Figure 14-13B).

7. Don gloves and compress the nipple to express any discharge (Figure 14-13C). If discharge is noted, palpate the breast along the wedge radii to determine from which lobe the discharge is originating.

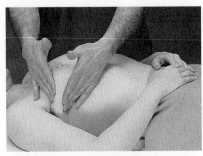

A. Palpation of the Glandular Tissue

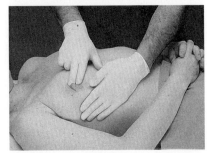

B. Palpation of the Areola

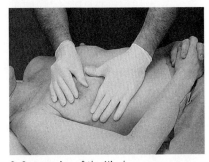

C. Compression of the Nipple

FIGURE 14-13 Palpation of the Breasts while Patient is Supine.

8. Repeat procedure on opposite breast.

N   See previous section on normal breast tissue findings upon palpation. The nipple should be elastic and return readily to its previous shape. No discharge should be expressed in the nonpregnant, nonlactating patient.

E   **Examination**   N   **Normal Findings**   A   **Abnormal Findings**   P   **Pathophysiology**

Refer to Table 14-1 for a description of breast masses. Table 14-2 offers a list of breast mass characteristics that are used to evaluate abnormal findings.

A Loss of nipple elasticity or nipple thickening.

P Tumour formation.

A Milky-white discharge in a nonpregnant, nonlactating patient.

P Nonpuerperal galactorrhea is either hormonally induced from lesions of the anterior pituitary gland or drug induced.

A Nonmilky discharge from the nipple, which may be green, brown, straw coloured, or grey.

P Benign or malignant breast disease such as duct ectasia.

A Bleeding from the nipple.

P Intraductal papilloma.

TABLE 14-2	Evaluation of Breast Mass Characteristics

If a mass is noted during palpation, the following information should be obtained regarding the mass.

Location

Identify the quadrant involved or visualize the breast with the face of a clock superimposed upon it. The nipple represents the centre of the clock. Note where the mass lies in relation to the nipple, for example, "3 cm from the nipple in the 3 o'clock position."

Size

Determine size in centimetres in all three planes (height, width, and depth).

Shape

Masses may be round, ovoid, matted, or irregular.

Number

Note if mass is singular or multiple. Note if one or both breasts are involved.

Consistency

Masses may be firm, hard, soft, fluid, or cystic.

Definition

Note if the mass borders are discrete or irregular.

Mobility

Determine if the mass is fixed or freely movable in relation to the chest wall.

Tenderness

Note if palpation elicits pain.

Erythema

Note any redness over involved area.

Dimpling or Retraction

Observe for dimpling or retraction as the patient raises arms overhead and presses her hands into her hips.

Lymphadenopathy

Note if the mass involves any of the regional lymph nodes, and indicate whether there is associated lymphadenopathy.

E Examination **N** Normal Findings **A** Abnormal Findings **P** Pathophysiology

Nursing Tip

Breast Self-Examination—The BSE steps are provided for the women who want to learn BSE.

Teaching BSE can be quick and simple.

1. BSE should be performed once a month, 8 days following menses or on any given fixed date. Advise the patient to avoid the time when her breasts might be tender due to menstruation or ovulation. Encourage her to put the BSE on her calendar and include her significant other in the process.

2. **B** (bed): Show the patient how to palpate her breast while supine in bed using the palmar surfaces of her fingers. She should start by placing her right arm over her head and palpating the right breast with the left hand, moving in concentric circles from the periphery inward, including the periphery, tail of Spence, and areola (Figure 14-14A). Finally, instruct her to squeeze the nipple to examine for discharge. Using the reverse procedure, she should examine the other breast.

3. **S** (standing): Instruct the patient to repeat the above palpation method while standing (Figures 14-14B and 14-14C).

4. **E** (examination before a mirror): The patient should stand in front of a mirror with her arms at her sides (Figure 14-14D), then with her arms raised over her head (Figure 14-14E), and finally with her hands pressed into her hips (Figure 14-14F). She should examine her breasts for symmetry, retractions, dimpling, inverted nipples, and nipple deviation.

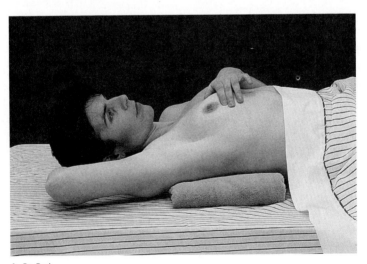

A. In Bed

FIGURE 14-14 Breast Self-Examination.

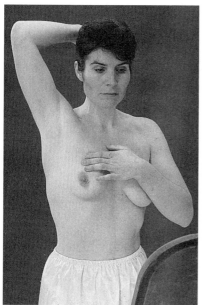

B. Standing

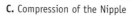

C. Compression of the Nipple

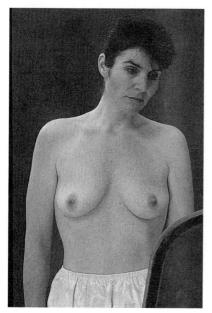

D. Before a Mirror: Arms at Side

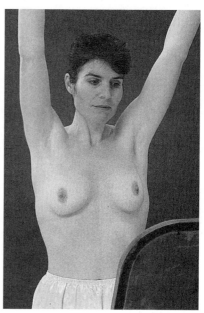

E. Before a Mirror: Arms Overhead

FIGURE 14-14 Breast Self-Examination *continues*

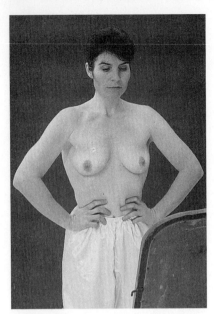

F. Before a Mirror: Hands Pressed into Hips

FIGURE 14-14 Breast Self-Examination
continues

Inspection and Palpation of the Male Breasts

Assessment of the male breasts is completed in essentially the same manner as that of the female breasts. Modify the technique for a smaller breast with less tissue bulk. Having the patient lean forward is usually not necessary unless gynecomastia is present. Males should perform a BSE every month and have clinical examinations of the breast every 1 to 3 years.

REFERENCES

[1]Canadian Cancer Society. (2006). *What causes breast cancer.* Retrieved May 27, 2006, from http://www.cancer.ca/ccs/internet/standard/ 0,3182,3172_10175_272579_langId-en, 00.html

[2]Health Canada. *Risks of developing breast cancer.* Retrieved May 27, 2006, from http://www.hc-sc.gc.ca/iyh-vsv/diseases- maladies/ breast-sein_e.html

15

Thorax and Lungs

The respiratory system extends from the nose to the alveoli (Figure 15-1). The normal air pathway is nose, pharynx, larynx, trachea, mainstem bronchus, right and left main bronchi, lobar/secondary bronchi, tertiary/segmental bronchi, terminal bronchioles, respiratory bronchioles, alveolar ducts, alveolar sacs, and alveoli.

The respiratory system is divided into the upper and lower tracts. The upper respiratory tract comprises the nose, pharynx, larynx, and the upper trachea. The nose and pharynx are discussed in Chapter 13. The lower respiratory tract is composed of the lower trachea to the lungs. This chapter deals only with those components of the respiratory system that are located in the thorax.

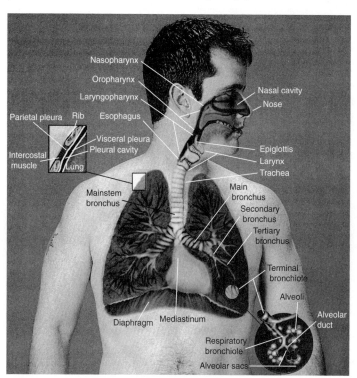

FIGURE 15-1 The Respiratory Tract.

ANATOMY

Thorax

The thorax is a cone-shaped structure (narrow at the top and wide at the bottom) that consists of bones, cartilage, and muscles. Of these, the bones are the supportive structure of the thorax. On the anterior thorax, these bones are the 12 pairs of ribs and the sternum. Posteriorly, there are the 12 thoracic vertebrae and the spinal column.

Sternum

The sternum, or breastbone, is a flat, narrow bone approximately 15 cm long. It is located at the median line of the anterior chest wall and is divided into three sections: the manubrium (the upper bone of the sternum that articulates with the clavicles and the first pair of ribs), the body, and the xiphoid process.

Ribs

The first seven pairs of ribs are articulated to the sternum via the costal cartilages and are called the vertebrosternal or true ribs. The false ribs, or rib pairs 8–10, articulate with the costal cartilages just above them. The remaining two pairs of ribs (11 and 12) are termed floating ribs and do not articulate at their anterior ends. The 10th rib is the lowest rib that can be palpated anteriorly. The 11th rib is palpated on the lateral thorax, and the 12th rib is palpated on the posterior thorax. All ribs articulate posteriorly to the vertebral column. When a rib is palpated, the costal cartilage cannot be distinguished from the rib itself (Figure 15-2).

Intercostal Spaces

Each area between the ribs is called an intercostal space (ICS). There are 11 ICSs.

Lungs

The lungs are cone-shaped organs that fill the lateral chamber of the thoracic cavity. The right lung is broader than the left lung because of the position of the heart. The right lung consists of three lobes (upper, middle, and lower), and the left lung has two lobes (upper and lower). The apex denotes the top of the lung, and the base refers to the bottom of the lung (Figure 15-3).

The lobes of the right and left lungs are divided by grooves called fissures. Figure 15-4 illustrates the right oblique (or diagonal) fissure, the right horizontal fissure, and the left oblique (or diagonal) fissure.

When assessing the thorax, it is helpful to envision it as a rectangular box, with the four sides being the anterior, posterior, right lateral, and left lateral thoraxes. Figure 15-5 illustrates the imaginary thoracic lines on each of the four sides.

Pleura

Each lung is encased in a serous sac, or pleura. The parietal pleura lines the chest wall and the superior surface of the diaphragm. The visceral pleura lines the external surface of the lungs.

Mediastinum

The mediastinum, or interpleural space, is the area between the right and left lungs. It extends from the sternum to the spinal column and

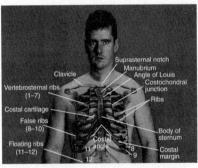

A. Anterior View

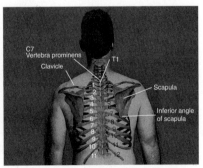

B. Posterior View

FIGURE 15-2 Thorax: Rib number is shown on the patient's right; intercostal space number is shown on the patient's left.

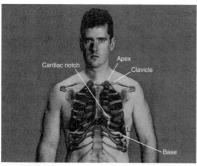
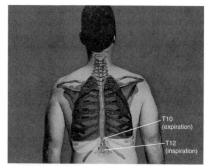

A. Anterior View

B. Posterior View

FIGURE 15-3 Lungs: RUL = Right Upper Lobe, RML = Right Middle Lobe, RLL = Right Lower Lobe, LUL = Left Upper Lobe, LLL = Left Lower Lobe.

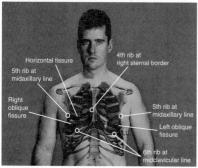
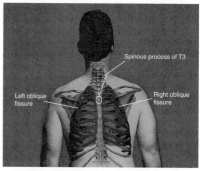

A. Anterior View

B. Posterior View

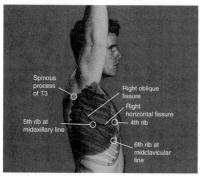
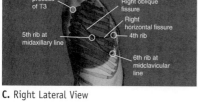
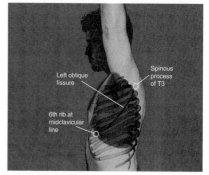

C. Right Lateral View

D. Left Lateral View

FIGURE 15-4 Lung Fissures.

contains the heart, great vessels, trachea, esophagus, and lymph vessels.

Bronchi

The trachea bifurcates into the left and right mainstem bronchi at the level of the fourth or fifth vertebral process posteriorly and the sternal angle anteriorly. The mainstem bronchi further divide into lobar or secondary bronchi. The bronchi transport gases as well as trap foreign particles in their mucus. Cilia aid in sweeping the foreign particles upward in the

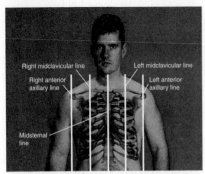

A. Anterior View

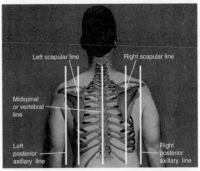

B. Posterior View

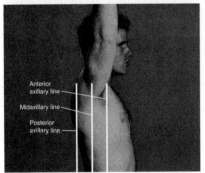

C. Right Lateral View

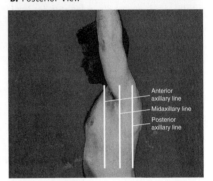

D. Left Lateral View

FIGURE 15-5 Imaginary Thoracic Lines.

respiratory tract for possible elimination. Culmination of the tracheobronchial tree is in the alveoli.

Alveoli

The alveoli are the smallest functional units of the respiratory system. It is here that gas exchange occurs.

Diaphragm

The diaphragm, which is innervated by the phrenic nerve, is a dome-shaped muscle that forms the inferior border of the thorax. The diaphragm is the principal muscle of respiration. Contraction of the diaphragm leads to an increase in volume in the thoracic cavity.

External Intercostal Muscles

The external intercostal muscles are located in the ICS. During inspiration, the external intercostal muscles elevate the ribs, thus increasing the size of the thoracic cavity. The internal intercostal muscles draw adjacent ribs together, thereby decreasing the size of the thoracic cavity during expiration.

Accessory Muscles

Accessory respiratory muscles are used to accommodate increased oxygen demand. Exercise and some diseases lead to the use of accessory muscles. The accessory muscles are the scalene, sternocleidomastoid, trapezius, and abdominal rectus.

PHYSIOLOGY

Ventilation

The primary function of the respiratory system is to deliver oxygen to the lungs and to remove carbon dioxide from the lungs. The breathing process includes inspiratory and expiratory phases. During inspiration, the pressure inside the lungs becomes subatmospheric when the

Nursing Alert

Personal Respiratory Protection (Masks) for Respiratory Infections Transmitted by Large Droplets or Contact[1]

- Suspected or possible respiratory tract infections include colds, pharyngitis, croup bronchiolitis, pneumonia and confirmed infections with adenovirus, influenza, parainfluenza virus, respiratory syncytial virus, metapneumovirus, rhinovirus, or coronavirus.
- Masks should be worn when within 1 metre of a coughing patient or when performing activities that are likely to generate splashes or sprays of blood, body fluids, or secretions.
- The patient should wear a surgical mask when not in a confined room.
- Carefully remove masks using the straps to avoid self-contamination; discard any mask that is crushed, wet, or contaminated by secretions, and wash hands after removing a mask.
- Masks should be changed if they become moist, hard to breathe in, physically damaged, or visibly soiled.
- High-risk patients should wear masks when in contact with people who have contagious diseases, and they should be tested regularly for TB.
- Disposable N95 respirators that have been fitted properly are used for airborne isolation precautions in patients with active TB or severe acute respiratory syndrome (SARS).

diaphragm and external intercostal muscles contract. The diaphragm lowers, and the ribs elevate, thus increasing the intrapulmonic volume. As a result of the negative intra-alveolar pressure, atmospheric air is pulled into the respiratory tract until intra-alveolar pressure equals atmospheric pressure. The lungs increase in size with the air.

Expiration is a passive process and occurs more rapidly than inspiration. During expiration, the diaphragm and external intercostal muscles relax, decreasing the volume of the thoracic cavity. The diaphragm rises. The intrapulmonic volume decreases and the intrapulmonic pressure increases above the atmospheric pressure. The lungs possess elastic recoil capabilities that allow air to be expelled until intrapulmonic pressure equals atmospheric pressure.

External Respiration

External respiration is the process by which gases are exchanged between the lungs and the pulmonary vasculature. Oxygen diffuses from the alveoli into the blood, and carbon dioxide diffuses from the blood to the alveoli. Diffusion is a passive process in which gases move across a membrane from an area of higher concentration to an area of lower concentration. In the lungs, the membrane is the alveolar–capillary network.

Internal Respiration

Internal respiration is the process by which gases are exchanged between the pulmonary vasculature and the body's tissues. Oxygen from the lungs diffuses from the blood into body tissue; carbon dioxide diffuses from the tissue into the

HEALTH HISTORY

Medical History	Asthma, bronchitis, croup, frequent coryza, CF, emphysema, epiglottitis, pleurisy, pneumonia, pneumothorax, pulmonary edema, pulmonary embolus, lung cancer, TB
Surgical History	Lobectomy, pneumonectomy, tracheostomy, wedge resection, bronchoscopy
Social History	**Tobacco use:** Cigarette smoking is the primary risk factor for chronic bronchitis, emphysema, and lung cancer, as well as other disorders.

continued

Social History	**Work environment:** Repeated exposure to materials in the workplace can create respiratory complications that range from minor problems to life-threatening events. Numerous categories of respiratory diseases have been identified from repeated exposure to toxic substances. These diseases are listed along with the industries and agents related to them.

Silicosis: glass making, tuning, stonecutting, mineral mining, insulation work, quarrying, cement work, ceramics, foundry work, semiconductor manufacturing

Asbestosis: mining, shipbuilding, construction

Coal worker's pneumoconiosis: coal mining

Pneumoconioses: tin and aluminum production, welding, insecticide manufacturing, rubber industry, fertilizer industry, ceramics, cosmetic industry

Occupational asthma: electroplating, grain working, woodworking, photography, printing, baking, painting

Chronic bronchitis: coal mining, welding, firefighting

Byssinosis: cotton mill dust, flax

Extrinsic allergic alveolitis (hypersensitivity pneumonia): animal hair, contamination of air conditioning or heating systems, mouldy hay, mouldy grains, mouldy dust, sugarcane

Toxic gases and fumes: welding, cigarette smoke, auto exhaust, chemical industries, firefighting, hair spray

Pulmonary neoplasms: radon gas, mustard gas, printing ink, asbestos

Pneumonitis: furniture polish, gasoline, or kerosene ingestion; mineral oil, olive oil, and milk aspiration

Home environment: Air pollution, cigarette smoke, wood-burning stoves, gas stoves and heaters, kerosene heaters, radon gas, pet hair and dander

Hobbie and leisure activities: Birds (bird breeder's lung), mushroom growers (mushroom grower's lung), scuba diving (lung rupture, oxygen toxicity, decompression sickness), high-altitude activities (skiing, climbing: pulmonary edema and pulmonary embolus)

blood. The blood is then carried back to the right side of the heart for reoxygenation.

Control of Breathing

Control of breathing is influenced by neural and chemical factors. The pons and medulla are the central nervous system structures primarily responsible for involuntary respiration. The stimulus for breathing is an increased carbon dioxide level, a decreased oxygen level, or an increased blood pH level.

EQUIPMENT

- Stethoscope
- Centimetre ruler or tape measure
- Washable marker
- Watch with second hand

◄ NURSING CHECKLIST ►

General Approach to Thorax and Lung Assessment

1. Greet the patient and explain the assessment techniques that you will be using.
2. Ensure that the examination room is at a warm, comfortable room temperature to prevent patient chilling and shivering.
3. Use a quiet room free from interruptions.
4. Ensure that the light in the room provides sufficient brightness to adequately observe the patient.
5. Instruct the patient to remove all street clothes from the waist up and to don an examination gown.
6. Place the patient in an upright sitting position on the examination table, or
6a. For patients who cannot tolerate the sitting position, rotate the supine, bedridden patient from side to side to gain access to the thorax.
7. Expose the entire area being assessed. Provide a drape that women can use to cover their breasts (if desired) when the posterior thorax is assessed.
8. When palpating, percussing, or auscultating the anterior thorax of female or obese patients, ask them to displace the breast tissue. Assessing directly over breast tissue is not an accurate indicator of underlying structures.
9. Visualize the underlying respiratory structures during the assessment process in order to accurately describe the location of any pathology.
10. Always compare the right and left sides of the anterior thorax and the posterior thorax to one another, as well as the right and left lateral thorax.
11. Use a systematic approach every time the assessment is performed. Proceed from the lung apices to the bases, right to left to lateral.

ASSESSMENT OF THE THORAX AND LUNGS

Inspection

Shape of Thorax

E 1. Stand in front of the patient.
2. Estimate visually the transverse diameter of the thorax.
3. Move to either side of the patient.
4. Estimate visually the width of the anteroposterior (AP) diameter of the thorax.
5. Compare the estimates of these two visualizations.

N In the normal adult, the ratio of the AP diameter to the transverse diameter is approximately 1:2 to 5:7. In other words, the normal adult is wider from side to

Nursing Alert

Risk Factors for Lung Cancer
- Smoking tobacco and second hand tobacco exposure
- Hereditary predisposition for some smokers
- Occupational or environmental exposure to known carcinogens (e.g., asbestos, radon, heavy metals)

side than from front to back. The normal thorax is slightly elliptical in shape. A barrel chest is normal in infants and sometimes in older adults. See Chapter 24 for a discussion of the pediatric patient.

E Examination	N Normal Findings	A Abnormal Findings	P Pathophysiology

Figure 15-6 illustrates the normal and abnormal configurations of the thorax.

A   In barrel chest, the ratio of the AP diameter to the transverse diameter is approximately 1:1. The patient's chest is circular or barrel-shaped in appearance.

P   COPD due to air trapping in the alveoli and subsequent lung hyperinflation.

A   Pectus carinatum, or pigeon chest, is a marked protrusion of the sternum.

P   Congenital anomaly; Vitamin D deficiency.

A   Pectus excavatum, or funnel chest, is a depression in the body of the sternum that can compress the heart and cause myocardial disturbances. The AP diameter of the chest decreases.

P   Congenital anomaly.

A   Kyphosis, or humpback, is an excessive convexity of the thoracic vertebrae. Gibbus kyphosis is an extreme deformity of the spine.

P   Idiopathic.

A. Normal Adult

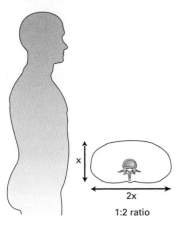

B. Barrel Chest

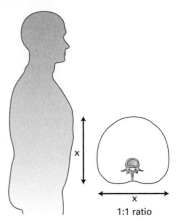

C. Pectus Carinatum

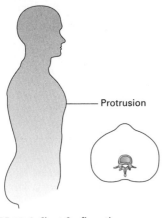

D. Pectus Excavatum

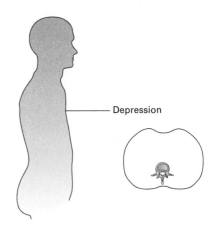

FIGURE 15-6 Chest Configurations.

E Examination	N Normal Findings	A Abnormal Findings	P Pathophysiology

A   Scoliosis is a lateral curvature of the thorax or lumbar vertebrae. See Chapter 18 for further discussion.

P   Idiopathic; neuromuscular diseases, connective tissue diseases, and osteoporosis.

Symmetry of Chest Wall

E
1. Stand in front of the patient.
2. Inspect the right and the left anterior thoraxes.
3. Note the shoulder height. Observe any differences between the two sides of the chest wall, such as the presence of masses.
4. Move behind the patient.
5. Inspect the right and the left posterior thoraxes, comparing right and left sides.
6. Note the position of the scapula.

N   The shoulders should be at the same height. Likewise, the scapula should be the same height bilaterally. There should be no masses.

A   Having one shoulder or scapula higher than the other.

P   Scoliosis.

A   Visible mass.

P   Mediastinal tumours or cysts.

Presence of Superficial Veins

E
1. Stand in front of the patient.
2. Inspect the anterior thorax for the presence of dilated superficial veins.

N   In the normal adult, dilated superficial veins are not seen.

A   Dilated superficial veins on the anterior chest wall.

P   Superior vena cava obstruction.

Costal Angle

E
1. Stand in front of the patient.
2. In a patient whose thoracic skeleton is easily viewed, visually locate the costal margins (medial borders created by the articulation of the false ribs).
3. Estimate the angle formed by the costal margins during exhalation and at rest. This is the costal angle.

4. In a heavy or obese patient, place your fingertips on the lower anterior borders of the thoracic skeleton.
5. Gently move your fingertips medially to the xiphoid process.
6. As your hands approach the midline, feel the ribs as they meet at the apex of the costal margins. Visualize the line that is created by your fingers as they move up the floating ribs toward the sternum. This is the costal angle. Approximate this angle.

N   The costal angle is less than 90° during exhalation and at rest. The costal angle widens slightly during inhalation due to the expansion of the thorax.

A   Costal angle greater than 90°.

P   Hyperinflation of the lungs (emphysema) or dilation of the bronchi (bronchiectasis).

Angle of the Ribs

E
1. Stand in front of the patient.
2. In a patient whose thoracic skeleton is easily viewed, visually locate the midsternal area.
3. Estimate the angle at which the ribs articulate with the sternum.
4. In a heavy or obese patient, place your fingertips on the midsternal area.
5. Move your fingertips along a rib laterally to the anterior axillary line. Visualize the line that is created by your hand as it traces the rib. Approximate this angle.

N   The ribs articulate at a 45° angle with the sternum.

A   An angle greater than 45°.

P   Emphysema, bronchiectasis, and CF.

Intercostal Spaces

E
1. Stand in front of the patient.
2. Inspect the ICS throughout the respiratory cycle.
3. Note any bulging of the ICS and any retractions.

N   There should be an absence of retractions and of bulging of the ICS.

A   The presence of retractions.

E Examination   N Normal Findings   A Abnormal Findings   P Pathophysiology

---

Nursing Alert

Respiratory Rate Emergencies

Extreme tachypnea (greater than 30 breaths per minute in an adult), bradypnea, and apnea are emergency conditions. Immediate intervention is necessary to prevent complications.

P Emphysema, asthma, tracheal or laryngeal obstruction, tumour.

A The presence of bulging.

P Obstruction to the free exhalation of air, such as in emphysema, asthma, an enlarged heart, aortic aneurysm, massive pleural effusion, tension pneumothorax, and tumours.

Muscles of Respiration

E 1. Stand in front of the patient.
   2. Observe the patient's breathing for a few respiratory cycles, paying close attention to the anterior thorax and the neck.
   3. Note all of the muscles that are being used by the patient.

N No accessory muscles are used in normal breathing.

A Use of accessory muscles.

P Patients experiencing hypermetabolic states such as exercise, fever, and infection, or hypoxic events such as COPD, pneumonia, pneumothorax, pulmonary edema, and pulmonary embolus.

Respirations

The inspection of the respiration process includes seven components: rate, pattern, depth, symmetry, audibility, patient position, and mode.

Rate

E 1. Stand in front of the patient or to the right side.
   2. Observe the patient's breathing without stating what you are doing—

the patient may change the respiratory rate (increase or decrease it) if aware that you are watching the chest rising and falling. This assessment can be conducted simultaneously with the pulse rate assessment.

   3. Count the number of respiratory cycles that the patient has for one full minute. A respiratory cycle consists of one inhaled and one exhaled breath.

N In the resting adult, the normal respiratory rate is 12–20 breaths per minute. This type of breathing is termed eupnea, or normal breathing.

A A respiratory rate greater than 20 breaths per minute.

P Tachypnea is present in hypermetabolic and hypoxic states. Tachypnea occurs in many disease states, such as pneumonia, bronchitis, asthma, and pneumothorax.

A A respiratory rate lower than 12 breaths per minute.

P Injury to the brain may cause bradypnea. Drug overdose (barbiturates, alcohol, and opiates).

A Apnea is the lack of spontaneous respirations for 10 or more seconds.

P Traumatic brain injury; central or obstructive sleep apnea.

Pattern (Figure 15-7)

E 1. Stand in front of the patient.
   2. While counting the respiratory rate, note the rhythm or pattern of the breathing for regularity or irregularity.

N Normal respirations are regular and even in rhythm.

A Cheyne-Stokes respirations occur in crescendo and decrescendo patterns interspersed between periods of apnea that can last 15–30 seconds (a normal finding in elderly patients and in young children).

P Central cerebral or high brain-stem lesions; sleep.

A Biot respirations, or ataxic respirations, is an example of an irregularly irregular respiratory pattern; deep and shallow

---

E **Examination** N **Normal Findings** A **Abnormal Findings** P **Pathophysiology**

1. Eupnea   (normal)
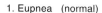
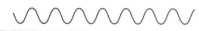

2. Tachypnea

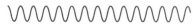

3. Bradypnea

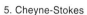

4. Apnea
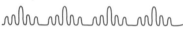

5. Cheyne-Stokes
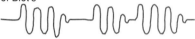

6. Biot's
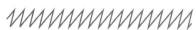

7. Apneustic

8. Agonal

9. Shallow

10. Hyperpnea
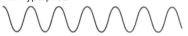

11. Air trapping
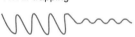

12. Kussmaul's
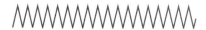

13. Sighing
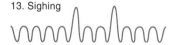

FIGURE 15-7 Respiratory Patterns.

breaths occur at random intervals interspersed with short and long pauses. Periods of apnea can be long and frequent.

P Damage to the medulla.

A Apneustic respirations are characterized by a prolonged gasping during inspiration followed by a very short, inefficient expiration (pauses can last 30–60 seconds).

P Injury to the upper portion of the pons.

A Agonal respirations are irregularly irregular respirations. They are of varying depths and patterns.

P Impending death, where there is little or no oxygen supplying the brain, or compression of the respiratory centre.

Depth

E 1. Stand in front of the patient.
2. Observe the relative depth with which the patient draws a breath during inspiration.

N The normal depth of inspiration is nonexaggerated and effortless.

A In hypoventilation, or shallow respirations, the chest wall is moved minimally during inspiration and expiration.

P Obesity, pain or recent abdominal or thoracic incision (due to the discomfort of moving the rib cage); pulmonary embolus, pneumonia, pneumothorax.

E   Examination   N   Normal Findings   A   Abnormal Findings   P   Pathophysiology

A   Hyperpnea is a breath that is greater in volume than the resting tidal volume. The respiratory rate is normal and the pattern is even.

P   Warm-up and cool-down periods of exercise; highly emotional states; high-altitude.

A   Air trapping with rapid, shallow respirations and forced expirations.

A   COPD; acute asthmatic attack.

A   Kussmaul's respirations: extreme increased depth and rate of respirations. These respirations are regular and the inspiratory and expiratory processes are both active.

P   Diabetic ketoacidosis, metabolic acidosis.

A   Sighing: normal respirations interrupted by a deep inspiration and followed by a deep expiration.

P   Central nervous system lesions.

Symmetry

E   1. Stand in front of the patient.
2. Observe the symmetry with which the chest rises and falls during the respiratory cycle.

N   The healthy adult's thorax rises and falls in unison in the respiratory cycle. There is no paradoxical movement.

A   Unilateral expansion of either side of the thorax.

P   Conditions in which the lung is absent or collapsed (pneumonectomy, pneumothorax); pulmonary fibrosis; acute pleurisy and massive atelectasis.

A   Paradoxical, or seemingly contradictory, chest wall movement.

P   Flail chest; broken ribs from trauma to the chest wall.

Audibility

E   1. Stand in front of the patient.
2. Listen for the audibility of the respirations.

N   A patient's respirations are normally heard by the unaided ear a few centimetres from the patient's nose or mouth.

A   Audible breathing when standing a few feet from the patient.

P   Any condition where air hunger exists (exercise, COPD, pneumonia, pneumothorax).

Patient Position

E   1. Ask the patient to sit upright for the respiratory assessment.
2. View the patient either before or after the assessment and note the assumed position for breathing. Ask if the assumed position is required for respiratory comfort.
3. Note if the patient can breathe normally when in a supine position.
4. Note if pillows are used to prop the patient upright to facilitate breathing.

N   The healthy adult breathes comfortably in a supine, prone, or upright position.

A   Orthopnea is difficulty breathing in positions other than upright.

P   COPD, congestive heart failure, and pulmonary edema.

Mode of Breathing

E   1. Stand in front of the patient.
2. Note whether the patient is using the nose, the mouth, or both, to breathe.
3. Note for which part of the respiratory cycle each is used.

N   Normal findings vary among individuals but generally, most patients inhale and exhale through the nose.

A   Continuous mouth breathing.

P   Any type of nasal or sinus blockage.

A   Pursed-lip breathing to prolong the expiration phase of the respiratory cycle.

P   COPD.

Sputum

E   1. Ask the patient to expectorate a sputum sample.
2. If the patient is unable to expectorate, ask the patient for a recent sputum sample from a handkerchief or tissue.
3. Note the colour, odour, amount, and consistency of the sputum.

N   A small amount of sputum is normal in every individual. The colour is light yellow or clear. Normal sputum is odourless. Depending on the hydration status of the patient, the sputum can be thick or thin.

| E | **Examination** | N | **Normal Findings** | A | **Abnormal Findings** | P | **Pathophysiology** |

A Colours of sputum that are abnormal are mucoid, yellow or green, rust or blood tinged, black, and pink (and frothy).

P Table 15-1 lists the pathologies that are associated with different colours of sputum.

A Foul-smelling sputum.

P Anaerobic infections.

A A large amount of sputum.

P Chronic bronchitis; pneumonia; pulmonary edema.

A Very thick sputum.

P Dehydration.

A Sputum has a thin consistency.

P Overhydration. In pulmonary edema, the sputum is thin, pink, and frothy.

Palpation

General Palpation

To perform anterior palpation:

E 1. Stand in front of the patient.
    2. Place the finger pads of your dominant hand on the apex of the right lung (above the clavicle).
    3. Using light palpation, assess the integument of the thorax in that area.
    4. Move the finger pads down to the clavicle and palpate.
    5. Proceed with the palpation, moving down to each rib and ICS of the right anterior thorax. Palpate any area(s) of tenderness last.
    6. Repeat the procedure on the left anterior thorax.

To perform posterior palpation:

E 1. Stand behind the patient.

    2. Place the finger pads of the dominant hand on the apex of the right lung (approximately at the level of T1).
    3. Using light palpation, assess the integument of the thorax in that area.
    4. Move the finger pads down to the first thoracic vertebra and palpate.
    5. Proceed with the palpation, moving down to each thoracic vertebra and ICS of the right posterior thorax.
    6. Repeat the procedure on the left posterior thorax.

To perform lateral palpation:

E 1. Stand to the patient's right side.
    2. Have the patient lift his or her arms overhead.
    3. Place the finger pads of your dominant hand beneath the right axillary fold.
    4. Using light palpation, assess the integument of the thorax in that area.
    5. Move the finger pads down to the first rib beneath the axillary fold.
    6. Proceed with the palpation, moving down to each rib and ICS of the right lateral thorax.
    7. Move to the patient's left side.
    8. Repeat steps 2–6 for the left lateral thorax.

Pulsations

N No pulsations should be present.

A The presence of pulsations on the thorax.

P Thoracic aortic aneurysm.

Masses

N No masses should be present.

TABLE 15-1	Pathologies Associated with Different Colours of Sputum	
SPUTUM COLOUR	**PATHOLOGY**	
Mucoid	Tracheobronchitis, asthma, coryza	
Yellow or green	Bacterial infection	
Rust or blood tinged	Pneumococcal pneumonia, pulmonary infarction, TB, lung cancer	
Black	Black lung disease	
Pink	Pulmonary edema	

E Examination   N Normal Findings   A Abnormal Findings   P Pathophysiology

A Thoracic mass.

P Thoracic tumour or cyst.

Thoracic Tenderness

N No thoracic tenderness should be present.

A Thoracic tenderness.

P Fractured ribs, infection, contusion from trauma.

Crepitus

N Crepitus should be absent.

A Fine beads of air escape the lung and are trapped in the subcutaneous tissue. As this area is palpated, a crackling sound may be heard. Crepitus is usually felt earliest in the clavicular region, but it can easily be found in the neck, face, and torso.

P Any condition that interrupts the integrity of the pleura and the lungs (pneumothorax, chest trauma, thoracic surgery, mediastinal emphysema, alveolar rupture, tearing of pleural adhesions).

Thoracic Expansion

Thoracic expansion assesses the extent of chest expansion and the symmetry of chest wall expansion. Anterior and posterior thoracic expansions can be assessed (Figure 15-8).

To perform anterior thoracic expansion:

E 1. Stand directly in front of the patient. Place the thumbs of both hands on the costal margins and pointing toward the xiphoid process. Gather a small fold of skin between your thumbs to help you see the results of this technique.

2. Lay your outstretched palms on the anterolateral thorax.

3. Instruct the patient to take a deep breath.

4. Observe the movement of your thumbs, both in direction and in distance.

5. Ask the patient to exhale.

6. Observe the movement of your thumbs as they return to the midline.

To perform posterior thoracic expansion:

E 1. Stand directly behind the patient. Place the thumbs of both hands at the level of the 10th spinal vertebra,

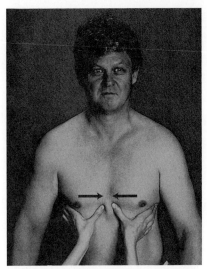

A. Anterior

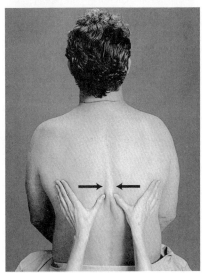

B. Posterior

FIGURE 15-8 Thoracic Expansion.

equidistant from the spinal column and approximately 2.5–7.5 cm apart. Gather a small amount of skin between your thumbs as directed for the anterior expansion.

E Examination **N** Normal Findings **A** Abnormal Findings **P** Pathophysiology

2. Place your outstretched palms on the posterolateral thorax.
3. Instruct the patient to take a deep breath.
4. Observe the movement of your thumbs, both in direction and in distance.
5. Ask the patient to exhale.
6. Observe the movement of your thumbs as they return to the midline.

N The thumbs separate an equal amount from the spinal column or xiphoid process (distance) and remain in the same plane of the 10th spinous vertebra or costal margin (direction). The normal distance for the thumbs to separate during thoracic expansion is 3–5 cm.

A Unilateral decreased thoracic expansion.

P Pneumothorax, pneumonia, atelectasis, lower lobe lobectomy, pleural effusion, bronchiectasis. In these conditions, the alveoli are either not present or not fully expanding on the affected side due to pathology inside or external to the lung.

A Bilateral decreased thoracic expansion.

P Bilateral disease external or internal to the lungs (hypoventilation, emphysema, pulmonary fibrosis, pleurisy).

A Displacement of thumbs from the 10th spinal vertebra region (thumbs will not meet in the midline when the patient exhales).

P Scoliosis.

Tactile Fremitus

Tactile or vocal fremitus is the palpable vibration of the chest wall that is produced by the spoken word and is useful in assessing the underlying lung tissue and pleura.

E
1. Firmly place the ulnar aspect of your open hand (or palmar base of the fingers or ulnar aspect of a closed fist) on the patient's right anterior apex (remember that this is above the clavicle).
2. Instruct the patient to say the words "99" or "1, 2, 3" with the same intensity every time you place your hand on the thorax.
3. Feel any vibration on the ulnar aspect of the hand as the patient

phonates. If no fremitus is palpated, ask the patient to speak more loudly.
4. Move your hand to the same location on the left anterior thorax.
5. Repeat steps 2 and 3.
6. Compare the vibrations palpated on the right and left apices.
7. Move your hand down 5–7.5 cm and repeat the process on the right and then on the left. Ensure that your hand is in the ICS in order to avoid the bony structures. Minimal or no fremitus will be felt over the ribs because they lie on top of the lungs.
8. Continue this process down the anterior thorax to the base of the lungs.
9. Repeat this procedure for the lateral chest wall and compare symmetry. Either do the entire right then the entire left thorax, or alternate right and left at each ICS.
10. Repeat this procedure for the posterior chest wall. Figure 15-9 illustrates the progression of the assessment.

N Normal fremitus is felt as a buzzing on the ulnar aspect of the hand. The fremitus will be more pronounced near the major bronchi (second ICS anteriorly, and T1 and T2 posteriorly) and the trachea, and will be less palpable in the periphery of the lung.

A Increased tactile fremitus.

P Diseases that involve consolidation (pneumonia, atelectasis, bronchitis) because solids conduct sound better than does air.

A Decreased or absent tactile fremitus.

P Pneumothorax, emphysema, asthma; pleural effusion (exudate is external to the alveoli and therefore acts as a blockade); large chest wall (obese patient).

Tracheal Position

To assess the position of the trachea:

E
1. Place the finger pad of your index finger on the patient's trachea in the suprasternal notch.
2. Move the finger pad laterally to the right and gently move the trachea in the space created by the border

---

E **Examination**   N **Normal Findings**   A **Abnormal Findings**   P **Pathophysiology**

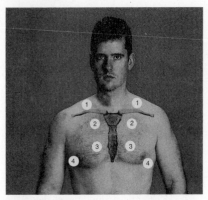

A. Anterior View

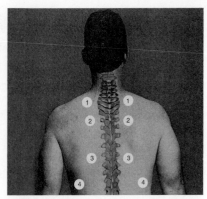

B. Posterior View

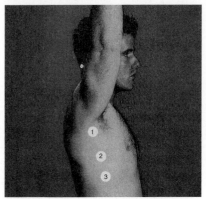

C. Right Lateral View

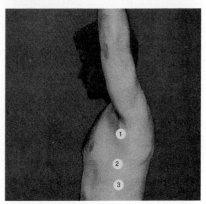

D. Left Lateral Thorax

FIGURE 15-9 Pattern for Tactile Fremitus.

of the inner aspect of the sterno-cleidomastoid muscle and the clavicle.

3. Move the finger pad laterally to the left and repeat the procedure.

The trachea can also be palpated by:

E 1. Gently placing the finger pad of your index finger in the midline of the suprasternal notch.

2. Palpate for the position of the trachea.

N The trachea is midline in the suprasternal notch.

A Tracheal deviation to the affected side.

P In atelectasis and pneumonia, alveoli are closed to some degree or filled with exudate. The trachea is slightly pushed by the healthy lung to the affected side, which contains less air.

A Tracheal deviation to the unaffected side.

P Tension pneumothorax, pleural effusion, tumour; enlarged thyroid.

Percussion

Indirect or mediate percussion is used to further assess the underlying structures of the thorax. Remember that percussion reverberates a sound that is generated from structures approximately 5 cm below the chest wall. Deep pathological conditions will not be revealed during the percussion process.

E **Examination**   N **Normal Findings**   A **Abnormal Findings**   P **Pathophysiology**

General Percussion

Figure 15-10 demonstrates the percussion pattern for the anterior, posterior, right lateral, and left lateral thoraxes.

To perform anterior thoracic percussion:

E
1. Place the patient in an upright sitting position with the shoulders back.
2. Percuss two or three strikes along the right lung apex.
3. Repeat this process at the left lung apex.
4. Note the sound produced from each percussion strike and compare the sounds from each. If different sounds are produced or if the sound is not resonant, then pathology is suggested.

5. Move down approximately 5 cm, or every other ICS, and percuss in that area.
6. Percuss in the same position on the contralateral side.
7. Continue to move down until the entire lung has been percussed.

To perform posterior thoracic percussion:

E
1. Place the patient in an upright sitting position with a slight forward tilt. Have the patient bend the head down and fold the arms in front at the waist. These actions move the scapula laterally and maximize the lung area that can be percussed.
2. Percuss the right lung apex located along the top of the shoulder.

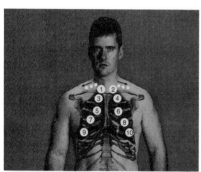

A. Anterior Thorax

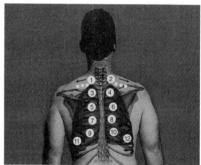

B. Posterior Thorax

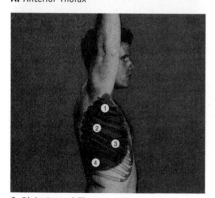

C. Right Lateral Thorax

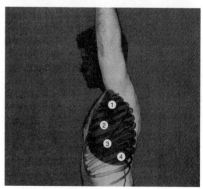

D. Left Lateral Thorax

FIGURE 15-10 Percussion Patterns.

E **Examination**   N **Normal Findings**   A **Abnormal Findings**   P **Pathophysiology**

Approximately three percussion strikes should be struck along this area.

3. Repeat the process on the left lung apex.

4. Note the sound produced from each percussion strike and compare the sounds from each. If different sounds are produced or if the sound is not resonant, then pathology is suggested.

5. Move down approximately 5 cm, or every other ICS, and percuss in that area.

6. Percuss in the same position on the contralateral side.

7. Continue to move down the thorax until the entire posterior lung field has been percussed.

To perform lateral thoracic percussion:

E   1. Place the patient in an upright sitting position, with arms raised directly overhead. This position allows for the greatest exposure of the thorax.

2. Either percuss the entire right lateral thorax and then the entire left lateral thorax, or alternate right and left sides. Start to percuss in the ICS directly below the axilla.

3. Note the sound produced from that strike.

4. Percuss approximately 5 cm below the original location, or about every other ICS.

5. Percuss down to the base of the lung.

N   Normal lung tissue produces a resonant sound. The diaphragm and the cardiac silhouette emit dull sounds. Rib sounds are flat. Hyperresonance is normal in thin adults and in patients with decreased musculature.

A   Hyperresonance.

P   Air-filled spaces (pneumothorax, emphysema, asthma, emphysematous bulla).

A   Dullness.

P   Solid or fluid-filled structures, pneumonia, atelectasis, pulmonary edema, pleural effusion, pulmonary fibrosis, hemothorax, empyema, tumours).

Diaphragmatic Excursion

Diaphragmatic excursion provides information on the patient's depth of ventilation by measuring the distance the diaphragm moves during inspiration and expiration.

To evaluate diaphragmatic excursion:

E   1. Position the patient for posterior thoracic percussion.

2. With the patient breathing normally, percuss the right lung from the apex (resonance in healthy adults) to below the diaphragm (dull). Note the level at which the percussion note changes quality to orient your assessment to the patient's percussion sounds. If full posterior thoracic percussion has already been performed, then this step can be eliminated.

3. Instruct the patient to inhale as deeply as possible and hold that breath.

4. With the patient holding the breath, percuss the right lung in the scapular line from below the scapula to the location where resonance changes to dullness.

5. Mark this location and tell the patient to exhale and breathe normally.

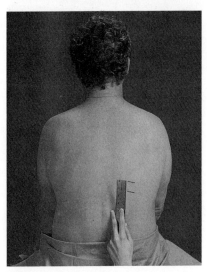

FIGURE 15-11 Diaphragmatic Excursion.

| E Examination | N Normal Findings | A Abnormal Findings | P Pathophysiology |

6. When the patient has recovered, instruct the patient to inhale as deeply as possible, exhale fully, and hold the exhaled breath.

7. Repercuss the right lung below the scapula in the scapular line in a caudal direction. Mark the spot where resonance changes to dullness.

8. Measure the distance between the two marks.

9. Repeat steps 1–8 for the left posterior thorax.

N The measured distance for diaphragmatic excursion is normally 3–5 cm. The level of the diaphragm on inspiration is T12, and T10 on expiration. The right side of the diaphragm is usually slightly higher than the left.

A A diaphragmatic excursion that is less than 3 cm.

P Conditions involving hypoventilation (pain, obesity, lung congestion, emphysema, asthma, pleurisy).

A A high diaphragm level.

P Lower lobe lobectomy, pneumonectomy (paralyzed diaphragm will move upward), space-occupying states such as ascites and pregnancy, atelectasis, pleural effusion in a lower lobe.

Auscultation

General Auscultation

To perform anterior thoracic auscultation:

E 1. Place the patient in an upright sitting position with the shoulders back.

2. Instruct the patient to breathe only through the mouth and inhale and exhale deeply and slowly.

3. Place the stethoscope on the apex of the right lung and listen for one complete respiratory cycle (one inhalation and one exhalation).

4. Note the sound that is auscultated.

5. Repeat on the left apex.

6. Note the breath sound auscultated in each area and compare one side to the other.

7. Continue to move the stethoscope down approximately 5 cm, or every other ICS, comparing contralateral sides.

To perform posterior thoracic auscultation:

E 1. Place the patient in an upright sitting position with a slight forward tilt, head bent down, and arms folded in front at the waist. These actions move the scapula laterally and maximize the lung area that can be auscultated.

2. Place the stethoscope firmly on the patient's right lung apex. Ask the patient to inhale and exhale deeply and slowly every time the stethoscope is felt on the back.

3. Repeat this process on the left lung apex.

4. Move the stethoscope down approximately 5 cm, or every other ICS, and auscultate in that area.

5. Auscultate in the same position on the contralateral side.

6. Continue to move inferiorly until the entire posterior lung has been assessed.

To perform lateral thoracic auscultation:

E 1. Place the patient in an upright sitting position with the hands and arms directly overhead.

2. Auscultate the entire right thorax first, then the entire left thorax, or auscultate the right and left lateral thoraxes by comparing side to side. The stethoscope should initially be placed in the ICS directly below the axilla.

3. Instruct the patient to breathe only through the mouth. Have the patient inhale and exhale deeply and slowly every time the stethoscope is felt on the lateral thorax.

4. Note the sound that is auscultated and continue to move the stethoscope inferiorly approximately every 5 cm, or every other ICS, until the entire thorax has been auscultated.

E Examination **N** Normal Findings **A** Abnormal Findings **P** Pathophysiology

Breath Sounds

N   Air rushing through the respiratory tract during inspiration and expiration generates different breath sounds in the normal patient. There are three distinct types of normal breath sounds (Table 15-2):
1. Bronchial (or tubular)
2. Bronchovesicular
3. Vesicular

Breath sounds that are not normal can be classified as either abnormal or adventitious breath sounds. Abnormal breath sounds are characterized by decreased or absent breath sounds. Adventitious breath sounds are superimposed sounds on the normal bronchial, bronchovesicular, and vesicular breath sounds. There are six adventitious breath sounds:

1. Fine crackle
2. Coarse crackle
3. Sonorous wheeze
4. Sibilant wheeze
5. Pleural friction rub
6. Stridor

Table 15-3 depicts general characteristics of adventitious breath sounds.

A   Decreased breath sounds.
P   A large chest, emphysema (due to the inability to inhale and exhale deeply), bronchial obstruction, atelectasis.
A   Absent breath sounds.
P   Pleural effusion, tumour, pulmonary fibrosis, empyema, hemothorax, hydrothorax, large pneumothorax, pneumonectomy, pulmonary edema, massive atelectasis, complete airway obstruction.

Voice Sounds

The assessment of voice sounds will reveal whether the lungs are filled with air or fluid, or are solid. This auscultation need be performed only if an abnormality is detected during the general auscultation, percussion, or palpation. There are three techniques by which voice sounds can be assessed:

1. Bronchophony
2. Egophony
3. Whispered pectoriloquy

Only one of these techniques needs to be performed because they all provide the same information. The voice sound findings will parallel those obtained during tactile fremitus. Thus, voice sounds will be heard loudest over the trachea and softest in the lung's periphery.

To perform bronchophony:
E   1. Position the patient for posterior, lateral, or anterior chest auscultation. The area to be auscultated will be that in which an abnormality was found during percussion or palpation or in which adventitious breath sounds were heard.
   2. Place the stethoscope in the appropriate location on the patient's chest.
   3. Instruct the patient to say the words "99" or "1, 2, 3" every time the stethoscope is placed on the chest or when told to do so.
   4. Auscultate the transmission of the patient's spoken word.

To perform egophony:
E   1. Repeat steps 1 and 2 from the bronchophony procedure.
   2. Instruct the patient to say the sound "ee" every time the stethoscope is placed on the chest or when told to do so.
   3. Auscultate the transmission of the patient's spoken word.

To perform whispered pectoriloquy:
E   1. Repeat steps 1 and 2 from the bronchophony procedure.
   2. Instruct the patient to whisper the words "99" or "1, 2, 3" every time the stethoscope is placed on the chest or when told to do so.
   3. Auscultate the transmission of the patient's spoken word.

N   The normal finding when performing tests for bronchophony, egophony, and whispered pectoriloquy is an unclear transmission or muffled sounds.
A   Positive (or present) voice sounds are: Bronchophony: clear transmission of "99" or "1, 2, 3" with increased intensity.

| E **Examination**   N **Normal Findings**   A **Abnormal Findings**   P **Pathophysiology** |

TABLE 15-2   Characteristics of Normal Breath Sounds

BREATH SOUND	PITCH	INTENSITY	QUALITY	RELATIVE DURATION OF INSPIRATORY AND EXPIRATORY PHASES	LOCATION
Bronchial	High	Loud	Blowing or hollow	I < E	Trachea
Bronchovesicular	Moderate	Moderate	Combination of bronchial and vesicular	I = E	Between scapulae, first and second ICS lateral to the sternum
Vesicular	Low	Soft	Gentle rustling or breezy	I > E	Peripheral lung

TABLE 15-3   Characteristics of Adventitious Breath Sounds

BREATH SOUND	RESPIRATORY PHASE	TIMING	DESCRIPTION	CLEAR WITH COUGH	ETIOLOGY	CONDITIONS
Fine crackle (rale)	Predominantly inspiration	Discontinuous	Dry, high-pitched crackling, popping, short duration; roll hair near ears between your fingers to simulate this sound	No	Air passing through moisture in small airways that suddenly reinflate	COPD, congestive heart failure (CHF), pneumonia, pulmonary fibrosis, atelectasis
Coarse crackle (coarse rale)	Predominantly inspiration	Discontinuous	Moist, low-pitched crackling, gurgling; long duration	Possibly	Air passing through moisture in large airways that suddenly reinflate	Pneumonia, pulmonary edema, bronchitis, atelectasis
Sonorous wheeze (rhonchi)	Predominantly expiration	Continuous	Low pitched; snoring	Possibly	Narrowing of large airways or obstruction of bronchus	Asthma, bronchitis, airway edema, tumour, bronchiolar spasm, foreign body obstruction
Sibilant wheeze (wheeze)	Predominantly expiration	Continuous	High pitched; musical	Possibly	Narrowing of large airways or obstruction of bronchus	Asthma, chronic bronchitis, emphysema, tumour, foreign body obstruction
Pleural friction rub	Inspiration and expiration	Continuous	Creaking, grating	No	Inflamed parietal and visceral pleura; can occasionally be felt on thoracic wall as two pieces of dry leather rubbing against each other	Pleurisy, tuberculosis, pulmonary infarction, pneumonia, lung abscess
Stridor	Predominantly inspiration	Continuous	Crowing	No	Partial obstruction of the larynx, trachea	Croup, foreign body obstruction, large airway tumour

Egophony: transformation of "ee" to "ay" with increased intensity; the voice has a nasal or bleating quality.

Whispered pectoriloquy: clear transmission of "99" or "1, 2, 3" with increased intensity.

P Any type of consolidation process, such as pneumonia.

A Voice sounds are absent or even more decreased than in the normal lung.

P Air-filled lungs (emphysema, asthma, pneumothorax).

Figure 15-12 lists assessment findings frequently associated with common lung conditions.

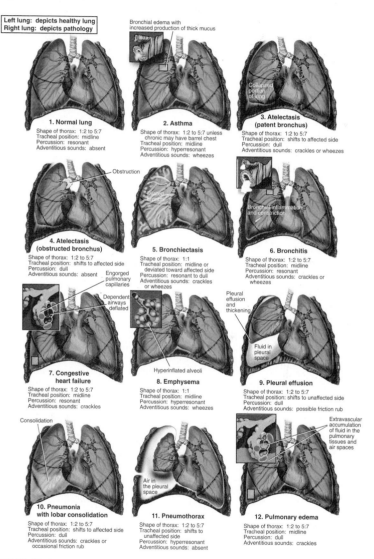

FIGURE 15-12 Comparison of Selected Respiratory Conditions.

E **Examination** N **Normal Findings** A **Abnormal Findings** P **Pathophysiology**

REFERENCES

[1]Health Canada—Public Health Agency. *Infection control precautions for respiratory infections transmitted by large droplet and contact: Infection control guidelines in a nonoutbreak setting.* Retrieved October 19, 2006, from http://www.phac-aspc.gc.ca/ sars-sras/pdf/sars-icg-nonoutbreak_e.pdf

16

Heart and Peripheral Vasculature

The heart is located in the thoracic cavity between the lungs and above the diaphragm in an area known as the mediastinum (Figure 16-1). The base of the heart is the uppermost portion, which includes the left and right atria as well as the aorta, pulmonary arteries, and the superior and inferior venae cavae. These structures lie behind the upper portion of the sternum. The apex, or lower portion of the heart, extends into the left thoracic cavity, causing the heart to appear as if it is lying on its right ventricle.

The heart is divided into four chambers: the right and left atria and the right and left ventricles.

The atrioventricular (A-V) valve between the right atrium and the right ventricle is known as the tricuspid valve; the A-V valve between the left atrium and the left ventricle is the bicuspid valve.

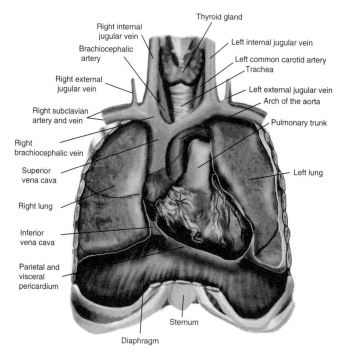

FIGURE 16-1 Position of the Heart in the Thoracic Cavity.

Anterior Aspect   Inferior Aspect

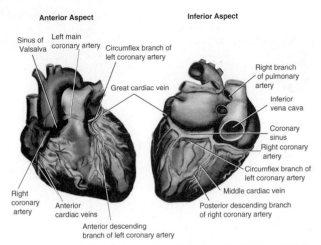

FIGURE 16-2 The Coronary Arteries and Major Veins of the Heart (Anterior and Inferior Views).

Blood flows from the right ventricle to the pulmonary vasculature for oxygenation by way of the pulmonic valve. Blood is pumped from the left ventricle into the systemic and coronary circulation through the aortic valve.

The myocardium is extremely dependent on a constant supply of oxygen that is delivered through the coronary arterial system (Figure 16-2). If the coronary blood supply is not sufficient to meet the needs of the heart, the result may be ischemia (local and temporary lack of blood supply to the heart), injury (beyond ischemia but still reversible), or an infarction (necrosis) of the heart muscle itself. Myocardial ischemia is often manifested as chest, neck, or arm pain known as angina pectoris.

The left main coronary artery branches into the left circumflex coronary artery and the left anterior descending (LAD) coronary artery.

The LAD supplies blood to the anterior wall and apex of the left ventricle as well as to the anterior portion of the interventricular septum. The smaller arterial branches that supply the septum also nourish the ventricular conduction system, including the bundle of His and the right and left bundle branches. The left circumflex (LCX) branch supplies arterial blood to the left atrium and to the lateral and posterior portions of the left ventricle. In some individuals, the sinoatrial (S-A) node and the A-V node are also supplied by this branch.

The right coronary artery (RCA) supplies nutrients and oxygen to the right atrium, the right

ventricle, and the inferior wall of the left ventricle. In most individuals, the RCA supplies the S-A and the A-V nodes as well as the posterior portion of the interventricular septum.

Venous drainage from the myocardium is carried by the coronary sinus, anterior cardiac veins, and thebesian veins. About 75% of the venous blood empties into the right atrium via the coronary sinus. The thebesian veins carry only a small portion of the unoxygenated blood that is emptied directly into all four chambers of the heart.

The cardiac cycle consists of two phases: systole and diastole. In systole, the myocardial fibres contract and tighten to eject blood from the ventricles (for the purpose of this chapter, any mention of systole will mean ventricular systole unless specifically called atrial systole). Diastole is a period of relaxation and reflects the pressure remaining in the blood vessels after the heart has pumped.

The electrocardiogram (ECG) shows the P, Q, R, S, and T waves. These waves are electrical voltages produced by the heart and recorded by ECG leads placed on the body. When the atria depolarize, the P wave is produced on the ECG. During this period, the pressure in the atria exceeds that in the ventricles, thus forcing the blood from the atria into the ventricles. Approximately 0.16 seconds after the appearance of the P wave, the QRS complex on the ECG occurs as the ventricles are electrically depolarized. As the ventricles begin to repolarize, the T wave appears on the ECG. The downslope of the T wave indicates the end of ventricular repolarization and the beginning of a relaxation period. Note that the ECG contains an isoelectric line, or flat line, after the T wave, indicating a period of electrical rest.

The sinoatrial (S-A) node is the normal pacemaker of the heart. It initiates a rhythmic impulse approximately 70 times per minute. The infranodal atrial pathways conduct the impulse initiated in the S-A node to the atrioventricular (A-V) node via the myocardium of the right atrium. The A-V node has its own intrinsic rate of 40 to 60 impulses per minute. The impulse then travels very rapidly from the A-V node to the bundle branch system via the bundle of His. The bundle branch system comprises the right bundle branch (RBB) and the left bundle branch (LBB). Finally, the Purkinje fibres arising from the distal portions of the bundle branches transmit the impulse into the subendocardial layers of both ventricles.

The circulatory system consists of arterial pathways, which are the distribution routes, and venous pathways, or the collection system that returns the blood to a central pumping station, the heart. Figure 16-3 demonstrates the journey of the blood through the systemic and pulmonary circuits.

EQUIPMENT

- Stethoscope
- Sphygmomanometer
- Watch with second hand
- Tape measure

ASSESSMENT OF THE PRECORDIUM

The cardiac landmarks (Figure 16-4) are defined as follows:

1. The aortic area is the second intercostal space (ICS) to the right of the sternum.
2. The pulmonic area is the second ICS to the left of the sternum.
3. The midprecordial area, Erb's point, is located in the third ICS to the left of the sternum.

4. The tricuspid area is the fifth ICS to the left of the sternum. Other terms for this area are the right ventricular area or the septal area.
5. The mitral area is the fifth ICS at the left midclavicular line. Other terms for this area are the left ventricular area or the apical area.

These cardiac landmarks are the locations where the heart sounds are heard best, not where the valves are actually located. The mitral area correlates anatomically with the apex of the heart; the aortic and pulmonic areas correlate anatomically with the base of the heart. Assessment of the heart should proceed in an orderly fashion from the base of the heart to the apex, or from the apex of the heart to the base.

Inspection
Aortic Area

E   1. Lightly place your index finger on the angle of Louis.
   2. Move your finger laterally to the right of the sternum to the rib. This is the second rib.
   3. Move your finger down beneath the second rib to the ICS. The aortic area is located in the second ICS to the right of the sternum.
N   No pulsations should be visible.
A   Pulsation.
P   Aortic root aneurysm.

Pulmonic Area

E   1. Lightly place your index finger on the left second ICS.
   2. The pulmonic area is located at the second ICS to the left of the sternum.
N   No pulsations should be visible.
A   Pulsation or bulge.
P   Pulmonary stenosis.

Midprecordial Area

E   1. Lightly place your index finger on the left second ICS.
   2. Continue to move your finger down the left rib cage, counting the third rib and the third ICS.

E Examination   N Normal Findings   A Abnormal Findings   P Pathophysiology

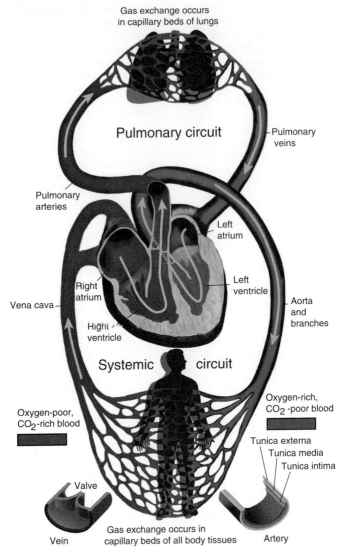

Gas exchange occurs
in capillary beds of lungs

Pulmonary circuit

Pulmonary
veins

Pulmonary
arteries

Left
atrium

Left
ventricle

Right
atrium

Vena cava

Aorta
and
branches

Right
ventricle

Systemic   circuit

Oxygen-poor,
CO_2-rich blood

Oxygen-rich,
CO_2-poor blood

Tunica externa
Tunica media
Tunica intima

Valve

Vein

Gas exchange occurs in
capillary beds of all body tissues

Artery

FIGURE 16-3 The Systemic and Pulmonary Circuits. The systemic pump consists of the left side of the heart, and the pulmonary circuit pump represents the right side of the heart.

3. The midprecordial area, or Erb's point, is located at the third ICS, left sternal border. Both aortic and pulmonic murmurs may be heard here.

A Pulsation or systolic bulge.
P Left ventricular aneurysm.
A Retraction in the midprecordial area.
P Pericardial disease.

N No pulsations should be visible.

E   Examination   N   Normal Findings   A   Abnormal Findings   P   Pathophysiology

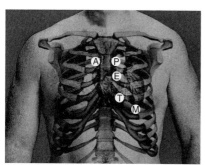

FIGURE 16-4 Figure 16-9 The Cardiac Landmarks.

A = Aortic Area; P = Pulmonic Area; E = Erb's Point; T = Tricuspid Area; M =Mitral Area

Tricuspid Area

E   1. Lightly place your index finger on the left third ICS.

2. Continue to move your finger down the left rib cage, counting the fourth rib, the fourth ICS, and the fifth rib followed by the fifth ICS.

3. The tricuspid area is located at the fifth ICS, left of the sternal border.

N   No pulsations should be visible.

A   Systolic pulsation.

P   Right ventricular enlargement secondary to increased stroke volume. Anxiety, hyperthyroidism, fever, and pregnancy produce an increased stroke volume.

Mitral Area

E   1. Lightly place your index finger on the left fifth ICS.

2. Move your finger laterally to the mid-clavicular line. This is the mitral landmark. In a large-breasted patient, have the patient displace the left breast upward and to the left so you can locate the mitral landmark.

N   Normally, there is no movement in the precordium except at the mitral area, where the left ventricle lies close enough

HEALTH HISTORY

Medical History	Abdominal aortic aneurysm (AAA), thoracic aortic aneurysm (TAA), angina, cardiogenic shock, cardiomyopathy, chest trauma, congenital anomalies, congestive heart failure (CHF), CAD, endocarditis, hyperlipoproteinemia, HTN, MI, myocarditis, pericarditis, peripheral vascular disease (PVD), rheumatic fever, valvular disease
Surgical History	Ablation of accessory pathways, aneurysm repair, cardiac catheterization, chest surgery for trauma, congenital heart repair, coronary artery bypass graft (CABG), coronary stents, directional coronary atherectomy (DCA), electrophysiology studies (EPS), heart transplant, implantable or internal cardioverter/defibrillator (ICD) placement, myotomy or myectomy, percutaneous laser myoplasty, pacemaker insertion, percutaneous transluminal coronary angioplasty (PTCA), pericardial window, pericardiectomy, pericardiotomy, peripheral vascular grafting and bypass, valve replacement
Medications	Antianginals, antidysrhythmics, anticoagulants, antihypertensives, antilipemics, diuretics, inotropics, thrombolytic enzymes, vasodilators
Communicable Diseases	Rheumatic fever (valvular dysfunction), untreated syphilis (aortic regurgitation, aortitis, and aortic aneurysm), viral myocarditis (cardiomyopathy)

continued

E	**Examination**	N	**Normal Findings**	A	**Abnormal Findings**	P	**Pathophysiology**

| Patient Classification | The Canadian Cardiovascular Society has outlined four classifications for patients with cardiac pathologies leading to angina. |

Grade I: *Ordinary physical activity does not cause angina* (walking or climbing stairs does not cause angina but strenuous or rapid or prolonged exertion does)

Grade II: *Slight limitation of ordinary activity* (angina occurs walking or stair climbing after meals, in cold, in wind, under emotional stress or only during the few hours after awakening, walking more than two blocks on a level surface or climbing more than one flight of ordinary stairs)

Grade III: *Marked limitation of ordinary activity* (angina occurs walking 1–2 blocks on a level surface or climbing one flight of stairs)

Grade IV: *Inability to carry on any physical activity without discomfort* (angina syndrome may be present at rest)

Nursing Alert

Risk Factors for Cardiovascular Disease

Unmodifiable
• Age, gender, race, family history

Modifiable
The Canadian Heart and Stroke Foundation asks that we help our patients *Know the Nine*. According to a Canadian-led global study,[1] the following nine factors collectively account for a full 90% of first heart attacks:

• cigarette smoking
• abnormal blood lipid ratios
• high blood pressure
• diabetes control
• abdominal obesity (waist circumference greater than 102 cm for men and 88 cm for women)
• stress
• lack of daily consumption of vegetables
• lack of daily consumption of fruit
• lack of daily exercise

---

to the skin's surface that it visibly pulsates during systole. The apical impulse at the mitral landmark is generally visible in about half of the adult population. This pulsation is also known as the point of maximal impulse (PMI) and occurs simultaneously with the carotid pulse.

A   Hypokinetic (decreased movement) pulsations.

P   Conditions that place more fluid between the left ventricle and the chest wall (pericardial effusion or cardiac tamponade), low output states such as shock, excess subcutaneous tissue.

A   Hyperkinetic (increased movement) pulsations.

P   High-output states such as mitral regurgitation, thyrotoxicosis, severe anemia, and left-to-right heart shunts.

Palpation

During palpation, assess for the apical impulse, pulsations, thrills (vibrations that feel similar

---

| E   Examination | N   Normal Findings | A   Abnormal Findings | P   Pathophysiology |

NURSING CHECKLIST

General Approach to Heart Assessment

1. Explain to the patient what you are going to do.
2. Ensure that the room is warm, quiet, and well lit.
3. Expose the patient's chest only as much as is needed for the assessment.
4. Position the patient in a supine or sitting position.
5. Stand to the patient's right side. The light should come from the opposite side of where you are standing so that shadows can be accentuated.

to what one feels when a hand is placed on a purring cat), and heaves (lifting of the cardiac area secondary to an increased workload and force of left ventricular contraction; also referred to as lift). The patient should be in a supine position for this portion of the assessment.

E   Palpate the cardiac landmarks for:

1. Pulsations: Using the finger pads, locate the cardiac landmark and palpate the area for pulsations.
2. Thrills: Using the palmar surface of the hand, at the base of the fingers (also known as the ball of the hand), locate the cardiac landmark and palpate the area for thrills.
3. Heaves: Follow step 2 and palpate the area for heaves.

Aortic Area

E   Palpate the aortic area for pulsations, thrills, and heaves.
N   No pulsations, thrills, or heaves should be palpated.
A   Thrill.

P   Aortic stenosis and aortic regurgitation create turbulent blood flow in the left ventricle.

Pulmonic Area

E   Palpate the pulmonic area for pulsations, thrills, and heaves.
N   No pulsations, thrills, or heaves should be palpated.
A   Thrill.
P   Pulmonic stenosis and pulmonic regurgitation create turbulent blood flow in the right ventricle.

Midprecordial Area

E   Palpate the midprecordial area for pulsations, thrills, and heaves.
N   No pulsations, thrills, or heaves should be palpated.
A   Pulsations.
P   Left ventricular aneurysm, enlarged right ventricle.

Tricuspid Area

E   Palpate the tricuspid area for pulsations, thrills, and heaves.
N   No pulsations, thrills, or heaves should be felt.
A   Thrill.
P   Tricuspid stenosis and tricuspid regurgitation.
A   Heave
P   Right ventricular enlargement (secondary to an increased workload).

Mitral Area

E   Palpate the mitral area for pulsations, thrills, and heaves. If a pulsation (apical impulse) is not palpable, turn the patient to the left side and palpate in this position. This position facilitates palpation because the heart shifts closer to the chest wall.
N   The apical impulse is palpable in approximately half of adults. It is felt as a light, localized tap that is 1 to 2 cm in diameter. The amplitude is small and it can be felt immediately after the first heart sound, lasting for about one-half of

| E **Examination** | N **Normal Findings** | A **Abnormal Findings** | P **Pathophysiology** |

◀ NURSING CHECKLIST ▶

General Approach to Heart Auscultation

1. Explain to the patient what you are going to do.
2. Expose the patient's chest only as much as is needed for the assessment. Never auscultate through any type of clothing.
3. Position the patient in a supine or sitting position. The left lateral position may be used for auscultation of the mitral and tricuspid areas. Also, the upright, leaning-forward position may be used for thorough auscultation of the aortic area.
4. Stand to the patient's right side.
5. Use the correct headpiece of the stethoscope. The diaphragm transmits high-frequency sounds whereas the bell is used for low-pitched sounds. Keep in mind when using the bell that it should rest lightly on the skin. If too much pressure is applied, the bell will act like a diaphragm.
6. Warm the headpiece in your hands prior to touching it to the patient.
7. Listen to all four of the valvular cardiac landmarks at least twice. During the first auscultation, identify S1 and S2, and then listen for a possible S3 and S4. During the second auscultation, listen for murmurs and friction rubs. As you gain expertise, you may be able to listen for S_1, S_2, S_3, S_4, murmurs, and friction rubs all at the same time.
8. Listen for at least a few cardiac cycles (10 to 15 seconds) in each area.

---

systole. This impulse may be exaggerated in young patients. A thrill is not found in the normal adult population. A heave is absent in the healthy adult.

A Thrill.

P Mitral stenosis and mitral regurgitation.

A A heave, or sustained apex beat, displaced laterally to the left sixth ICS at the anterior axillary line.

P Left ventricular hypertrophy produces a laterally displaced apical impulse because of the increased size of the left ventricle in the thorax and the subsequent shifting of the heart (aortic stenosis, systemic hypertension, and idiopathic hypertrophic subaortic stenosis).

A Hypokinetic pulsations.

P Pericardial effusion, cardiac tamponade, obesity, shock, decreased myocardial contractility.

A Hyperkinetic pulsations, usually greater than 1 to 2 cm in diameter.

P High-output states (mitral regurgitation, thyrotoxicosis, severe anemia, left-to-right heart shunts).

Auscultation

Aortic Area

E Place the diaphragm of the stethoscope on the aortic landmark and listen for S_2.

N S_2 is caused by the closure of the semilunar valves. S_2 corresponds to the "dub" sound in the phonetic "lub-dub" representation of heart sounds. S_2 heralds the onset of diastole. S_2 is louder than S_1 at this landmark.

A A greatly intensified or diminished A_2.

P Arterial hypertension, which increases the pressure in the aorta, may be suspected in the case of a greatly intensified A_2. Aortic stenosis, where the aortic

---

| E Examination | N Normal Findings | A Abnormal Findings | P Pathophysiology |

valve is calcified or thickened, may be the cause of a diminished A_2.

A Ejection click.

P Aortic stenosis (calcified valve).

Pulmonic Area

E Place the diaphragm of the stethoscope on the chest wall at the pulmonic landmark and listen for S_2.

N S_2 is heard in the pulmonic area. S_2 is louder than S_1 at this landmark. It is softer than the S_2 auscultated in the aortic area because the pressure on the left side of the heart is greater than that on the right. There is a normal physiological splitting of S_2 that is heard best at the pulmonic area. The components of a split S_2 are A_2 (aortic) and P_2 (pulmonic). The aortic component occurs slightly before the pulmonic component during inspiration. The physiology of a split S_2 is that during inspiration, because of the more negative intrathoracic pressure, the venous return to the right side of the heart increases. Thus, pulmonic closure is delayed because of the extra time needed for the increased blood volume to pass through the valve. Normally, the A_2 component of the split S_2 is louder than the P_2 component because of the greater pressures in the left side of the heart.

A When a split S_2 occurs that is abnormally wide, the aortic valve closes early and the pulmonic valve closes late. There is a split on both inspiration and expiration, but a wider split on inspiration.

P Delay in the electrical stimulation of the right ventricle.

A Fixed splitting, a wide splitting that does not change with inspiration or expiration. The pulmonic valve consistently closes later than the aortic valve.

P Right ventricular failure, atrial septal defect.

A In paradoxical splitting, the aortic valve closes after the pulmonic valve because of the delay in left ventricular systole. This occurs during expiration and disappears with inspiration.

P Left bundle branch block, aortic stenosis, patent ductus arteriosus, severe hypertension, left ventricular failure.

A Pulmonic ejection click.

P Opening of a diseased pulmonic valve.

A P_2 louder than or equal in volume to A_2.

P Pulmonary hypertension.

Midprecordial Area

Both aortic and pulmonic murmurs may be auscultated at Erb's point. Refer to the discussion on murmurs later in this chapter for additional information.

Tricuspid Area

E Place the diaphragm of the stethoscope on the chest wall at the tricuspid landmark to listen for S_1.

N S_1 in the tricuspid area is softer than the S_1 auscultated in the mitral area because the pressure in the left side of the heart is greater than that in the right. S_1 is louder than S_2 at this landmark. There is a normal physiological splitting of S_1 that is best heard in the tricuspid area. This split occurs because the mitral valve closes slightly before the tricuspid valve due to greater pressures in the left side of the heart. The components of a split S_1 are M_1 (mitral) and T_1 (tricuspid). Physiological splitting disappears when the patient holds his or her breath.

A Abnormally wide split (split is wider than usual during inspiration and is still heard on expiration).

P Electrical malfunctions (right bundle branch block), mechanical problems (mitral stenosis).

Mitral Area

E 1. Place the diaphragm of the stethoscope over the mitral area to identify S_1.

2. If you are unable to distinguish S_1 from S_2, palpate the carotid artery with the hand closest to the head while auscultating the mitral landmark. You will hear S_1 with each carotid pulse beat.

E **Examination** N **Normal Findings** A **Abnormal Findings** P **Pathophysiology**

N S_1 is heard the loudest in the mitral area. S_1 is caused by the closure of the mitral and tricuspid valves. S_1 corresponds to the "lub" sound in the phonetic "lub-dub" representation of heart sounds. S_1 is louder than S_2 at this landmark. S_1 also heralds the onset of systole. At normal or slow heart rates, systole (the time occurring between S_1 and S_2) is usually shorter than diastole. Diastole constitutes two-thirds of the cardiac cycle and systole constitutes the other third. The intensity of S_1 depends on:
1. The adequacy of the A-V cusps in halting the ventricular blood flow
2. The mobility of the cusps
3. The position of the cusps and the rate of ventricular contraction

A An abnormally loud S_1.

P Mitral stenosis, short PR interval syndrome (0.11 to 0.13 second), high-output states such as tachycardia, hyperthyroidism, and exercise.

A A soft S_1.

P Rheumatic fever, where the mitral valve has only limited motion.

A A variable abnormal S_1.

P Complete heart block, atrial fibrillation.

A An opening snap is an early diastolic sound that is high-pitched.

P Mitral stenosis.

A Tachycardia.

P Exercise, fever, anxiety, pregnancy, heart failure.

Mitral and Tricuspid Area (S_3)

Auscultation of the mitral and tricuspid areas is repeated for low-pitched sounds, specifically an S_3 (otherwise known as a ventricular diastolic gallop, or extra heart sound). An S_3 is an early diastolic filling sound that originates in the ventricles and is therefore heard best at the apex of the heart. A right-sided S_3 (tricuspid area) is heard louder during inspiration because the venous return to the right side of the heart increases with a more negative intrathoracic pressure. An S_3 sound occurs just after an S_2.

E
1. Place the bell of the stethoscope lightly over the mitral landmark. When the S_3 originates in the left ventricle, it is heard best with the patient in a left lateral decubitus position and exhaling.
2. When originating in the right ventricle, an S_3 can best be heard by placing the bell of the stethoscope lightly over the third or fourth ICS at the left sternal border.
3. Auscultate for 10 to 15 seconds for a left- or right-sided S_3.

N An S_3 heart sound can be a normal physiological sound in children and in young adults. After the age of 30, a physiological S_3 is very infrequent. An S_3 can also be normal in high-output states such as the third trimester of pregnancy.

A S_3 in a non gravid adult.

P Ventricular dysfunction, excessively rapid early diastolic ventricular filling, and restrictive myocardial or pericardial disease; congestive heart failure and fluid overload.

Mitral and Tricuspid Area (S_4)

An S_4 heart sound, or atrial diastolic gallop, is a late diastolic filling sound associated with atrial contraction. An S_4 can be either left- or right-sided and is therefore heard best in the mitral or tricuspid area. An S_4 is a late diastolic filling sound that occurs just before S_1.

Sometimes, the S_3 and the S_4 heart sounds can occur simultaneously in mid-diastole, thus creating one loud diastolic filling sound. This is known as a summation gallop.

E
1. Place the bell of the stethoscope lightly over the mitral area.
2. Place the bell of the stethoscope lightly over the tricuspid area.
3. Auscultate for 10 to 15 seconds for a left- or right-sided S_4.

N An S_4 heart sound may occur with or without any evidence of cardiac decompensation. A left-sided S_4 is usually louder on expiration. A right-sided S_4 is usually louder on inspiration.

A Presence of an S_4.

E Examination	**N Normal Findings**	**A Abnormal Findings**	**P Pathophysiology**

Conditions that increase the resistance to filling because of a poorly compliant ventricle (MI, CAD, CHF, cardiomyopathy), conditions that result in systolic overload (HTN, aortic stenosis, hyperthyroidism).

Murmurs

Murmurs are distinguished from heart sounds by their longer duration. Murmurs may be classified as innocent (which are always systolic and are not associated with any other abnormalities), functional (which are associated with high-output states), or pathological (which are related to structural abnormalities). Murmurs are produced by turbulent blood flow in the following situations:

1. Flow across a partial obstruction
2. Increased flow through normal structures
3. Flow into a dilated chamber
4. Backward or regurgitant flow across incompetent valves
5. Shunting of blood out of a high-pressure chamber or artery through an abnormal passageway

When assessing for a murmur, analyze the murmur according to the following seven characteristics:

1. Location: area where the murmur is heard the loudest (e.g., mitral, pulmonic, etc.).
2. Radiation: transmission of sounds from the specific valves to other adjacent anatomic areas. For example, mitral murmurs can often radiate to the axilla.
3. Timing: phase of the cardiac cycle in which the murmur is heard. Murmurs can be either systolic or diastolic. If the murmur occurs simultaneously with the pulse, it is a systolic murmur. If it does not, it is a diastolic murmur. Murmurs can further be characterized as pansystolic or holosystolic, meaning that the murmur is heard throughout all of systole. Murmurs can also be characterized as early, mid-, or late-systolic or diastolic murmurs.
4. Intensity: See Table 16-1 for the six grades of loudness or intensity. The murmur is recorded with the grade over the roman

TABLE 16-1	Grading Heart Murmurs
GRADE	**CHARACTERISTICS**
I	Very faint; heard only after a period of concentration
II	Faint; heard immediately
III	Moderate intensity
IV	Loud; may be associated with a thrill
V	Loud; stethoscope must remain in contact with the chest wall in order to hear; thrill palpable
VI	Very loud; heard with stethoscope off of chest wall; thrill palpable

numeral "VI" to show the scale being used (e.g., III/VI).

5. Quality: harsh, rumbling, blowing, or musical.
6. Pitch: high, medium, or low. Low-pitched murmurs should be auscultated with the bell of the stethoscope whereas high-pitched murmurs should be auscultated with the diaphragm of the stethoscope.
7. Configuration: pattern that the murmur makes over time (Figure 16-5). The configuration of a murmur can be described as crescendo (soft to loud), decrescendo (loud to soft), crescendo-decrescendo (soft to loud to soft), and plateau (sound is sustained).

E 1. The patient should be in the same position for murmur auscultation as that which was used for the first auscultation (i.e., supine or sitting).
2. Auscultate each of the following cardiac landmarks for 10 to 15 seconds:
   a. Aortic and pulmonic areas, with the diaphragm of the stethoscope
   b. Mitral and tricuspid areas, with the diaphragm of the stethoscope
   c. Mitral and tricuspid areas, with the bell of the stethoscope

E **Examination** N **Normal Findings** A **Abnormal Findings** P **Pathophysiology**

A. Crescendo

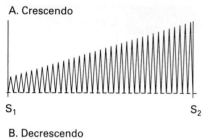

S_1 S_2

B. Decrescendo

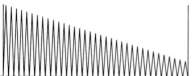

S_1 S_2

C. Crescendo-decrescendo

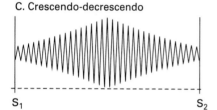

S_1 S_2

D. Plateau

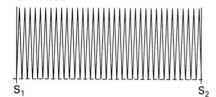

S_1 S_2

FIGURE 16-5 Characteristic Patterns of Murmurs.

3. Label the murmur using the characteristics of location, radiation, timing, configuration, intensity, pitch, and quality.

N   No murmur should be heard; however, a physiological or functional murmur in children and adolescents may be innocent. These murmurs are usually systolic, short, grade I or II, vibratory, heard at the left sternal border, and do not radiate. No cardiac symptoms accompany the murmur.

A   Murmurs of stenosis (Table 16-2).

P   Valve that should be open remains partially closed. It produces an increased afterload, or pressure overload (rheumatic fever, congenital defects of the valves, calcification associated with the aging process).

A   Murmurs of regurgitation or insufficiency (Table 16-2).

P   Valve that should be closed remains partially open. An insufficient valve causes volume overload, or increased preload (rheumatic fever, congenital defects of the valves).

Pericardial Friction Rub

E   1. Position the patient so that he or she is reclining in the sitting position, in the knee-chest position, or leaning forward.

2. Auscultate from the sternum (third to fifth ICS) to the apex (mitral area) with the diaphragm of the stethoscope for 10 to 15 seconds.

3. Characterize any sound according to its location, radiation, timing, quality, and pitch.

N   No pericardial friction rub should be auscultated.

A   Pericardial friction rub (Table 16-2).

P   Caused by the rubbing together of the inflamed visceral and parietal layers of the pericardium (pericarditis), renal failure.

Prosthetic Heart Valves

N   Prosthetic heart valves can be located in any of the four heart valves, although mitral and aortic valve replacements are the most common. Refer to the aortic and mitral valve auscultation discussions.

A   Prosthetic heart valves produce abnormal heart sounds. Furthermore, mechanical prosthetic valve sounds can sometimes be heard without the use of a stethoscope.

P   Mechanical prosthetic valves (caged-ball, tilting disk, and bileaflet valves) produce "clicky" opening and closing sounds. Homograft (human tissue) and heterograft (animal tissue) valves produce

---

E Examination   N Normal Findings   A Abnormal Findings   P Pathophysiology

TABLE 16-2	Murmurs and Pericardial Friction Rub		
HEART SOUND	**LOCATION/RADIATION**	**QUALITY/PITCH**	**CONFIGURATION**
Systolic Murmurs			
Aortic stenosis	Second right ICS; may radiate to neck or left sternal border	Harsh/medium	Crescendo/decrescendo
Pulmonic stenosis	Second or third left ICS; radiates toward shoulder and neck	Harsh/medium	Crescendo/decrescendo
Mitral regurgitation	Apex; fifth ICS, left midclavicular line; may radiate to left axilla and back	Blowing/high	Holosystolic/plateau
Tricuspid regurgitation	Lower left sternal border; may radiate to right sternum	Blowing/high	Holosystolic/plateau
Diastolic Murmurs			
Aortic regurgitation	Second right ICS and Erb's point; may radiate to left or right sternal border	Blowing/high	Decrescendo
Pulmonic regurgitation	Second left ICS; may radiate to left lower sternal border	Blowing/high	Decrescendo
Mitral stenosis	Apex; fifth ICS, left midclavicular line; may get louder with patient on left side; does not radiate	Rumbling/low	Crescendo/decrescendo
Tricuspid stenosis	Fourth ICS, at sternal border	Rumbling/low	Crescendo/decrescendo
Pericardial Friction Rub	Third to fifth ICS, left of sternum; does not radiate	Leathery, scratchy, grating/high	Three components: 1. Ventricular systole 2. Ventricular diastole 3. Atrial systole

Note: Timing is described as systolic or diastolic; intensity is described in Table 16-5.

sounds that are similar to those of the human valves; however, they usually produce a murmur.

ASSESSMENT OF THE PERIPHERAL VASCULATURE

Inspection of the Jugular Venous Pressure

Identify the internal and external jugular veins (Figure 16-6) with the patient in a supine position with the head elevated to 30° or 45° so that the jugular veins are visible. The external jugular veins are more superficial than the internal jugular (IJ) veins and traverse the neck diagonally from the centre of the clavicle to the angle of the jaw. The IJ veins are larger and are located deep below the sternocleidomastoid muscle adjacent to the carotid arteries. The pulsations of the IJ veins can be difficult to identify visually because the veins are deep and the pulsations can be confused with the adjacent carotid arteries.

E   1.   To indirectly estimate a patient's JVP:
   a.   Place the patient at a 30° to 45° angle (the highest position where the neck veins remain visible).

   b.   Measure the vertical distance in centimetres from the patient's sternal angle to the top of the distended neck vein. This will give you the JVP.
   c.   Knowing that the sternal angle is roughly 5 cm above the right atrium, take the JVP measurement obtained in the previous step and add 5 cm to get an estimate of the CVP. For example, a JVP of 2 cm at a 45° angle estimated on a patient's right side is equivalent to a CVP of 5 + 2, or 7, cm.

N   A JVP reading less than 4 cm is considered normal. Normally, the jugular veins are:
   1.   Most distended when the patient is flat because gravity is eliminated and the jugular veins fill
   2.   1 to 2 cm above the sternal angle when the head of the bed is elevated to a 45° angle
   3.   Absent when the head of the bed is at a 90° angle

A   A JVP greater than 4 cm.

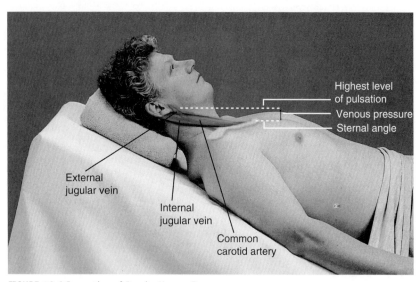

FIGURE 16-6 Inspection of Jugular Venous Pressure.

E   Examination   **N   Normal Findings**   **A   Abnormal Findings**   **P   Pathophysiology**

P   Increased right ventricular pressure, increased blood volume, obstruction to right ventricular flow.
A   Bilateral jugular venous distension (JVD).
P   Increased JVP.
A   Unilateral JVD.
P   Local vein blockage.
A   JVD with the head of the bed elevated to a 90° angle.
P   Severe right ventricular failure, constrictive pericarditis, cardiac tamponade.

Inspection of the Hepatojugular Reflux

Hepatojugular reflux is a test that is very sensitive in detecting right ventricular failure. This procedure is performed if the CVP is normal but right ventricular failure is suspected.

E   1. Place the patient flat in bed, or elevated to a 30° angle if the jugular veins are visible. Remind the patient to breathe normally.
    2. Using single or bimanual deep palpation, press firmly on the right upper quadrant for 30 to 60 seconds. Press on another part of the abdomen if this area is tender.
    3. Observe the neck for an elevation in JVP (Figure 16-7).
N   Normally, this pressure should not elicit any change in the jugular veins.
A   A rise of more than 1 cm in JVP.
P   Right-sided congestive heart failure; fluid overload.

Palpation and Auscultation of Arterial Pulses

E   1. The arterial pulse assessment is best facilitated with the patient in a supine position with the head of the bed elevated at 30° to 45°. If the patient cannot tolerate such a position, then the supine position alone is acceptable.
    2. Using your dominant hand, palpate the pulses with the pads of the index

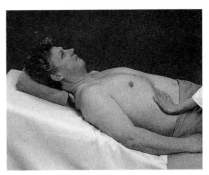

FIGURE 16-7 Hepatojugular Reflux.

and middle fingers. The number of fingers used will be determined by the amount of space where the pulse is located.
3. Evaluate the pulse in terms of:
    a. Rate
    b. Rhythm: If there is an irregularity in the pulse rate, then auscultate the heart.
    c. Amplitude: Refer to Table 9-2 for grading scales.
    d. Symmetry: Palpate the pulses on both sides of the patient's body simultaneously (with the exception of the carotid pulses).
4. Using the bell of the stethoscope, auscultate the temporal, carotid, and femoral pulses for bruits, which are blowing sounds heard when blood flow becomes turbulent as it rushes past an obstruction. Ask the patient to hold his or her breath during auscultation of the carotid pulse because respiratory sounds can interfere with auscultation.

N   Refer to Chapter 9, for normal pulse rate, rhythm, and amplitude. When assessing symmetry, the pulses should be equal bilaterally. No bruits should be auscultated in the carotid or femoral pulses.
A/P Figure 16-8 illustrates abnormal pulses with possible etiologies.
A   Bruits at the temporal, carotid, and femoral areas.

E   Examination   N   Normal Findings   A   Abnormal Findings   P   Pathophysiology

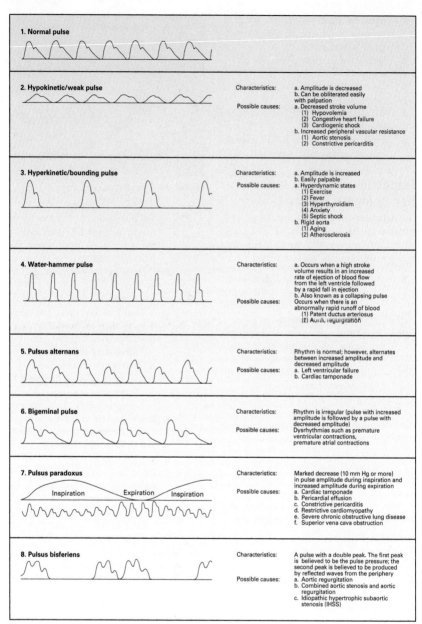

1. Normal pulse

2. Hypokinetic/weak pulse

Characteristics:
a. Amplitude is decreased
b. Can be obliterated easily with palpation

Possible causes:
a. Decreased stroke volume
  (1) Hypovolemia
  (2) Congestive heart failure
  (3) Cardiogenic shock
b. Increased peripheral vascular resistance
  (1) Aortic stenosis
  (2) Constrictive pericarditis

3. Hyperkinetic/bounding pulse

Characteristics:
a. Amplitude is increased
b. Easily palpable

Possible causes:
a. Hyperdynamic states
  (1) Exercise
  (2) Fever
  (3) Hyperthyroidism
  (4) Anxiety
  (5) Septic shock
b. Rigid aorta
  (1) Aging
  (2) Atherosclerosis

4. Water-hammer pulse

Characteristics:
a. Occurs when a high stroke volume results in an increased rate of ejection of blood flow from the left ventricle followed by a rapid fall in ejection
b. Also known as a collapsing pulse

Possible causes:
Occurs when there is an abnormally rapid runoff of blood
  (1) Patent ductus arteriosus
  (2) Aortic regurgitation

5. Pulsus alternans

Characteristics:
Rhythm is normal; however, alternates between increased amplitude and decreased amplitude

Possible causes:
a. Left ventricular failure
b. Cardiac tamponade

6. Bigeminal pulse

Characteristics:
Rhythm is irregular (pulse with increased amplitude is followed by a pulse with decreased amplitude)

Possible causes:
Dysrhythmias such as premature ventricular contractions, premature atrial contractions

7. Pulsus paradoxus

Inspiration   Expiration   Inspiration

Characteristics:
Marked decrease (10 mm Hg or more) in pulse amplitude during inspiration and increased amplitude during expiration

Possible causes:
a. Cardiac tamponade
b. Pericardial effusion
c. Constrictive pericarditis
d. Restrictive cardiomyopathy
e. Severe chronic obstructive lung disease
f. Superior vena cava obstruction

8. Pulsus bisferiens

Characteristics:
A pulse with a double peak. The first peak is believed to be the pulse pressure; the second peak is believed to be produced by reflected waves from the periphery

Possible causes:
a. Aortic regurgitation
b. Combined aortic stenosis and aortic regurgitation
c. Idiopathic hypertrophic subaortic stenosis (IHSS)

FIGURE 16-8 Alterations in Arterial Pulses.

P   Obstruction related to atherosclerotic plaque formation, jugular vein–carotid artery fistula, high-output states such as anemia or thyrotoxicosis.

Inspection and Palpation of Peripheral Perfusion

E   1. Inspect the fingers, toes, or points of trauma on the feet and legs for ulceration. Inspect the sides of the ankles for ulceration.

N   No ulcerations should be noted.

A   Arterial ulcerations.
   1. Location: occurs at toes or points of trauma on the feet or the legs.
   2. Characteristics: well-defined edges; black or necrotic tissue; a deep, pale base and lack of bleeding; hairlessness or disruption of the hair along with shiny, thick, waxy skin.
   3. Pain: exceedingly painful; claudication related to chronic arterial insufficiency is relieved by rest; pain at rest is relieved by dependency.

P   Inadequate arterial flow (peripheral vascular disease, diabetes mellitus), Raynaud's disease.

A   Venous ulcerations.
   1. Location: occurs at the sides of the ankles.
   2. Characteristics: uneven edges and ruddy granulation of tissue; thin, shiny skin that lacks the support of subcutaneous tissue; disruption of hair pattern, or hairlessness.
   3. Pain: deep muscular pain (associated with inadequate venous flow) with acute DVT; aching and cramping are relieved with elevation.

P   Inadequate venous flow.

REFERENCES

[1]Yusuf, S; Hawken, S., Ôunpuu, S., & Dans, T. (2004). Effect of potentially modifiable risk factors associated with myocardial infarction in 52 countries. *Lancet*, 364 (9438): 937–52.

| E **Examination** | N **Normal Findings** | A **Abnormal Findings** | P **Pathophysiology** |

17

Abdomen

ANATOMY AND PHYSIOLOGY

The abdomen is the largest cavity of the body. It is located between the diaphragm and the symphysis pubis (Figure 17-1).

Anatomic maps serve as a frame of reference during assessment of the abdomen (Figures 17-2 and Tables 17-1 and 17-3). The organs of the abdomen include the stomach, small intestine, large intestine, liver, gallbladder, pancreas, spleen, vermiform appendix, kidneys, ureters, and bladder.

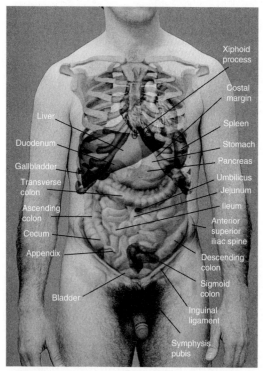

FIGURE 17-1 Structures of the Abdomen: Anterior View.

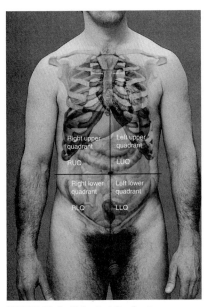

FIGURE 17-2 Abdominal Quadrants.

EQUIPMENT

- Drapes
- Small pillow for under knee
- Tape measure or small ruler with centimetre markings
- Marking pencil
- Gooseneck lamp for tangential lighting
- Stethoscope
- Sterile safety pin or sterile needle

ASSESSMENT OF THE ABDOMEN

The order of abdominal assessment is inspection, auscultation, percussion, and palpation. Auscultation is performed second because percussion and palpation can alter bowel sounds.

Inspection

Contour

E   View the contour of the patient's abdomen from the costal margin to the symphysis pubis.

TABLE 17-1	Four-Quadrant Anatomic Map
RIGHT UPPER QUADRANT (RUQ) • Liver • Gallbladder • Pylorus • Duodenum • Pancreas (head) • Portion of right kidney and adrenal gland • Hepatic flexure of colon • Section of ascending and transverse colons	**LEFT UPPER QUADRANT (LUQ)** • Left lobe of liver • Stomach • Spleen • Pancreas (body) • Portion of left kidney and adrenal gland • Splenic flexure of colon • Sections of transverse and descending colons
RIGHT LOWER QUADRANT (RLQ) • Appendix • Cecum • Lower pole of right kidney • Right ureter • Right ovary (female) • Right spermatic cord (male)	**LEFT LOWER QUADRANT (LLQ)** • Sigmoid colon • Section of descending colon • Lower pole of left kidney • Left ureter • Left ovary (female) • Left spermatic cord (male)

E   Examination   N   Normal Findings   A   Abnormal Findings   P   Pathophysiology

TABLE 17-2	Etiologies of Abdominal Pain: Anatomical Regions Where They Are Perceived

RIGHT UPPER QUADRANT

Biliary stone
Cholecystitis
Cholelithiasis
Duodenal ulcer
Gastric ulcer
Hepatic abscess
Hepatitis
Hepatomegaly
Pancreatitis
Pneumonia

EPIGASTRIUM

Abdominal aortic
  aneurysm
Appendicitis (early)
Biliary stone
Cholecystitis
Diverticulitis
Gastroesophageal
  reflux disease
Hiatal hernia

LEFT UPPER QUADRANT

Gastric ulcer
Gastritis
Myocardial infarction
Pneumonia
Splenic enlargement
Splenic rupture

PERIUMBILICAL

Abdominal aortic aneurysm
Appendicitis (early)
Diverticulitis
Intestinal obstruction
Irritable bowel syndrome
Pancreatitis
Peptic ulcer
Recurrent abdominal pain
  (in children)
Volvulus

RIGHT LOWER QUADRANT

Appendicitis
Crohn's disease

Diverticulitis
Ectopic pregnancy (ruptured)
Endometriosis
Hernia (strangulated)
Irritable bowel syndrome
Mittelschmerz

Ovarian cyst
Pelvic inflammatory disease
Renal calculi
Salpingitis

LEFT LOWER QUADRANT

Diverticulitis
Ectopic pregnancy
  (ruptured)
Endometriosis
Hernia (strangulated)
Irritable bowel syndrome
Mittelschmerz
Ovarian cyst
Pelvic inflammatory
  disease
Renal calculi
Salpingitis
Ulcerative colitis

DIFFUSE
Gastroenteritis
Peritonitis

N   In the normal adult, the abdominal contour is flat (straight horizontal line from costal margin to symphysis pubis) or rounded (convexity of abdomen from costal margin to symphysis pubis).

A   Large convex symmetrical profile from the costal margin to the symphysis pubis.

P   Refer to 7 Fs of Abdominal Distension Nursing Tip.

E Examination	N Normal Findings	A Abnormal Findings	P Pathophysiology

HEALTH HISTORY

Medical History Malignancies, peritonitis, cholecystitis, appendicitis, pancreatitis, small bowel obstruction, ulcerative colitis, hepatitis, hiatal hernia, diverticulitis, diverticulosis, peptic ulcer disease, Crohn's disease, acute renal failure, chronic renal failure, gallstones, kidney stone, irritable bowel syndrome, gastroesophageal reflux disease, urinary tract infection, parasitic infections, food poisoning, cirrhosis, infectious mononucleosis, hyper- or hypoadrenalism, malabsorption syndromes

Surgical History Cholecystectomy, gastrectomy, Billroth I or II, ileostomy, colostomy, appendectomy, colectomy, nephrectomy, pancreatectomy, ileal conduit, portal caval shunt, splenectomy, hiatal hernia repair, umbilical hernia repair, femoral or inguinal hernia repair, removal of renal calculi, liver transplant, renal transplant, bariatric surgery

Social History

Alcohol Use Altered nutrition, impaired gastric absorption, at risk for upper and lower gastrointestinal bleeding, cirrhosis of liver

---

A A concave symmetrical profile from the costal margin to the symphysis pubis.

P A scaphoid abdomen reflects a decrease in fat deposits, a malnourished state, or flaccid muscle tone.

Symmetry

E 1. View the symmetry of the patient's abdomen from the costal margin to the symphysis pubis.

2. Move to the foot of the examination table and recheck the symmetry of the patient's abdomen.

N The abdomen should be symmetrical bilaterally.

A Asymmetrical abdomen.

P Tumour, cysts, bowel obstruction, enlargement of abdominal organs, scoliosis. Bulging at the umbilicus can indicate an umbilical hernia.

Rectus Abdominis Muscles

E 1. Instruct the patient to raise the head and shoulders off the examination table.

2. Observe the rectus abdominis muscles for separation.

N The symmetry of the abdomen remains uniform; no ridge is observed parallel to the umbilicus or between the rectus abdominis muscles.

A A ridge between the rectus abdominis muscles.

P Diastasis recti abdominis and is attributed to marked obesity or past pregnancy.

Pigmentation and Colour

E View the colour of the patient's abdomen from the costal margin to the symphysis pubis.

N The abdomen should be uniform in colour and pigmentation.

Nursing Tip

7 Fs of Abdominal Distension

Seven possible causes of abdominal distension are:
- Fat
- Fluid (ascites)
- Flatus
- Feces
- Fetus
- Fatal growth (malignancy)
- Fibroid tumour

E **Examination** N **Normal Findings** A **Abnormal Findings** P **Pathophysiology**

◀ NURSING CHECKLIST ▶

General Approach to Abdominal Assessment

1. Greet the patient and explain the assessment technique.
2. Ensure that the room is at a warm, comfortable temperature to prevent patient chilling and shivering.
3. Use a quiet room that will be free from interruptions.
4. Utilize an adequate light source. This includes both a bright overhead light and a freestanding lamp for tangential lighting.
5. Ask the patient to urinate before the exam.
6. Drape the patient from the xiphoid process to the symphysis pubis, and then expose the patient's abdomen.
7. Position the patient comfortably in a supine position with knees flexed over a pillow or position the patient so that the arms are either folded across the chest or at the sides to ensure abdominal relaxation.
8. Stand to the right side of the patient for the examination.
9. Visualize the underlying abdominal structures during the assessment process in order to accurately describe the location of any pathology.
10. Have the patient point to tender areas; assess these last. Mark these and other significant findings (scars, dullness, and so on) on the body diagram in the patient's chart.
11. Watch the patient's face closely for signs of discomfort or pain.
12. Help the patient relax by using an unhurried approach, diverting attention with questions, and so on.
13. Ensure that your hands and the stethoscope are warm to promote patient comfort.

A Uneven skin colour or pigmentation.
P Jaundice suggests liver dysfunction.
P Blue tint at the umbilicus suggests free blood in the peritoneal cavity, known as Cullen's sign.
Irregular patches of tan skin pigmentation (café au lait spots) may be attributed to von Recklinghausen's disease.
A Engorged abdominal veins (caput medusae).
P Circulatory obstruction of the superior or the inferior vena cava.

Scars

E Inspect the abdomen for scars from the costal margin to the symphysis pubis.
N There should be no abdominal scars present.

A Scar(s).
P Traumatic injuries or burns, surgery.

Striae

E Observe the abdominal skin for striae (stretch marks), or abdominal atrophic lines or scars.
N No evidence of striae is present.
A Striae.
P Rapid or prolonged stretching of the skin (abdominal tumours, obesity, ascites, pregnancy).

Respiratory Movement

E Observe the abdomen for smooth, even respiratory movement.

E **Examination**   N **Normal Findings**   A **Abnormal Findings**   P **Pathophysiology**

N There is no evidence of respiratory retractions. Normally, the abdomen rises with inspiration and falls with expiration.

A Abnormal respiratory movements and retractions.

P Appendicitis with local peritonitis, pancreatitis, biliary colic, or perforated ulcer.

Masses or Nodules

E Observe the abdominal skin for nodules or masses.

N No masses or nodules are present.

A Abdominal masses or nodules.

P Tumours, metastases of an internal malignancy, or pregnancy.

Visible Peristalsis

E Observe the abdominal wall for surface motion.

N Ripples of peristalsis may be observed in thin patients. Peristalsis movement slowly traverses the abdomen in a slanting downward direction.

A Strong peristaltic contractions.

P Intestinal obstruction.

Pulsation

E Inspect the epigastric area for pulsations.

N In the patient with a normal build, a non-exaggerated pulsation of the abdominal aorta may be visible in the epigastric area. In heavier patients, pulsation may not be visible.

A Marked, strong abdominal pulsations.

P Aortic aneurysm, aortic regurgitation, right ventricular hypertrophy.

Umbilicus

E 1. Observe the umbilicus in relation to the abdominal surface.
2. Ask the patient to flex the neck. Perform the valsalva manoeuvre.
3. Observe for protrusion of the intestine through the umbilicus.

N The umbilicus is depressed and beneath the abdominal surface.

Nursing Alert

Hepatitis A–Risk Factors

- Overcrowded living quarters
- Poor personal hygiene (poor handwashing, especially after defecation)
- Poor sanitation (sewage disposal)
- Food and water contamination
- Ingestion of shellfish caught in contaminated water
- Travel to endemic area (many developing countries)
- Those in close personal contact with infected individual
- Day care centres, especially those with children wearing diapers

Hepatitis B–Risk Factors

- Injection drug use with shared needles
- Receipt of multiple transfusions of blood and blood products (oncology and hemodialysis patients, hemophiliacs)
- Frequent contact with blood (health care workers such as nurses, doctors)
- Heterosexual activities such as having multiple heterosexual partners
- Sex with hepatitis B–infected individuals
- Male homosexual activity
- Perinatal transmission
- Travel to endemic areas (e.g., China)
- Sharing blood-contaminated toothbrushes, razors

E Examination   N Normal Findings   A Abnormal Findings   P Pathophysiology

A   The umbilicus protrudes above the abdominal surface.

P   Umbilical hernia, abdominal carcinoma with metastasis (Sister Mary Joseph's nodule), ascites, masses, pregnancy.

Auscultation

Bowel Sounds

E   1.   Place the diaphragm lightly on the abdominal wall beginning at the RLQ.

 2.   Listen to the frequency and character of the bowel sounds. It is necessary to listen for at least five minutes in an abdominal quadrant before concluding that bowel sounds are absent.

 3.   Move diaphragm to RUQ, LUQ, LLQ.

N   Bowel sounds are heard as intermittent gurgling sounds throughout the abdominal quadrants. Usually, they are high-pitched sounds and occur 5 to 30 times per minute. Bowel sounds result from the movement of air and fluid through the gastrointestinal tract. Normally, bowel sounds are always present at the ileocecal valve area (RLQ).

Normal hyperactive bowel sounds are called borborygmi. They are loud, audible, gurgling sounds. Borborygmi may be due to hyperperistalsis ("stomach growling") or the sound of flatus in the intestines.

A   Absent bowel sounds.

P   Late intestinal obstruction.

A   Hypoactive bowel sounds.

P   Decreased motility of the bowel (peritonitis, non-mechanical obstruction, inflammation, gangrene, electrolyte imbal-

ances, intraoperative manipulation of the bowel).

A   Hyperactive bowel sounds.

P   Increased motility of the bowel (gastroenteritis, diarrhea, laxative use, subsiding ileus).

A   High-pitched tinkling.

P   Partial obstruction.

Vascular Sounds

E   1.   Place the bell of the stethoscope over the abdominal aorta, renal arteries, iliac arteries, and femoral arteries (Figure 17-3).

 2.   Listen for bruits over each area .

N   No audible bruits are auscultated.

A   Audible bruits.

P   A bruit over an abdominal vessel indicates turbulence of blood flow (abdominal aortic aneurysm, renal stenosis, femoral stenosis).

Venous Hum

E   Using the bell of the stethoscope, listen for a venous hum, or a continuous, medium-pitched sound, in all four quadrants.

N   Venous hums are normally not present in adults.

A   A continuous pulsing or fibrillary sound.

P   Obstructed portal circulation.

Friction Rubs

E   1.   Using the diaphragm of the stethoscope, listen for friction rubs over the right and left costal margins, the liver, and the spleen.

 2.   Listen for friction rubs in all four quadrants.

N   No friction rubs should be present.

A   Friction rubs are high-pitched sounds that resemble the sound produced by two pieces of sandpaper being rubbed together. The sound increases with inspiration.

P   Tumours, inflammation, or infarct cause the visceral layers of the peritoneum to rub together over the liver and the spleen.

Nursing Alert

Palpation Contraindication

Never palpate over areas where bruits are auscultated. Palpation may cause rupture. Refer the patient immediately.

E   **Examination**   N   **Normal Findings**   A   **Abnormal Findings**   P   **Pathophysiology**

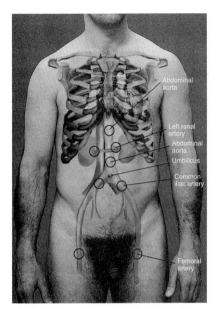

FIGURE 17-3 Stethoscope Placement for Auscultating Abdominal Vasculature.

Percussion

General Percussion

E 1. Percuss all four quadrants in a systematic manner. Begin percussion in the RLQ, moving upward to the RUQ, crossing over to the LUQ, and moving down to the LLQ.
   2. Visualize each organ in the corresponding quadrant; note when tympany changes to dullness.

N Tympany is the predominant sound heard because air is present in the stomach and in the intestines. It is a high-pitched sound of long duration. In obese patients it may be difficult to elicit tympany due to the quantity of adipose tissue. Dullness is normally heard over organs such as the liver or a distended bladder. Dull sounds are high pitched and of moderate duration.

A Dullness over areas where tympany normally occurs, such as over the stomach and intestines.

P Mass, tumour, pregnancy, ascites, full intestine.

Liver Span

E 1. Stand to the right side of the patient.
   2. Begin at the right midclavicular line below the umbilicus and percuss upward to determine the lower border of the liver (Figure 17-18A).
   3. With a marking pen, mark where the sound changes from tympany to dullness.
   4. Then, at the right midclavicular line, percuss downward from an area of lung resonance to one of dullness.
   5. With a tape measure or ruler, measure the two marks in centimetres.

N Normally, the distance between the two marks is 6 to 12 cm in the midclavicular line. There is a direct correlation between body size and the size of the liver. The mean span for a man is 10.5 cm and for a woman it is 7.0 cm.

A A liver span greater than 12 cm or less than 6 cm.

P The liver span is increased when the liver becomes enlarged. Hepatomegaly can occur with hepatitis, cirrhosis, cardiac or renal congestion, cysts, or metastatic tumours.

P The liver span can be falsely increased when the upper border is obscured by the dullness of lung consolidation or pleural effusion.

P The liver span can be decreased in the later stages of cirrhosis (liver atrophy), gas in the colon, tumours, or pregnancy push the lower border of the liver upward.

Liver Descent

E 1. Percuss the liver descent by asking the patient to take a deep breath and to hold it (because on inspiration, the diaphragm moves downward).
   2. Again, percuss the lower border of the liver at the right midclavicular line by percussing from tympany to dullness. Have the patient exhale.
   3. Repercuss the liver–lung border.

E **Examination**   N **Normal Findings**   A **Abnormal Findings**   P **Pathophysiology**

4. Mark where the change in sound takes place.

5. Measure the difference in centimetres between the two lower borders of the liver.

N Normally, the area of lower border dullness descends 2 to 3 cm.

A Liver descent greater or less than 2 to 3 cm.

P The liver descent is greater than 2 to 3 cm due to hepatomegaly, as in cirrhosis.

P The liver descent is less than 2 cm due to abdominal tumours, pregnancy, or ascites.

Spleen

E 1. Percuss the lower level of the left lung slightly posterior to the midaxillary line and continue downward (Figure 17-4).

2. Percuss downward until dullness is ascertained. In some individuals, the spleen is positioned too deeply to be discernable by percussion.

N Normally, the upper border of dullness is found 6 to 8 cm above the left costal margin. Splenic dullness may be heard from the sixth to the tenth rib.

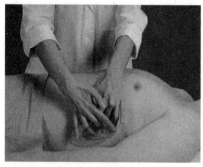

FIGURE 17-4 Percussion of the Spleen.

A Dullness beyond the 8 cm line is indicative of splenic enlargement.

P Portal hypertension resulting from liver disease; mononucleosis, thrombosis, stenosis, atresia, angiomatous deformities of the portal or splenic vein, cysts, aneurysm of the splenic artery.

Stomach

E Percuss for a gastric air bubble in the LUQ at the left lower anterior rib cage and left epigastric region.

N The tympany of the gastric air bubble is lower in pitch than the tympany of the intestine.

A An increase in size of the gastric air bubble.

P Gastric dilation.

Fist Percussion

Fist percussion is done over the kidneys and liver to check for tenderness.

Kidney

E 1. Place the patient in a sitting position.

2. Strike the costovertebral angle with a closed fist (direct fist percussion, Figure 17-5A) or

2A. Place the palmar surface of one hand over the costovertebral angle (CVA). Strike that hand with the ulnar surface of the fist of the other hand (indirect fist percussion, Figure 17-5B).

3. Ask the patient what was felt. Observe the patient's reaction.

4. Repeat on the other side.

N No tenderness should be elicited.

E Examination   **N** Normal Findings   **A** Abnormal Findings   **P** Pathophysiology

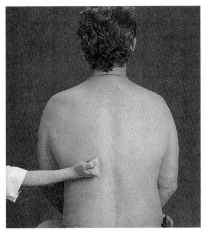

A. Direct Fist Percussion of the Left Kidney

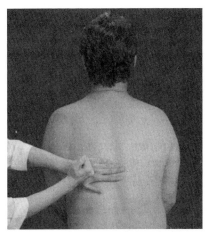

B. Indirect Fist Percussion of the Left Kidney

FIGURE 17-5 Percussion Patterns.

A   Tenderness or pain over the costovertebral angle.
P   Pyelonephritis.

Liver

E   1. Place the patient in a supine position.
    2. Place the palmar surface of one hand over the lower right rib cage (where the liver was percussed).
    3. Strike that hand with the ulnar surface of the fist of the other hand (Figure 17-6).
    4. Ask the patient what was felt. Observe the patient's reaction.
N   No tenderness should be elicited.
A   Tenderness or pain elicited over the liver.
P   Cholecystitis, hepatitis.

Bladder

E   1. Percuss upward from the symphysis pubis to the umbilicus.
    2. Note where the sound changes from dullness to tympany.
N   A urine-filled bladder is dull to percussion. A recently emptied bladder should not be percussable above the symphysis pubis.
A   It is abnormal to percuss a bladder that has recently been emptied.

P   Inability to completely empty the bladder occurs in the elderly, in postoperative, bedridden, and acutely ill patients, and in patients with neurogenic bladder dysfunction. Prostatic hypertrophy, urethral pathology, and some medications (antipsychotics: phenothiazine; anticholinergics: atropine; antihypertensives: hydralazine).

Palpation

Light Palpation

E   1. With your hands and forearm on a horizontal plane, use the pads of the

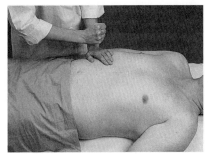

FIGURE 17-6 Indirect Fist Percussion of the Liver.

E **Examination**   N **Normal Findings**   A **Abnormal Findings**   P **Pathophysiology**

approximated fingers to depress the abdominal wall 1 cm (Figure 17-7).

2. Avoid short, quick jabs.
3. Lightly palpate all four quadrants in a systematic manner.

N The abdomen should feel smooth with consistent softness.

A Changes in skin temperature, tenderness, or large masses.

P Inflammation. Tumours, feces, or enlarged organs.

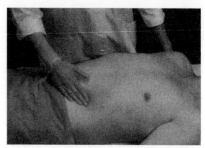

FIGURE 17-7 Light Palpation of the Abdomen.

Abdominal Muscle Guarding

To determine whether muscle guarding is involuntary:

E 1. Perform light palpation of the rectus muscles during expiration.
   2. Note muscle tensing.

N Muscle guarding, or tensing of the abdominal musculature, is absent during expiration. The abdomen is soft. Normally, during expiration the patient cannot exercise voluntary muscle tensing.

A Muscle guarding of the rectus muscles occurs during expiration.

P Irritation of the peritoneum, as in peritonitis.

Deep Palpation

In performing deep palpation of all four quadrants, you can use either a one-handed or a two-handed method.

E 1. With the one-handed method, use the palmar surface of the extended

fingers to depress the skin approximately 5 to 8 cm in the RLQ (Figure 17-8A).

2. A two-handed approach is used when palpation is difficult because of obesity or muscular resistance. With the bimanual technique, the non-dominant hand is placed on top of the dominant hand. The bottom hand is used for sensation, and the top hand is used to apply pressure (Figure 17-8B).

3. Identify any masses and note location, size, shape, consistency, tenderness, pulsation, and degree of mobility.

4. Continue palpation of RUQ, LUQ, and LLQ.

N No organ enlargement should be palpable, nor should there be any abnormal masses, bulges, or swelling. Normally, only the aorta and the edge of the liver are palpable. When the large colon or the bladder is full, palpation is possible.

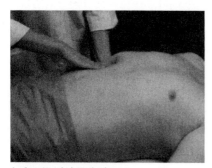

A. One-Handed Method

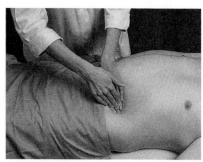

B. Bimanual Method

FIGURE 17-8 Deep Palpation.

| **E** Examination | **N** Normal Findings | **A** Abnormal Findings | **P** Pathophysiology |

A The gallbladder, liver, spleen, fecal-filled colon, or flatus-filled cecum should not be palpable. Masses, bulges, and swellings are considered abnormal.

P Organomegaly (cholecystitis, hepatitis, cirrhosis); masses, bulges, or swelling can be due to tumours, fluids, feces, flatus, fat.

Liver

Liver palpation can be performed by one of two methods: the bimanual method or the hook method.

Bimanual Method

E 1. Stand at the patient's right side, facing the patient's head.
   2. Place the left hand under the patient's right flank at about the 11th or 12th rib.
   3. Press upward with the left hand to elevate the liver toward the abdominal wall.
   4. Place the right hand parallel to the midline at the right midclavicular line below the right costal margin or below the level of liver dullness.
   5. Instruct the patient to take a deep breath.
   6. Push down deeply and under the costal margin with your right fingers. On inspiration, the liver will descend and contact the hand (Figure 17-9A).
   7. Note the level of the liver.
   8. Note the size, shape, consistency, and any masses.

Hook Method

E 1. Stand at the patient's right side, facing the patient's feet.
   2. Place both hands side by side on the right costal margin below the border of liver dullness.
   3. Hook the fingers in and up toward the costal margin and ask the patient to take a deep breath and hold it.
   4. Palpate the liver's edge as it descends (Figure 17-9B).
   5. Note the level of the liver.

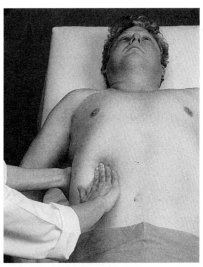

A. Bimanual Method

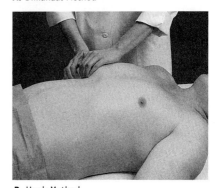

B. Hook Method

FIGURE 17-9 Palpation of the Liver.

E Examination   **N** Normal Findings   **A** Abnormal Findings   **P** Pathophysiology

6. Note the size, shape, consistency, and any masses.

N A normal liver edge presents as a firm, sharp, regular ridge with a smooth surface. Normally, the liver is not palpable, although it may be felt in extremely thin adults.

A Liver palpable below the costal margin both medially and laterally.

P Congestive heart failure, hepatitis, encephalopathy, cirrhosis, cysts, cancer.

A Enlarged and has an irregular border and nodules, hard.

P Liver malignancy.

Spleen

Use the bimanual technique to palpate the spleen.

E 1. Stand at the patient's right side.
 2. Reach across and place the left hand beneath the patient and over the left costovertebral angle. Press upward to lift the spleen anteriorly toward the abdominal wall
 3. With the right hand, press inward along the left costal margin while asking the patient to take a deep breath (Figure 17-10).
 3A. The procedure can be repeated with the patient lying on the right side, with the hips and knees flexed. This position will facilitate the spleen coming forward and to the right because the spleen is located retroperitoneally.

4. Note the size, shape, consistency, and any masses.

N The spleen should not be palpable.

A Splenomegaly.

P Inflammation, congestive heart failure, cancer, cirrhosis, mononucleosis.

Kidneys

E 1. Stand at the patient's right side.
 2. Place one hand on the right costovertebral angle on the patient's back.
 3. Place the other hand below and parallel to the costal margin.
 4. As the patient takes a deep breath, press hands firmly together and try to feel the lower pole of the kidney (Figure 17-11).
 5. At the peak of inspiration, press the fingers together with greater pressure from above than from below.
 6. Ask the patient to exhale and to hold the breath briefly.
 7. Release the pressure of your fingers.
 8. If the kidney has been "captured," it can be felt as it slips back into place.
 9. Note the size, shape, and consistency. Note any masses.
 10. For the left kidney, reach across the patient and place the left hand under the patient's left flank.
 11. Apply downward pressure with the right hand below the left costal margin and repeat steps 4 to 9.

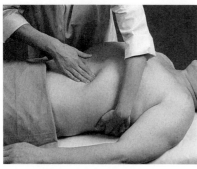

FIGURE 17-10 Deep Palpation.

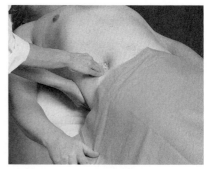

FIGURE 17-11 Palpation of the Right Kidney.

| E **Examination** | N **Normal Findings** | A **Abnormal Findings** | P **Pathophysiology** |

N   The kidneys should not be palpable in the normal adult. However, the lower pole of the right kidney may be felt in very thin individuals. Kidneys are more readily palpable in the elderly due to loss of muscle tone and muscle bulk.

A   Enlarged kidneys.

P   Hydronephrosis, neoplasms, polycystic kidney disease.

Aorta

E   1. Press the upper abdomen with one hand on each side of the abdominal aorta, slightly to the left of the midline.

    2. Assess the width of the aorta (Figure 17-12).

N   The aorta width is 2.5 to 4.0 cm, and the aorta pulsates in an anterior direction.

A   Aorta width greater than 4.0 cm. Lateral pulsation.

P   Abdominal aortic aneurysm.

Bladder

E   1. Using deep palpation, palpate the abdomen at the midline, starting at the symphysis pubis and progressing upward to the umbilicus (Figure 17-13).

    2. If the bladder is located, palpate the shape, size, and consistency.

N   An empty bladder is not usually palpable. A moderately full bladder is smooth and round, and it is palpable above the symphysis pubis. A full bladder is palpated above the symphysis pubis, and it may be close to the umbilicus.

A   Nodular or asymmetrical bladder.

P   Malignancy (tumour in the bladder or an abdominal tumour that is compressing the bladder).

Inguinal Lymph Nodes

E   1. Place the patient in a supine position, with the knees slightly flexed.

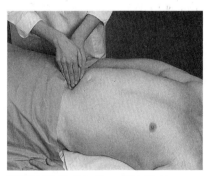

FIGURE 17-12 Palpation of the Aorta.   **FIGURE 17-13** Palpation of the Bladder.

E Examination	N Normal Findings	A Abnormal Findings	P Pathophysiology

2. Drape the genital area.
3. Using the finger pads of the second, third, and fourth fingers, apply firm pressure and palpate with a rotary motion in the right inguinal area.
4. Palpate for lymph nodes in the left inguinal area.

N   It is normal to palpate small, movable nodes less than 1 cm in diameter. Palpable nodes are non-tender.

A   Lymph nodes greater than 1 cm in diameter or elicitation of non-movable, tender lymph nodes is abnormal.

P   Large, palpable nodes can be attributed to localized or systemic infections. More serious pathology includes processes associated with cancer or lymphomas.

18

Musculoskeletal System

ANATOMY AND PHYSIOLOGY

The musculoskeletal system supports body position, promotes mobility, protects underlying soft organs, allows for mineral storage, and produces select blood components (platelets, red blood cells, and white blood cells).

The adult human skeleton comprises 206 bones (Figure 18-1). Bone is ossified connective tissue. The skeleton is divided into the central axial skeleton (facial bones, skull, auditory ossicles, hyoid bone, ribs, sternum, and vertebrae) and the peripheral appendicular skeleton (limbs, pelvis, scapula, and clavicle).

There are over 600 muscles in the human body, and they can be characterized as one of three types. Cardiac and smooth muscles are involuntary, meaning that the individual has no conscious control over the initiation and termination of the muscle contraction. The largest type of muscle, and the only type of voluntary muscle, is called skeletal muscle. Skeletal muscle provides for mobility by exerting a pull on the bones near a joint. Figure 18-2 illustrates the major muscles.

Bursae are sacs filled with fluid. Bursae act as cushions between two nearby surfaces (e.g., between tendon and bone or between tendon and ligament) to reduce friction. They can also develop in response to prolonged friction or pressure.

Joints secure the bones firmly together but allow for some degree of movement between the two bones. Terms used for joint range of motion are described in Table 18-1.

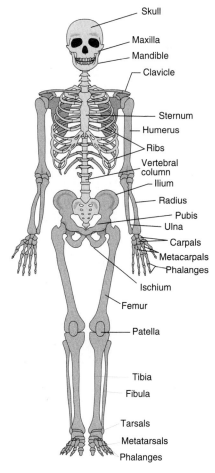

FIGURE 18-1 Adult Skeleton: Anterior View.

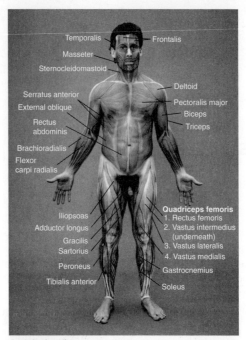

A. Anterior View

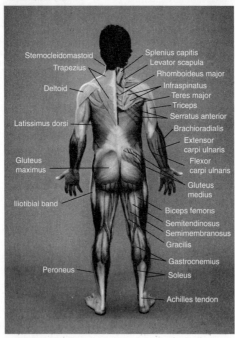

B. Posterior View

FIGURE 18-2 Muscles of the Body.

TABLE 18-1	Descriptive Terms for Joint Range of Motion	

TERM	DESCRIPTION	CHANGE IN JOINT ANGLE
Flexion	Bending of a joint so that the articulating bones on either side of the joints are moved closer together	Decreased
Extension	Bending the joint so that the articulating bones on either side of the joint are moved farther apart	Increased
Hyperextension	Extension beyond the neutral position	Increased beyond the angle of extension
Adduction	Moving the extremity medially and toward the midline of the body	Decreased
Abduction	Moving the extremity laterally and away from the midline of the body	Increased
Internal rotation	Rotating the extremity medially along its own axis	No change
External rotation	Rotating the extremity laterally along its own axis	No change
Circumduction	Moving the extremity in a conical fashion so that the distal aspect of the extremity moves in a circle	No change
Supination	Rotating the forearm laterally at the elbow so that the palm of the hand turns laterally to face upward	No change
Pronation	Rotating the forearm medially at the elbow so that the palm of the hand turns medially to face downward	No change
Opposition	Moving the thumb outward to touch the little finger of the same hand	No change
Eversion	Tilting the foot inward, with the medial side of the foot lowered	No change
Inversion	Tilting the foot outward, with the lateral side of the foot lowered	No change
Dorsiflexion	Flexing the foot at the ankle so that the toes move toward the chest	Decreased
Plantar flexion	Moving the foot at the ankle so that the toes move away from the chest	Increased
Elevation	Raising a body part in an upward direction	No change
Depression	Lowering a body part	No change
Protraction	Moving a body part anteriorly along its own axis (parallel to the ground)	No change
Retraction	Moving a body part posteriorly along its own axis (parallel to the ground)	No change
Gliding	One joint surface moves over another joint surface in a circular or angular nature	No change

HEALTH HISTORY

Medical History	Rheumatoid arthritis, osteoarthritis, osteoporosis, Paget's disease, gout, ankylosing spondylitis, osteogenesis imperfecta, loosening or malfunction of joint prosthesis, aseptic necrosis, chronic low back pain, herniated nucleus pulposus, chronic muscle spasms or cramps, scoliosis, poliomyelitis, polymyalgia rheumatica, osteomalacia, rickets, Marfan's syndrome, scleroderma, spina bifida, congenital deformity, MD, MS, myasthenia gravis, ALS, Guillain-Barré syndrome, Reiter's syndrome, carpal tunnel syndrome, paralysis
Surgical History	Joint aspiration, therapeutic joint arthroscopy, joint arthroplasty, joint replacement, synovectomy, meniscectomy, arthrodesis, open reduction and internal fixation (ORIF), discectomy, laminectomy, spinal fusion, Harrington rod placement or other spinal instrumentation, repair of torn rotator cuff, debridement, limb or digit amputation, reattachment of a limb or digit
Injuries and Accidents	Fracture, dislocation, subluxation, tendon tear, tendonitis, muscle contusion, joint strain or sprain, spinal cord injury, torn rotator cuff, traumatic amputation of a digit or limb, crush injury, back injury (including herniated vertebral disc), sports-related injury (e.g., golf elbow, pitcher's shoulder), cartilage damage.
Special Needs	Amputation, hemiplegia, paraplegia, quadriplegia, need for brace or splint, limb in a cast, need for supportive devices, muscle atrophy
Work Environment	Manual movement of heavy objects (lifting, pushing, pulling), duties requiring repetitive motions (e.g., keyboard use), duties requiring prolonged standing or walking, use of hazardous equipment, availability and use of safety equipment (e.g., lifting equipment, availability of back support vest or brace)

EQUIPMENT

- Measuring tape: cloth tape measure that will not stretch
- Goniometer: protractor-type instrument with two movable arms to measure the angle of a skeletal joint during range of motion
- Sphygmomanometer and blood pressure cuff
- Felt-tip marker

ASSESSMENT OF THE MUSCULOSKELETAL SYSTEM

General Assessment

Overall Appearance

E   1. Obtain height and weight. Refer to Chapter 7.

2. Observe the patient's ability to tolerate weight bearing on the lower limbs during standing and walking. Assess the amount of weight bearing placed on each of the lower limbs.

3. Identify obvious structural abnormalities (e.g., atrophy, scoliosis, kyphosis, amputated limbs, contractures).

4. Note indications of discomfort (e.g., restricted weight bearing or movement, frequent shifting of position, facial grimacing, excessive fatigue).

N   The Body Mass Index is in the normal range (see Chapter 7). The patient should be able to enter the assessment area via independent walking. Structural defects

E Examination	N Normal Findings	A Abnormal Findings	P Pathophysiology

◀ NURSING CHECKLIST ▶

General Approach to Musculoskeletal Assessment

1. Assist the patient to a comfortable position.
2. Offer pillows or folded blankets to support a painful body part.
3. If necessary because of a painful body part or limited mobility, provide the patient assistance in disrobing. Allow the patient extra time to remove clothing.
4. To maximize patient comfort during the physical assessment, maintain a warm temperature in the exam room.
5. Be clear in your instructions to the patient if you are asking the patient to perform a certain body movement or to assume a certain position. Demonstrate the desired movement if necessary.
6. Notify the patient before touching or manipulating a painful body part.
7. Inspection, palpation, range of motion, and muscle testing are performed on the major skeletal muscles and joints of the body in a cephalocaudal, proximal-to-distal manner. Always compare paired muscles and joints.
8. Examine non-affected body parts before examining affected body parts.
9. Avoid unnecessary or excessive manipulation of a painful body part. If the patient complains of pain, stop the aggravating motion.
10. If necessary because of a painful body part or limited mobility, provide the patient assistance in dressing after the physical assessment. Allow the patient extra time to get dressed.
11. Some musculoskeletal disorders may affect the patient more during certain times of the day. Arrange for the follow-up appointment to be during the patient's time of optimal function.

should be absent. There should be no outward indications of discomfort during rest, weight bearing, or joint movement. There should be a distinct and symmetrical relationship among the limbs, torso, and pelvis.

A An excessively tall or short, or overweight or underweight patient.

P Marfan's syndrome, dwarfism, severe osteoporosis, ankylosing spondylitis, obesity.

A Any weight-bearing status other than full weight bearing.

P Low back pain may cause a patient to lean forward or toward the affected side.

A Structural defects.

P Acromegaly, congenital defect, surgery, trauma, scoliosis, kyphosis.

Posture

E 1. Stand in front of the patient.
   2. Instruct the patient to stand with the feet together.
   3. Observe the structural and spatial relationship of the head, torso, pelvis, and limbs. Assess for symmetry of the shoulders, scapulae, and iliac crests.
   4. Ask the patient to sit; observe posture.

N In the standing position, the torso and head are upright. The head is midline and perpendicular to the horizontal line of the shoulders and pelvis. The shoulders and hips are level, with symmetry of the scapulae and iliac crests. The arms hang freely from the shoulders. The feet are

---

E **Examination**   N **Normal Findings**   A **Abnormal Findings**   P **Pathophysiology**

aligned and the toes point forward. The extremities are proportional to the overall body size and shape, and the limbs are also symmetrical with each other. The knees face forward, with symmetry of the level of the knees. There is usually less than a 5 cm interval between the knees when the patient stands with the feet together, facing forward. When full growth is reached, the arm span is equal to the height. In the sitting position, both feet should be placed firmly on the floor surface, with toes pointing forward.

A   Forward slouching of the shoulders.
P   Poor posture habits.

Gait and Mobility

E   1. Instruct the patient to walk normally across the room.
    2. Ask the patient to walk on toes and then on the heels of the feet.
    3. Ask the patient to walk by placing one foot in front of the other, in a "heel to-toe" fashion (tandem walking).
    4. Instruct the patient to walk forward, then backward.
    5. Ask the patient to side step to the left, then to the right.
    6. Instruct the patient to ambulate forward a few steps with the eyes closed.
    7. Observe the patient during transfer between the standing and sitting position.

N   Walking is started in one smooth, rhythmic fashion. The foot is lifted 2.5 to 5 cm off the floor and then propelled 30 to 45 cm forward in a straight path. As the heel strikes the floor, body weight is then shifted onto the ball of that foot. The heel of the foot is then lifted off the floor before the next step forward. The patient remains erect and balanced during all stages of gait. Step height and length are symmetrical for each foot. The arms swing freely at the side of the torso but in opposite direction to the movement of the legs. The lower limbs are able to bear full body weight during standing and walking. Prior to turning, the head

and neck turn toward the intended direction, followed by the rest of the body. The patient should be able to transfer easily to various positions.

A/P   Table 18-2 provides examples of abnormal gait patterns.

Inspection
Muscle Size and Shape

E   1. Survey the overall appearance of the muscle mass.
    2. Ask the patient to contract the muscle without inducing movement (isometric muscle contraction), relax the muscle, and then repeat the muscle contraction.
    3. Look for any obvious muscle contraction.

N   Muscle contour will be affected by the exercise and activity patterns of the individual. Muscle shape may be accentuated in certain body areas (e.g., the limbs and upper torso) but should be symmetrical. There may be hypertrophy in the dominant hand. During muscle contraction, you should be able to visualize sudden tautness of the muscle area. Muscle relaxation will be associated with termination of muscle tautness. There is no involuntary movement.

A   Atrophy describes a reduction in muscle size and shape.
P   Prolonged immobility, sedentary lifestyle, hemiparesis, paraplegia, quadriplegia, following the removal of a limb cast or splint.
A   Involuntary muscle movement.
P   See Table 18-3.

Joint Contour and Periarticular Tissue

E   1. Observe the shape of the joint while the joint is in its neutral anatomic position.
    2. Visually inspect the 5 to 7.5 cm of skin and subcutaneous tissue surrounding that joint. Assess the periarticular area for erythema, swelling, bruising, nodules, deformities, masses, skin atrophy, or skin breakdown.

E Examination   N Normal Findings   A Abnormal Findings   P Pathophysiology

TABLE 18-2 Examples of Abnormal Gait Patterns

TYPE OF ABNORMAL GAIT	ETIOLOGY	DESCRIPTION
Antalgic	Degenerative joint disease of the hip or knee	Limited weight bearing is placed on an affected leg in an attempt to limit discomfort.
Short leg	Discrepancy in leg length, flexion contracture of the hip or knee, congenital hip dislocation	A limp is present during ambulation unless shoes have been adapted to compensate for length discrepancy.
Spastic hemiplegia	Cerebral palsy, unilateral upper motor neuron lesion (e.g., stroke)	Extension of one lower extremity with plantar flexion and foot inversion; arm is flexed at the elbow, wrist, and fingers. The patient walks by swinging the affected leg in a semicircle. The foot is not lifted off the floor. The affected arm does not swing with the gait.
Scissors	Multiple sclerosis, bilateral upper motor neuron disease	Adduction at the knee level produces short, slow steps. Gait is uncoordinated, stiff, and jerky. The foot is dragged across the floor in a semicircle.
Cerebellar ataxia	Cerebellar disease	Gait is broad based and uncoordinated, and the patient appears to stagger and sway during ambulation.
Sensory ataxia	Disorders of peripheral nerves, dorsal roots, and posterior column that interfere with proprioceptive input	Stance is broad based. Patient lifts feet up too high and abruptly slaps them on the floor, heel first. The patient watches the floor carefully to help ensure correct foot placement because the patient is unaware of position in space.

TABLE 18-2   Examples of Abnormal Gait Patterns *continued*

TYPE OF ABNORMAL GAIT	ETIOLOGY	DESCRIPTION
Festinating	Parkinson's disease	Decreased step height and length, but increased step speed, resulting in "shuffling" (feet barely clearing the floor). Patient's posture is stooped and patient appears to hesitate both in initiation and in termination of ambulation. Rigid body position, with flexion of the knees during standing and ambulation.
Steppage or footdrop	Peroneal nerve injury, paralysis of the dorsiflexor muscles, damage to spinal nerve roots L5 and S1 from poliomyelitis	Hip and knee flexion are needed for step height in order to lift the foot off the floor. Instead of placing the heel of the foot on the floor first, the whole sole of the foot is slapped on the floor at once. May be unilateral or bilateral.
Apraxic	Alzheimer's disease, frontal lobe tumors	Patient has difficulty with walking despite intact motor and sensory systems. The patient is unable to initiate walking, as if stuck to the floor. After walking is initiated, the gait is slow and shuffling.
Trendelenburg	Developmental dysplasia of hip, muscular dystrophy	During ambulation, pelvis of the unaffected side drops when weight bearing is performed on the affected side. When both hips are affected, a "waddling" gait may be evident.

Source: Reprinted with permission from *Orthopedic Nursing* (3rd ed.), A. Maher, S. Salmond, & T. Pellino, Copyright 2002, Philadelphia: Elsevier.

TABLE 18-3	Involuntary Muscle Movements

TYPE	DESCRIPTION
Fasciculation	Visible twitching of a group of muscle fibers that may be stimulated by the tapping of a muscle.
Fibrillation	Ineffective, uncoordinated muscle contraction that resembles quivering.
Spasm	Sudden muscle contraction. A cramp is a muscle spasm that is strong and painful. Clonic muscle spasms are contractions that alternate with a period of muscle relaxation. A tonic muscle spasm is a sustained contraction with a period of relaxation.
Tetany	Paroxysmal tonic muscle spasms, usually of the extremities. The face and jaw may also be affected by spasm. Tetany may be associated with discomfort.
Chorea	Rapid, irregular, and jerky muscle contractions of random muscle groups. It is unpredictable and without purpose. It can involve the face, upper trunk, and limbs. Sometimes, the patient tries to incorporate the movement into voluntary movement, which may appear grotesque and exaggerated. The patient may have difficulty with chewing, speaking, and swallowing.
Tremors	A period of continuous shaking due to muscle contractions. Although the quality of the tremors will be influenced by the cause, the amplitude and the frequency should remain the same. Tremors may be fine or coarse, rapid or slow, continuous or intermittent. They may be exacerbated during rest and attempts at purposeful movements, or by certain body positions.
Tic	Sudden, rapid muscle spasms of the upper trunk, face, or shoulders. The action is often repetitive and may decrease during purposeful movement. It can be persistent or limited in nature.
Ballism	Jerky, twisting movements due to strong muscle contraction.
Athetosis	Slow, writhing, twisting type of movement. The patient is unable to sustain any part of the body in one position. The movements are most often in the fingers, hands, face, throat, and tongue, although any part of the body can be affected. The movements are generally slower than in chorea.
Dystonia	Similar to athetosis but differing in the duration of the postural abnormality, and involving large muscles such as the trunk. The patient may present with an overflexed or overextended posture of the hand, pulling of the head to one side, torsion of the spine, inversion of the foot, or closure of the eyes along with a fixed grimace.
Myoclonus	A rapid, irregular contraction of a muscle or group of muscles, such as the type of jerking movement that occurs when drifting off to sleep.
Tremors at rest	Asymmetrical and coarse movements that disappear or diminish with action. They tend to diminish or cease with purposeful movement.
Action tremors	Symmetrical or asymmetrical movements that increase in states of fatigue, weakness, drug withdrawal, hypocalcemia, uremia, or hepatic disease. This type of tremor may be induced in a normal individual when he or she is required to maintain a posture that demands extremes of power or precision. Action tremors are also called postural tremors.
Intention tremors	These tremors may appear only on voluntary movement of a limb and may intensify on termination of movement.
Asterixis	This is a variant of a tremor. The rate of limb flexion and extension is irregular, slow, and of wide amplitude. The outstretched limb temporarily loses muscle tone.

N   Joint contour should be somewhat flat in extension, and smooth and rounded in flexion. You should be unable to detect any difference between periarticular tissue, the skin, and subcutaneous tissue. Bilateral joints should be symmetrical in position and appearance. There should be no observable erythema, swelling, bruising, nodules, deformities, masses, skin atrophy, or skin breakdown.

A   Enlargement of the joint.

P   Joint inflammation from inflammatory disorders such as rheumatoid arthritis and gout, trauma.

A   Deformity of the joint capsule.

P   Joint contractures, joint destruction, joint dislocation or subluxation.

A   Alteration in periarticular skin and subcutaneous tissue.

P   Joint trauma (strain, sprain, contusion, dislocation, subluxation, fracture within or near the joint capsule).

Palpation

Muscle Tone

E   1. Palpate the muscle by applying light pressure with the finger pads of the dominant hand.

2. Note the change in muscle shape as the muscle belly tapers off to become a tendon.

3. Ask the patient to alternately perform muscle relaxation and isometric muscle contraction. Note the change in palpable muscle tone between relaxation and isometric contraction.

4. Palpate the muscle belly during contraction induced by voluntary movement of a nearby joint.

5. Perform passive range of motion to all extremities and note whether these movements are smooth and sustained.

N   Muscle tone refers to the partial muscle contraction state that is maintained in order for the muscle to respond quickly to the next stimulus. On palpation, the muscle should feel smooth and firm, even

during the phase of muscle relaxation. Normal muscle tone provides light resistance to passive stretch. During muscle contraction, especially against moderate external resistance to nearby joint movement, you will be able to palpate a significant overall increase in the firmness of the muscle belly. Muscle tone increases during anxiety or excitable states. Tone decreases during rest and sleep. You will be able to palpate the muscle belly and detect a change in its shape as it tapers down to become a tendon. The hypertrophied muscle will have a distinctive contour. You will detect muscle tautness even during the phase of relaxation.

A   Hypotonicity (flaccidity) is a decrease in muscle tone.

P   Diseases involving the muscles, anterior horn cells, or peripheral nerves.

P   Spasticity refers to an increase in muscle tension on passive stretching.

P   Upper motor neuron dysfunction.

A   Muscle spasm represents persistent muscle contraction without relaxation.

P   Fracture, paralysis, electrolyte imbalance, peripheral vascular disease, cerebral palsy.

A   Crepitus refers to a grating or crackling sensation caused by two rough musculoskeletal surfaces rubbing together.

P   Shaft fracture due to trauma or loss of bone density.

A   Muscle masses.

P   Muscle rupture, tendon rupture, displaced fracture, complete dislocation.

Joints

E   1. With the joint in its neutral anatomic position, begin palpating the joint by applying light pressure with the finger pads of the dominant hand 5 to 7 cm away from the centre of the joint.

2. Palpate from the periphery inward to the centre of the joint.

3. Note any swelling, pain, tenderness, warmth, or nodules.

N   When the major skeletal joints are palpated in their neutral anatomic positions,

---

E   **Examination**   N   **Normal Findings**   A   **Abnormal Findings**   P   **Pathophysiology**

the external joint contour will feel smooth, strong, and firm. The shape of the joint corresponds to that specific joint type. The area surrounding the joint (periarticular tissue) is free from swelling, pain, tenderness, warmth, or nodules. As the joint is moved through its normal range of motion, it should be able to articulate in proper alignment without any visible or palpable deformity. Palpation of joint movement produces a smooth sensation, without tactile detection of grating or popping.

A Bony enlargement or bony deformities.

P Urate deposits associated with gout.

A Subcutaneous nodules.

P Rheumatoid arthritis, tophi nodules in chronic gout.

A Crepitus.

P Acute rheumatoid arthritis, degenerative joint disease.

A Any tenderness felt on light touch or joint palpation.

P Septic arthritis, increased joint capsule pressure with a joint effusion, joint contusion, infection, synovitis.

A Periarticular warmth.

P Joint inflammation, gout.

Range of Motion (ROM)

E 1. Ask the patient to move the joint through each of its various ROM movements.
2. Note angle of each joint movement.
3. Note any pain, tenderness, or crepitus.
4. If the patient is unable to perform active ROM, then passively move each joint through its ROM.
5. Always stop if the patient complains of pain, and never push a joint beyond its anatomic angle.

N Refer to the specific sections on joints for the ROM for each joint movement (see Table 18-1).

A Abnormalities of joint function are indicated by the inability of the patient to voluntarily and comfortably move a joint in the directions and to the degrees that are considered the norms for that joint.

P Degenerative joint disease, rheumatoid arthritis, and joint trauma are some of the many musculoskeletal disorders that prevent the affected joint from moving through its normal ROM.

Muscle Strength

Each muscle group is assessed for strength via the same movements as are performed in range of motion.

E 1. Note whether muscle groups are strong and equal.
2. Always compare right and left sides of paired muscle groups.
3. Note involuntary movements.

N Normal muscle strength allows for complete voluntary range of joint motion against both gravity and moderate to full resistance. Muscle strength is equal bilaterally. There is no observed involuntary muscle movement.

A A decrease in skeletal muscle strength is significant if complete range of joint motion is either impossible or possible only without resistance or gravity.

P Local decrease in muscle strength will accompany muscle atrophy of the limbs secondary to disuse.

P Diffuse reduction in muscle strength is associated with general atrophy, severe fatigue, malnutrition, muscle relaxant medications, long-term steroid use, and deteriorating neuromuscular disorders. (ALS, MD, MS, myasthenia gravis, and Guillain-Barré syndrome).

A One-sided muscle weakness or paralysis.

P Unilateral weakness or paralysis is indicative of hemiparesis (hemiplegia) from a cerebrovascular accident, brain tumour, or head trauma.

Examination of Joints

Temporomandibular Joint

E 1. Stand in front of the patient.
2. Inspect the right and left temporomandibular joints.

E **Examination**   N **Normal Findings**   A **Abnormal Findings**   P **Pathophysiology**

3. Palpate the temporomandibular joints.
   a. Place your index and middle fingers over the joint.
   b. Ask the patient to open and close the mouth.
   c. Feel the depression into which your fingers move with an open mouth.
   d. Note the smoothness with which the mandible moves.
   e. Note any audible or palpable click as the mouth opens.
4. Assess ROM. Ask the patient to:
   a. Open the mouth as wide as possible.
   b. Push out the lower jaw.
   c. Move the jaw from side to side.
5. Palpate the strength of the masseter and temporalis muscles as the patient clenches the teeth. This assesses cranial nerve V.

N It is normal to hear or palpate a click when the mouth opens. The mouth can normally open 3 to 6 cm with ease. The lower jaw protrudes without deviating to the side and moves 1 to 2 cm with lateral movement.

A Pain, limited ROM, crepitus.

P Temporomandibular joint dysfunction secondary to malocclusion, arthritis, dislocation, poorly fitting dentures, myofacial dysfunction, trauma.

Cervical Spine

E 1. Stand behind the patient.
2. Inspect the position of the cervical spine.
3. Palpate the spinous processes of the cervical spine and the muscles of the neck.
4. Stand in front of the patient.
5. Assess the ROM of the cervical spine. Ask the patient to:
   a. Touch the chin to the chest (flexion).
   b. Look up at the ceiling (hyperextension).
   c. Move each ear to the shoulder on its respective side without

elevating the shoulder (lateral bending).
   d. Turn the head to each side to look at the shoulder (rotation).
6. Assess strength of the cervical spine by repeating the movements in step 5d while applying opposing force. This also assesses the function of cranial nerve XI.

N The cervical spine's alignment is straight and the head is held erect. The normal ROM for the cervical spine is flexion—45°, hyperextension—55°, lateral bending—40° to each side, rotation—70° to each side. Hypertrophy of the neck muscles due to weight-lifting exercises will produce the appearance of a thick neck.

A A neck that is not erect and straight.

P Degenerative joint disease of the cervical vertebrae, torticollis.

A A change in the size of the neck.

P Klippel-Feil syndrome (congenital absence of one or more cervical vertebrae along with fusion of the upper cervical vertebrae and bilateral elevation of the scapulae, resulting in a shortened neck appearance).

A Inability of the patient to perform ROM, and pain and tenderness on palpation.

P Osteoarthritis, neck injury, disc degeneration (among aging patients or from occupational stress), spondylosis.

Shoulders

E 1. Stand in front of the patient.
2. Inspect the size, shape, and symmetry of the shoulders.
3. Move behind the patient and inspect the scapula for size, shape, and symmetry.
4. Palpate the shoulders and surrounding muscles.
   a. Move from the sternoclavicular joint along the clavicle to the acromioclavicular joint.
   b. Palpate the acromion process, subcromial area, greater tubercle of the humerus, the anterior aspect of the glenohumeral joint, and the biceps groove.

| **E Examination** | **N Normal Findings** | **A Abnormal Findings** | **P Pathophysiology** |

5. Assess ROM of the shoulders. Ask the patient to:
   a. Place arms at the side, elbows extended, and move the arms forward in an arc (forward flexion).
   b. Move the arms backward in an arc as far as possible (hyperextension).
   c. Place arms at side, elbows extended, and move both arms out to the sides in an arc until the palms touch together overhead (abduction).
   d. Move one arm at a time in an arc toward the midline and cross it as far as possible (adduction).
   e. Place hands behind the back and reach up, trying to touch the scapula (internal rotation).
   f. Place both hands behind the head with elbows flexed (external rotation).
   g. Shrug the shoulders. This assesses cranial nerve XI function.
6. Assess strength of the shoulders by applying opposing force to the ROM movement in step 5g.

N The shoulders are equal in height. There is no fluid palpable in the shoulder area. Crepitus is absent. The normal ROM for the shoulder is forward flexion—180°, hyperextension—50°, abduction—180°, adduction—50°, internal rotation—90°, external rotation—90°.

A Increased outward prominence of the scapula (winging).

P Serratus anterior muscle injury or weakness.

A Decreased movement, pain with movement, swelling from fluid, and asymmetry.

P Immobility, osteoarthritis, injury, frozen shoulder (adhesive capsulitis), bursitis, acromioclavicular joint separation, shoulder subluxation, dislocation.

Elbows

E 1. Stand to the side of the elbow being examined.
   2. Support the patient's forearm on the side that is being examined (approximately 70°).

3. Inspect the elbow in flexed and extended positions. Note the olecranon process and the grooves on each side of the olecranon process.
4. Using your thumb and middle fingers, palpate the elbow. Note the olecranon process, the olecranon bursa, the groove on each side of the olecranon process, and the medial and lateral epicondyles of the humerus.
5. Assess ROM of the elbows. Ask the patient to:
   a. Bend the elbow (flexion).
   b. Straighten the elbow (extension).
   c. Hold the arm straight out, bent at the elbow, and turn the palm upward toward the ceiling (supination).
   d. Turn the palm downward toward the floor (pronation).
6. Assess strength of the elbow:
   a. Stabilize the patient's arm at the elbow with your non-dominant hand. With your dominant hand, grasp the patient's wrist.
   b. Ask the patient to flex the elbow (pulling it toward the chest) while you apply opposing resistance.
   c. Ask the patient to extend the elbow (pushing it away from the chest) while you apply opposing resistance.

N The elbows are at the same height and are symmetrical in appearance. The normal ROM for the elbow is flexion—160°, extension—0°, supination—90°, pronation—90°.

A Elbows that are not symmetrical. Pain is present.

P Dislocation or a subluxation of the elbow.

A Localized tenderness and pain with elbow flexion, extension, or both.

P Epicondylitis from repetitive motions, radial head fractures.

A Red, warm, swollen, and tender areas in the grooves beside the olecranon process.

P Inflammatory processes such as gouty arthritis, rheumatoid arthritis, SLE.

| E **Examination** | N **Normal Findings** | A **Abnormal Findings** | P **Pathophysiology** |

Wrists and Hands

E 1. Stand in front of the patient.
   2. Inspect the wrists and the palmar and dorsal aspects of the hands. Note the shape, position, contour, and number of fingers.
   3. Inspect the thenar eminence (the rounded prominence at the base of the thumb).
   4. Support the patient's hand in your two hands, with your fingers underneath the patient's hands and your thumbs on the dorsum of the patient's hand.
   5. Palpate the joints of the wrists by moving your thumbs from side to side. Feel the natural indentations.
   6. Palpate the joints of the hand:
      a. Use your thumbs to palpate the metacarpophalangeal joints, which are immediately distal to and on each side of the knuckle.
      b. Between your thumb and index finger, gently pinch the sides of the proximal and distal interphalangeal joints.
   7. Assess the ROM of the wrists and hands. Ask the patient to:
      a. Straighten the hand (extension) and bend it up at the wrist toward the ceiling (hyperextension).
      b. Bend the hand down at the wrist toward the floor (flexion).
      c. Bend the fingers up at the metacarpophalangeal joint toward the ceiling (hyperextension).
      d. Bend the fingers down at the metacarpophalangeal joint toward the floor (flexion).
      e. Place the hands on a flat surface and move them side to side (radial deviation is movement toward the thumb, and ulnar deviation is movement toward the little finger) without moving the elbow.
      f. Ask the patient to make a fist with the thumb on the outside of the clenched fingers.
      g. Spread the fingers apart.
      h. Touch the thumb to each fingertip. Touch the thumb to the base of the little finger.
   8. Assess the strength of the wrists. Ask the patient to:
      a. Place the arm on a table with the forearm supinated. Stabilize the forearm by placing your non-dominant hand on it.
      b. Flex the wrist while you apply resistance with your dominant hand.
      c. Extend the wrist while you apply resistance.
   9. Assess the strength of the fingers. Ask the patient to:
      a. Spread the fingers apart while you apply resistance.
      b. Push the fingers together while you apply resistance.
   10. Assess the strength of the hand grasp. Ask the patient to:
      a. Grasp your dominant index and middle fingers in the patient's dominant hand and your non-dominant index and middle fingers in the patient's non-dominant hand.
      b. Squeeze your fingers as hard as possible.
      c. Release the grasp.

N There are five fingers on each hand. The normal range of motion for the wrists is extension—0°, hyperextension—70°, flexion—90°, radial deviation—20°, ulnar deviation—55°. The normal range of motion for the metacarpophalangeal joints is hyperextension—30° and flexion—90°.

A Extra fingers, loss of fingers, or webbing between fingers.

P Polydactyly is the congenital presence of extra digits. Syndactyly is the congenital webbing or fusion of fingers or toes.

A Bony enlargement or bony deformities of the joints of the hand.

P Osteoarthritis is associated with bony enlargement of the proximal interphalangeal joint (Bouchard's node) and the

---

E **Examination**   N **Normal Findings**   A **Abnormal Findings**   P **Pathophysiology**

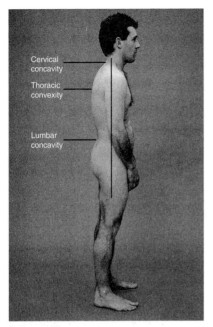

A. Lateral View

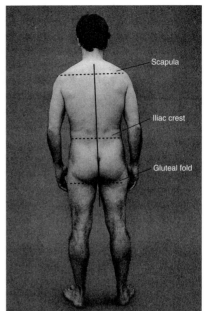

B. Posterior View

FIGURE 18-3 Alignment of Spinal Landmarks.

distal interphalangeal joint (Heberden's node) of the finger, rheumatoid arthritis results in ulnar deviation.
A A round, cystic growth near the tendons of the wrist or joint capsule.
P Ganglion (benign growth)—etiology is unknown.
A Flexion of the fingers.
P Dupuytren's contracture.
A Muscular atrophy of the thenar eminence.
P Median nerve compression such as in carpal tunnel syndrome.
A Severe flexion ankylosis of the wrist.
P Rheumatoid arthritis or severe disuse.
A Tenderness over the distal radius.
P Colles fracture or fracture of the distal radius.
A Wrist drop, inability to flex wrist.
P Radial nerve injury may.
A Inability to prevent moving of spread fingers together.
P Ulnar nerve injury.

A Weakness of opposition of thumb.
P Median nerve disorders, such as carpal tunnel syndrome.

Hips

E **1.** While the patient is standing, inspect the iliac crests, size and symmetry of the buttocks, and number of gluteal folds.
   2. Observe the patient's gait.
   3. Assist the patient to a supine position on the examination table with the legs straight and the feet pointing toward the ceiling.
   4. Palpate the hip joints.
   5. Assess ROM of the hips. Ask the patient to:
      a. Raise the leg straight off the examination table with the knee extended (hip flexion with knee straight). The other leg should remain on the table.

| E Examination | N Normal Findings | A Abnormal Findings | P Pathophysiology |

b. With the knee flexed, raise the leg off the examination table toward the chest as far as possible (hip flexion with knee flexed). The other leg should remain on the table. This is called the Thomas test.

c. Flex the hip and knee. Move the flexed leg medially as the foot moves outward (internal rotation).

d. Flex the hip and knee. Move the flexed leg laterally as the foot moves medially (external rotation).

e. With the knee straight, swing the leg away from the midline (abduction).

f. With the knee straight, swing the leg toward the midline (adduction).

g. Roll over onto the abdomen and assume a prone position.

h. From the hip, move the leg back as far as possible while maintaining the pelvis on the table (hyperextension). This can also be performed while the patient is standing.

6. Assist the patient to a supine position.

7. Assess strength of the hips.

a. Place the palm of your hand on the anterior thigh, above the knee. Instruct the patient to raise the leg against your resistance. Repeat on the other leg.

b. Place the palm of your hand posteriorly above and behind the knee. Instruct the patient to lower the leg against your resistance. Repeat on the other leg.

c. Place your hands on the lateral aspects of the patient's legs at the level of the knee. Instruct the patient to move the legs apart against your resistance.

d. Place your hands on the medial aspects of the patient's legs just above the knee. Instruct the patient to move the legs together against your resistance.

N The normal ROM for the hips is flexion with knee straight—90°, flexion with knee flexed—120°, internal rotation—40°, external rotation—45°, abduction—45°, adduction—30°, hyperextension—15°.

A Leg is externally rotated and painful on movement.

P Hip fractures, which usually result from falls.

A A positive Thomas test, when the patient is unable to flex one knee and hip while simultaneously maintaining the other leg in full extension.

P Flexion contractures of the hip joint (degenerative joint diseases).

Knees

E **1.** With the patient standing, note the position of the knees in relation to each other and in relation to the hips, thighs, ankles, and feet.

2. Ask the patient to sit on the examination table with the knees flexed and resting at the edge of the table.

3. Inspect the contour of the knees. Note the normal depressions around the patella.

4. Inspect the suprapatellar pouch and the prepatellar bursa.

5. Note the quadriceps muscle, located on the anterior thigh.

6. Palpate the knees. The patient may assume a supine position if this is more comfortable.

a. Grasp the anterior thigh approximately 10 cm above the patella, with your thumb on one side of the knee and the other four fingers on the other side of the knee.

b. As you palpate, gradually move your hand down the suprapatellar pouch.

7. Palpate the tibiofemoral joints. It is best to have the knee flexed to 90° when performing this assessment.

E **Examination** **N** **Normal Findings** **A** **Abnormal Findings** **P** **Pathophysiology**

a. Place both thumbs on the knee, with the fingers wrapped around the knee posteriorly.

b. Press in with the thumbs as you palpate the tibial margins.

c. Palpate the lateral collateral ligament.

8. Assess ROM of the knees. Ask the patient to stand and:

a. Bend the knee (flexion).

b. Straighten the knee (extension). The patient may also be able to hyperextend the knee during this movement.

9. Assess strength of the knees with the patient seated and the legs hanging off the table.

a. Ask the patient to bend the knee. Place your non-dominant hand under the knee and place your other hand over the ankle.

b. Instruct the patient to straighten the leg against your resistance.

c. Ask the patient to place the foot on the bed and the knee at approximately 45° of flexion. Place one hand under the knee and place the other hand over the ankle.

d. Instruct the patient to maintain the foot on the table despite your attempts to straighten the leg.

N The knees are in alignment with each other and do not protrude medially or laterally. The normal ROM for the knees is flexion—130°, extension—0°; in some cases, hyperextension is possible up to 15°.

A Alteration in lower limb alignment.

P Genu valgum (knock knees), genu varum (bow legs).

A Knee effusion.

P Baker cyst.

Ankles and Feet

E 1. Inspect the ankles and feet as the patient stands, walks, and sits (bearing no weight).

2. Inspect the alignment of the feet and toes with the lower leg.

3. Inspect the shape and position of the toes.

4. Assist the patient to a supine position on the examination table.

5. Stand by the patient's feet.

6. Palpate the ankle and foot.

a. Grasp the heel with the fingers of both hands. Palpate the posterior aspect of the heel at the calcaneus.

b. Use your thumbs to palpate the medial malleolus (bony prominence on the distal medial aspect of the tibia) and the lateral malleolus (bony prominence on the distal lateral aspect of the fibula).

c. Move your hands forward and palpate the anterior aspects of the ankle and foot, particularly at the joints.

d. Palpate the inferior aspect of the foot over the plantar fascia.

e. Use your finger pads to palpate the Achilles tendon.

f. Palpate with your thumb and index finger each metatarsophalangeal joint.

g. Between your thumb and index finger, palpate the medial and lateral surfaces of each interphalangeal joint.

7. Assess ROM of the ankles and feet. Ask the patient to:

a. Point the toes toward the chest by moving the ankle (dorsiflexion).

b. Point the toes toward the floor by moving the ankle (plantar flexion).

c. Turn the soles of the feet outward (eversion).

d. Turn the soles of the feet inward (inversion).

e. Curl the toes toward the floor (flexion).

E **Examination**   N **Normal Findings**   A **Abnormal Findings**   P **Pathophysiology**

f. Spread the toes apart (abduction).

g. Move the toes together (adduction).

8. Assess strength of the ankles and feet.

a. Assist the patient to a supine position on the examination table with the legs extended and the feet slightly apart.

b. Stand at the foot of the examination table.

c. Place your left hand on top of the patient's right foot and place your right hand on top of the patient's left foot.

d. Ask the patient to point the toes toward the chest (dorsiflexion) despite your resistance.

e. Place your left hand on the sole of the patient's right foot and place your right hand on the sole of the patient's left foot.

f. Ask the patient to point the toes down (plantar flexion) despite your resistance.

N   The foot is in alignment with the lower leg. The foot has a longitudinal arch. There is no pain over the plantar fascia. The normal ROM for the ankles and feet is dorsiflexion—20°, plantar flexion—45°, eversion—20°, inversion—30°, abduction—30°, and adduction—10°.

A   Alteration in the shape and the position of the foot.

P   Pes varus describes a foot that is turned inward toward the midline.

P   Pes valgus occurs when the foot is turned laterally away from the midline.

P   Pes planus (flat foot) refers to a foot with a low longitudinal arch.

P   Pes cavus refers to a foot with an exaggerated arch height.

P   In hallux valgus (bunion), the big toe is deviated laterally while the first metatarsal is deviated medially.

P   In hammertoe, there is a flexion of the proximal interphalangeal joint and hyperextension of the distal metatarsophalangeal joint.

A   Pain over the plantar fascia.

P   Plantar fasciitis (heel-spur syndrome).

A   Swollen, red, warm, and painful metatarsophalangeal joint.

P   Acute gouty arthritis.

A   Decreased ROM of the ankle.

P   Ankle sprain or fracture secondary to injury or trauma.

Spine

E   1. Ask the patient to stand and to leave the back of the gown open.

2. Stand behind the patient so that you can visualize the posterior anatomy.

3. Inspect the position and alignment of the spine from a posterior and a lateral position.

4. Draw an imaginary line:

a. From the head down through the spinous processes (Figure 18-3A).

b. Across the top of the scapula (Figure 18-3B).

c. Across the top of the iliac crests.

d. Across the bottom of the gluteal folds.

5. Palpate the spinous processes with your thumb.

6. Palpate the paravertebral muscles.

7. Assess ROM of the spine. Ask the patient to bend forward from the waist and touch the toes (flexion).

8. If necessary, stabilize the patient's pelvis with your hands during the ROM assessment. Ask the patient to:

a. Bend to each side (lateral bending).

b. Bend backward (hyperextension).

c. Twist the shoulders to each side (rotation).

N   The normal spine has a cervical concavity, a thoracic convexity, and a lumbar concavity. An imaginary line can be drawn from the head straight down the spinous processes to the gluteal cleft. The imaginary lines drawn from the scapula, iliac crests, and gluteal folds are symmetrical with each other. The normal ROM of the spine is flexion—90°, hyperexten-

---

E   **Examination**   N   **Normal Findings**   A   **Abnormal Findings**   P   **Pathophysiology**

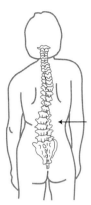 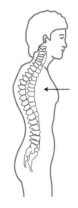 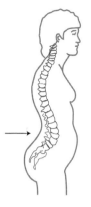 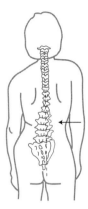

A. Scoliosis   **B.** Kyphosis   **C.** Lordosis   **D.** List

FIGURE 18-4 Abnormalities of the Spine.

sion—30°, lateral bending—35°, and rotation—30°. As the patient flexes forward, the concavity of the lumbar spine disappears and the entire back assumes a convex C shape.

A Scoliosis (lateral curvature of the thoracic or lumbar vertebrae) (Figure 18-4A).

P Structural scoliosis occurs most frequently in adolescence, especially in females. Functional scoliosis, which manifests itself only in a standing position, is due to unequal leg length or poor posture.

A Kyphosis, an excessive convexity of the thoracic spine (Figure 18-4B).

P Osteoporosis, ankylosing spondylitis, Paget's disease.

A Lordosis, an excessive concavity of the lumbar spine (Figure 18-4C).

P Obesity, pregnancy.

A A list, a leaning of the spine (Figure 18-4D).

P Herniated vertebral disc, paravertebral muscle spasms.

A Iliac crests that are unequal in height.

P Scoliosis and congenital or acquired limb length discrepancies.

A Decreased ROM.

P Back injury, osteoarthritis, ankylosing spondylitis.

E Examination   N Normal Findings   A Abnormal Findings   P Pathophysiology

19

Mental Status and Neurological Techniques

The nervous system controls all body functions and thought processes. The complex interrelationships among the various divisions of the nervous system permit the body to maintain homeostasis; receive, interpret, and react to stimuli; and control voluntary and involuntary processes, including cognition.

ANATOMY AND PHYSIOLOGY
Meninges

There are three layers of meninges (protective membranes), known as the dura mater, arachnoid mater, and pia mater, located between the brain and the skull. The dura mater is the thick, tough outermost layer. The arachnoid mater lies between the dura mater and the pia mater. Below the arachnoid mater is the subarachnoid space, where cerebrospinal fluid (CSF) is circulated. The pia mater is thin and vascular. It is the innermost layer of the meninges.

Central Nervous System

The brain and the spinal cord make up the central nervous system (CNS). The brain is divided into four main components: the cerebrum, the diencephalon, the cerebellum, and the brain stem (Figure 19-1).

The cerebrum is incompletely divided into right and left hemispheres. The two hemispheres are connected by the corpus callosum, which serves as a communication link. The cerebral cortex, or the outermost layer of the cerebrum, is involved in memory storage and recall, conscious understanding of sensation, vision, hearing, and motor function.

The diencephalon, a relay centre for the brain, is composed of the thalamus, the epithalamus, and the hypothalamus. The hypothalamus is important in body temperature regulation, pituitary hormone control, and autonomic nervous system responses. It also plays a role in behaviour via its connections with the limbic system.

The cerebellum is divided into two lateral lobes and a medial part called the vermis. The vermis is the part of the cerebellum concerned primarily with maintenance of posture and equilibrium. Each cerebellar hemisphere is responsible for coordination of movement of the ipsilateral (same) side of the body.

The brain stem is located immediately below the diencephalon and is divided into the midbrain, the pons, and the medulla oblongata. The midbrain contains the nuclei of cranial nerves III (oculomotor) and IV (trochlear), which are associated with control of eye movements. Sensory and motor nuclei of cranial nerves V (trigeminal), VI (abducens), VII (facial), and VIII (acoustic) are located in the pons. The medulla oblongata contains the nuclei of cranial nerves IX (glossopharyngeal), X (vagus), XI (spinal accessory), and XII (hypoglossal).

The spinal cord is a continuation of the medulla oblongata (Figure 19-2). A cross-section of the spinal cord shows that the central part of the cord is grey matter. The grey matter is in the shape of an H and is surrounded by white matter.

There are three motor pathways in the CNS: the corticospinal or pyramidal tract, the extrapyramidal tract, and the cerebellum.

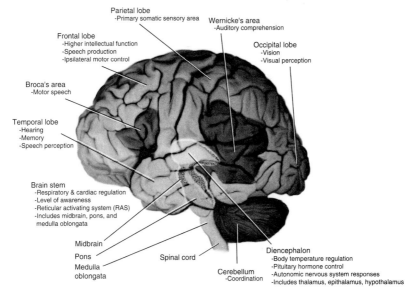

FIGURE 19-1 The Locations and Functions of the Cerebral Lobes, Diencephalon, Cerebellum, and Brain Stem.

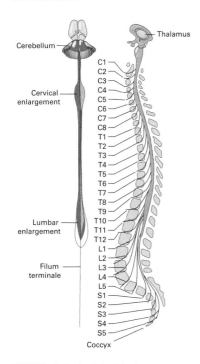

FIGURE 19-2 The Spinal Cord.

Blood is supplied to the brain by two pairs of arteries, the internal carotid arteries (anterior circulation) and the vertebral arteries (posterior circulation).

Peripheral Nervous System

The peripheral nervous system consists of nervous tissue found outside the CNS, including the spinal nerves, cranial nerves, and the autonomic nervous system. The 31 pairs of spinal nerves include 8 cervical, 12 thoracic, 5 lumbar, 5 sacral, and 1 coccygeal. There are 12 pairs of cranial nerves. Table 19-1 summarizes the functions of the cranial nerves.

The autonomic nervous system (ANS) is divided into two functionally different subdivisions: the sympathetic and parasympathetic nervous systems. The ANS functions without voluntary control to maintain the body in a state of homeostasis. See Table 19-2 for specific system responses to autonomic stimulation.

Reflexes

Reflexes are classified into three main categories: muscle stretch, or deep tendon reflexes (DTR); superficial reflexes; and pathological reflexes.

TABLE 19-1	The 12 Cranial Nerves and Their Functions

NAME AND NUMBER	FUNCTION
Olfactory (I)	Smell
Optic (II)	Visual acuity, visual fields, funduscopic examination
Oculomotor (III)	Cardinal fields of gaze (EOM movement), eyelid elevation, pupil reaction, doll's eyes phenomenon
Trochlear (IV)	EOM movement
Trigeminal (V)	Motor: strength of temporalis and masseter muscles Sensory: light touch, superficial pain and temperature to face, corneal reflex
Abducens (VI)	EOM movement
Facial (VII)	Motor: facial movements Sensory: taste anterior two-thirds of tongue *Parasympathetic: tears and saliva secretion
Acoustic (VIII)	Cochlear: gross hearing, Weber and Rinne tests Vestibular: vertigo, equilibrium, nystagmus
Glossopharyngeal (IX)	Motor: soft palate and uvula movement, gag reflex, swallowing, guttural and palatal sounds Sensory: taste posterior one-third of tongue *Parasympathetic: carotid reflex, chemoreceptors
Vagus (X)	Motor and Sensory: same as CN IX *Parasympathetic: carotid reflex, stomach and intestinal secretions, peristalsis, involuntary control of bronchi, heart innervation
Spinal Accessory (XI)	Sternocleidomastoid and trapezius muscle movements
Hypoglossal (XII)	Tongue movement, lingual sounds

*Cannot be directly assessed.   EOM = extraocular muscle; CN = cranial nerve.

TABLE 19-2	Sympathetic versus Parasympathetic Response

SYSTEM	SYMPATHETIC RESPONSE	PARASYMPATHETIC RESPONSE
Neurological	Pupils dilated Heightened awareness	Pupils normal size
Cardiovascular	Increased heart rate Increased myocardial contractility Increased blood pressure	Decreased heart rate Decreased myocardial contractility
Respiratory	Increased respiratory rate Increased respiratory depth Bronchial dilation	Bronchial constriction
Gastrointestinal	Decreased gastric motility Decreased gastric secretions Increased glycogenolysis Decreased insulin production Sphincter contraction	Increased gastric motility Increased gastric secretions Sphincter dilatation
Genitourinary	Decreased urine output Decreased renal blood flow	Normal urine output

HEALTH HISTORY

Medical History	Amyotrophic lateral sclerosis (ALS), multiple sclerosis (MS), tumours, Guillain-Barré syndrome, cerebral aneurysm, arteriovenous malformations (AVM), stroke (brain attack), migraines, Alzheimer's disease, myasthenia gravis, congenital defects, metabolic disorders, childhood seizures, head trauma, neuropathies, peripheral vascular disease, Parkinson's disease
Surgical History	Craniotomy, laminectomy, carotid endarterectomy, transsphenoidal hypophysectomy, cordotomy, aneurysmectomy or repair
Medications	Antidepressants, antiseizure medications, narcotics, antianxiety medications, antipsychotic medications
Injuries and Accidents	Closed head injury, chronic subdural hematoma, spinal cord injury, peripheral nerve damage
Family Health History	Congenital defects such as neural tube defects, hydrocephalus, arteriovenous malformation (AVM), headaches, epilepsy, Alzheimer's disease, Huntington's chorea, muscular dystrophies, lipid storage diseases, Gaucher's disease, Niemann-Pick's disease
Alcohol Use	Patients suffering from chronic alcoholism may exhibit the following abnormal findings: Korsakoff's psychosis, polyneuropathy, Wernicke's encephalopathy, tremor

Nursing Alert

Brain Attack (Stroke, Cerebrovascular Accident)–Risk Factors[1]

Unmodifiable
Age
• Over 2/3 of all strokes occur in people over 65 years.

Gender
• Men have a higher risk than women.

Ethnicity
• Aboriginal Canadians and people of African, Hispanic, South Asian, and Black descent have higher rates of high blood pressure and diabetes—conditions that can lead to stroke.

Family History
• Risk of having a stroke is higher if a parent or sibling had a stroke before the age of 65.

Modifiable
Hypertension
• High blood pressure is the single most important modifiable risk factor for stroke.

Diabetes Mellitus
Smoking
High Blood Cholesterol
Inactivity
Excessive alcohol consumption   *continued*

Signs and symptoms (any one of the following can be significant)
- Weakness, numbness, or paralysis
- Difficulty speaking or understanding
- Blurred vision or loss of vision
- Dizziness or loss of consciousness
- Sudden, severe headache

If a patient experiences any of these signs or symptoms he or she must seek prompt assessment.

EQUIPMENT

- Cotton wisp
- Cotton-tipped applicators
- Penlight
- Tongue blade
- Tuning fork: 128 Hz or 256 Hz
- Reflex hammer
- Sterile needle, either a 22-gauge needle or a sterile safety pin
- Familiar small objects (coins, key, paperclip)
- Vials containing odorous materials (coffee, orange extract, vinegar)
- Vials containing hot and cold water
- Vials with solutions for tasting: quinine (bitter), glucose solution (sweet), lemon or vinegar (sour), saline (salty)
- Snellen chart or Rosenbaum pocket screener
- Pupil gauge in millimetres

ASSESSMENT OF THE NEUROLOGICAL SYSTEM

A complete neurological assessment includes an assessment of mental status, sensation, cranial nerves, motor function, cerebellar function, and reflexes. For patients with minor or intermittent symptoms, a rapid screening assessment may be used as outlined in Table 19-3.

Mental Status

Much of the mental status assessment should be done during the interview, with the patient comfortably positioned facing you. Mental status may also be assessed throughout the neurological assessment. Assess physical appearance and behaviour, communication, level of consciousness, cognitive abilities, and mentation while talking with the patient.

Physical Appearance and Behaviour
Posture and Movements

E 1. Observe the patient's ability to wait patiently.
   2. Note if patient's posture is relaxed, slumped, or stiff.
   3. Observe the patient's movements for control and symmetry.
   4. Observe the patient's gait (see Chapter 18).

N The patient should appear relaxed with the appropriate amount of concern for the assessment. The patient should exhibit erect posture, a smooth gait, and symmetrical body movements.

A Restlessness, tenseness, pacing.
P Anxiety, metabolic disorders.
A Slumped posture, slow gait, poor eye contact, and slow responses.
P Depression.
A Stooped, flexed, or rigid posture, drooping neck, deformities of the spine, and tics.
P Kyphosis, scoliosis, Parkinson's disease, cerebral palsy, osteoporosis, schizophrenia, muscular atrophy, myasthenia gravis, stroke.

Dress, Grooming, and Personal Hygiene

E 1. Note the appearance of the patient's clothing, specifically:
   a. Cleanliness
   b. Condition

| E | **Examination** | N | **Normal Findings** | A | **Abnormal Findings** | P | **Pathophysiology** |

TABLE 19-3	Neurological Screening Assessment	

ASSESSMENT PARAMETER	ASSESSMENT SKILL	COMMENTS
Mental status	Note general appearance, affect, speech content, memory, logic, judgment, and speech patterns during the history.	If any abnormalities or inconsistencies are evident, perform full mental status assessment.
	Perform Glasgow Coma Scale (GCS) with motor assessment component and pupil assessment.	If GCS <15, perform full assessment of mental status and consciousness. If motor assessment is abnormal or asymmetrical, perform complete motor and sensory assessment.
Sensation	Assess pain and vibration in the hands and feet, light touch on the limbs.	If deficits are identified, perform a complete sensory assessment.
Cranial nerves	Assess CN II, III, IV, VI: visual acuity, gross visual fields, funduscopic examination, pupillary reactions, and extra-ocular movements. Assess CN VII, VIII, IX, X, XII: facial expression, gross hearing, voice, and tongue.	If any abnormalities exist, perform complete assessment of all 12 cranial nerves.
Motor system	• Muscle tone and strength • Abnormal movements • Grasps	If deficits are noted, perform a complete motor system assessment.

Cerebellar function	Observe the patient's:
	1. Gait on arrival
	2. Ability to:
	  • Walk heel-to-toe
	  • Walk on toes
	  • Walk on heels
	  • Hop in place
	  • Perform shallow knee bends
	
	3. Check Romberg's test
	4. Finger-to-nose test
	5. Fine repetitive movements with hands
		If any abnormalities exist, perform complete cerebellar assessment.

Reflexes	Assess the deep tendon reflexes and the plantar reflex.	If an abnormal response is elicited, perform a complete reflex assessment.

c. Age appropriateness
d. Weather appropriateness
e. Appropriateness for the patient's socioeconomic group

2. Observe the patient's personal grooming (hair, skin, nails, teeth) for:
a. Adequacy
b. Symmetry
c. Odour

E Examination	N Normal Findings	A Abnormal Findings	P Pathophysiology

◄ NURSING CHECKLIST ►

General Approach to Neurological Assessment

1. Greet the patient and explain the assessment techniques that you will be using.
2. Maintain a quiet, unhurried, self-confident demeanour to help relieve any feelings of anxiety or discomfort, and to help the patient relax during the assessment.
3. Provide a warm, quiet, and well-lit environment.
4. After the mental status examination, instruct the patient to remove all street clothes, and provide an examination gown for the patient to put on.
5. Begin the assessment with the patient in a comfortable upright sitting position, or for the patient on bed rest, position the patient comfortably, preferably with the head of the bed elevated, or flat, whichever is tolerated best or is within activity orders for the patient.

N   The patient should be clean and well groomed, and should wear appropriate clothing for age, weather, and socioeconomic status.

A   Poor personal hygiene such as uncombed hair, body odour, or unkempt clothing.

P   Depression, schizophrenia, dementia.

A   Excessive, meticulous care and attention to clothing and grooming.

P   Obsessive-compulsive behaviour.

A   One-sided differences in grooming and dressing or the use of only one side of the body.

P   Stroke in the parietal lobe.

Facial Expression

E   Observe for appropriateness of, variations in, and symmetry of facial expressions.

N   Facial expressions should be appropriate to the content of the conversation and should be symmetrical.

A   Extreme, inappropriate, or unchanging facial expressions, or asymmetrical facial movements.

P   Anxiety, depression, the unchanging facial expression of a patient with Parkinson's disease, lesion in the facial nerve (CN VII).

Affect

E   1. Observe the patient's interaction with you, paying particular atten-

tion to both verbal and non-verbal behaviours.

2. Note if the patient's affect appears labile, blunted, or flat.

3. Note the variations in the patient's affect with a variety of topics.

4. Note any extreme emotional responses during the interview.

N   The appropriateness and degree of affect should vary with the topics and the patient's cultural norms, and be reasonable, or eurhythmic (normal).

A   Blunted affect, manifested by the patient shuffling into the examination room, slumping into a chair, moving slowly and not making eye contact.

P   Depression.

A   Unresponsive, inappropriate affect.

P   Depression or schizophrenia.

A   Anger, hostility, paranoia.

P   Paranoid schizophrenic.

A   Euphoric, dramatic, disruptive, irrational, elated behaviours.

P   Bipolar disorder.

Communication

E   1. Note voice quality, which includes voice volume and pitch.

2. Assess articulation, fluency, and rate of speech by engaging the patient

---

E   **Examination**   N   **Normal Findings**   A   **Abnormal Findings**   P   **Pathophysiology**

in normal conversation. Ask the patient to repeat words and sentences after you or to name objects you point out.

3. Note the patient's ability to carry out requests during the assessment, such as pointing to objects within the room as requested. Ask questions that require "yes" and "no" responses.

4. Write simple commands for the patient to read and perform, for example "point to your nose" or "tap your right foot." Reading ability may be influenced by the patient's educational level or visual impairment.

5. Ask the patient to write the name, birthday, a sentence the patient composes, or a sentence that you dictate. Note the patient's spelling, grammatical accuracy, and logical thought process.

N The patient should be able to produce spontaneous, coherent speech. The speech should have an effortless flow with normal inflections, volume, pitch, articulation, rate, and rhythm. Content of the message should make sense. Comprehension of language should be intact. The patient's ability to read and write should match the patient's educational level. Non-native speakers may exhibit some hesitancy or inaccuracy in written and spoken language.

A Aphasia, an impairment of language functioning.

P See Table 19-4.

A Dysarthria, a disturbance in muscular control of speech.

P Ischemia affecting motor nuclei of CN X and CN XII; defects in the premotor or motor cortex that provide motor input for the face, throat, and mouth; cerebellar disease.

A Dysphonia, difficulty making laryngeal sounds can progress to aphonia (total loss of voice).

P Lesions of CN X, swelling and inflammation of the larynx.

A Apraxia, the inability to convert the intended speech into the motor act of speech.

P Dysfunction in the precentral gyrus of the frontal lobe.

A Agraphia, the loss of the ability to write.

P Lesions of Broca's and Wernicke's areas in the dominant side of the brain.

A Alexia, the inability to grasp the meaning of written words and sentences.

P Lesion of the angular gyrus and the occipital lobe.

Level of Consciousness (LOC)

E 1. Observe the patient's eyes when entering the room (environmental stimuli). Note whether the patient's eyes are open or whether they open when you enter the room (prior to any verbalization). Note the patient's response to any general environmental stimuli, such as noises or lights.

2. If the patient's eyes are closed, call out the patient's name (verbal stimuli). Observe whether the patient's eyes open, whether the patient responds verbally and appropriately, and whether the patient follows verbal commands.

3. If the patient does not respond to verbal stimuli, lightly touch the patient's hand or gently shake the patient awake.

4. If the patient is not responding to environmental or verbal stimuli, proceed to the application of a painful stimulus.
   a. Apply pressure with a pen to the nailbed of each extremity, or
   b. Firmly pinch the trapezius muscle, or
   c. Apply pressure to the supraorbital ridge or the manubrium.

5. Observe the patient's reaction to the painful stimulus. Note whether the patient's eyes open.

6. Observe whether the patient can localize the painful stimulus by

---

E Examination   N Normal Findings   A Abnormal Findings   P Pathophysiology

TABLE 19-4	Classification of Aphasias		
APHASIA	**PATHOPHYSIOLOGY**	**EXPRESSION**	**CHARACTERISTICS**
Broca's aphasia	Motor cortex lesion, Broca's area	Expressive Nonfluent	Speech slow and hesitant, the patient has difficulty in selecting and organizing words. Naming, word and phrase repetition, and writing impaired. Subtle defects in comprehension.
Wernicke's aphasia	Left hemisphere lesion in Wernicke's area	Receptive Fluent	Auditory comprehension impaired, as is content of speech. Patient unaware of deficits. Naming severely impaired.
Anomic aphasia	Left hemisphere lesion in Wernicke's area	Amnesic Fluent	Patient unable to name objects or places. Comprehension and repetition of words and phrases intact.
Conduction aphasia	Lesion in the arcuate fasciculus, which connects and transports messages between Broca's and Wernicke's areas	Central Fluent	Patient has difficulty repeating words, substitutes incorrect sounds for another (e.g., dork for fork).
Global aphasia	Lesions in the frontal-temporal area	Mixed Fluent	Both oral and written comprehension severely impaired; naming, repetition of words and phrases, ability to write impaired.
Transcortical sensory aphasia	Lesion in the periphery of Broca's and Wernicke's areas (watershed zone)	Fluent	Impairment in comprehension, naming, and writing. Word and phrase repetition intact.
Transcortical motor aphasia	Lesion anterior, superior, or lateral to Broca's area	Nonfluent	Comprehension intact. Naming and ability to write impaired. Word and phrase repetition intact.

reaching for the area being stimulated. Strength of the patient's extremities can be assessed by the strength and distance of movement during his attempt to reach the painful stimulus. Note any abnormal motor responses.

7. Compare the motor responses and strength of the responses of right versus left sides of the patient.

8. Note whether the patient responds verbally to the painful stimulus.

9. Assess orientation by asking questions related to person, place, and time:
   a. Person: name of the patient, name of spouse or significant other

   b. Place: where the patient is now (what town, what province), where the patient lives
   c. Time: the time of day, month, year, season

10. Determine the Glasgow Coma Scale (GCS) (Figure 19-3) score, an international method for grading neurological responses of the injured or severely ill patient. It is monitored in patients who have the potential for rapid deterioration in level of consciousness. The GCS assesses three parameters of consciousness: eye opening, verbal response, and motor response.

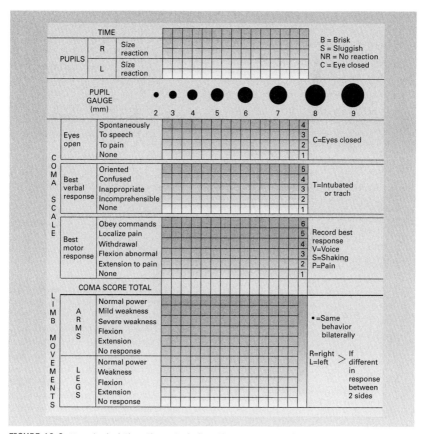

FIGURE 19-3 Neurological Flow Sheet, including Glasgow Coma Scale.

| E Examination | N Normal Findings | A Abnormal Findings | P Pathophysiology |

N The patient's best response to each of these categories is recorded. The sum of the three categories is the total GCS score. The highest score of responsiveness is 15 and the lowest is 3. A score of 15 would indicate a fully alert, oriented individual.

A/P See Table 19-5.

Cognitive Abilities and Mentation

Assessment of cognitive function includes testing for attention, memory, judgment, insight, spatial perception, calculation, abstraction, thought processes, and thought content.

Attention

E 1. Pronounce a list of numbers slowly (approximately one second apart), starting with a list of two numbers and progressing to a series of five or six numbers. For example: 2, 5; 3, 7, 8; 1, 9, 4, 3; 1, 5, 4, 9, 0.
   2. Ask the patient to repeat the numbers in correct order, both forward and backward.
   3. Give the patient a different series of the same number of digits if the patient is unable to repeat the first series correctly. Stop after two misses of any length series.
   4. Serial 7s is another way of assessing attention and concentration. Instruct the patient to begin with the number 100 and to count backward by subtracting 7 each time: 100, 93, 86, 79, 72, 65, etc.
   5. The patient may also try serial 3s (counting backward from 100 by threes) if unable to perform serial 7s.

N The patient should be able to correctly repeat the series of numbers up to a series of five numbers. The patient should be able to recite serial 7s or serial 3s accurately to at least the 40s or 50s from 100 within one minute.

A Short attention span.

P Dementia, neurological injury or disease, mental retardation.

Memory

E 1. Assess immediate recall in conjunction with attention span as discussed previously.
   2. Give a list of three items that the patient is to remember and repeat in five minutes. Have the patient repeat the items to check initial understanding. During the five minutes, carry on conversation as usual. Ask the patient to repeat the items again after the five-minute time frame.
   3. If the patient is unable to remember one or more of the objects, show a list containing the objects along with others, and check recognition.
   4. Record the number of objects remembered over the number of objects given.
   5. Long-term memory is memory that is retained for at least 24 hours. Commonly asked questions for testing long-term memory include name of spouse, spouse's birthday, mother's maiden name, name of the prime minister, or the patient's birthday.

N The patient should be able to correctly respond to questions and identify all the objects as requested.

A Memory loss.

P Nervous system infection, trauma, stroke, tumours, Alzheimer's disease, seizure disorders, alcohol, drug toxicity.

Judgment

E 1. During the interview, assess whether the patient is responding appropriately to social, family, and work situations that are discussed.
   2. Note whether the patient's decisions are based on sound reasoning and decision making.
   3. Present hypothetical situations and ask the patient to make decisions as to what his or her responses would be. For example: "What would you do if followed by a police car with

| E Examination   N Normal Findings   A Abnormal Findings   P Pathophysiology |

TABLE 19-5	Levels of Consciousness: Abnormalities and Pathophysiology			
LOC	**GCS**	**RESPONSE TO STIMULI**	**PUPIL RESPONSE**	**PATHOPHYSIOLOGY**	**PROGNOSIS**
Confusion	14	Spontaneous but may be inappropriate Memory faulty Reflexes intact	Normal	Metabolic derangements Diffuse brain dysfunction	Good chance of recovery Must treat primary cause
Lethargy	13–14	Requires stimulus to respond (verbal, touch) Reflexes intact	Normal to unequal	Metabolic derangements Medications Increased ICP	Good chance of recovery Must treat primary cause
Stupor	12–13	Requires vigorous, continuous stimuli to respond Reflexes intact	Normal, unequal, or sluggish	Metabolic derangements Medications Increased ICP	Good chance of recovery Must treat primary cause
Permanent vegetative state	8–10	Responds to pain No cognitive response Reflexes abnormal	Normal	Anoxic ischemic insults	Irreversible
Locked-in syndrome	6	Awake and aware	Normal	Lesion in ventral pons All four extremities and lower cranial nerves paralyzed Myasthenia gravis Acute polyneuritis	Poor prognosis
Coma	3–6	Abnormal Varied response to pain Reflexes abnormal or absent	Abnormal Dilated or pinpoint	Anoxia Traumatic injury Space-occupying lesion Cerebral edema	Prognosis dependent on length of time in coma
Brain death	3	No response Reflexes abnormal or absent	Abnormal Dilated or pinpoint	Anoxia Structural damage	Irreversible

LOC = level of consciousness; GCS = Glasgow Coma Scale; ICP = intracranial pressure.

flashing lights?" or "What would you do if you saw a house burning?"

4. Interview the patient's family or directly observe the patient to assess judgment more carefully.

N The patient should be able to evaluate and act appropriately in situations requiring judgment.

A Impaired judgment.

P Frontal lobe damage, dementia, psychotic states, mental retardation.

Insight

Insight is the ability to realistically understand oneself.

E 1. Ask the patient to describe personal health status, reason for seeking health care, symptoms, current life situation, and general coping behaviours.

2. If the patient describes symptoms, ask what life was like prior to the appearance of the symptoms, what life changes the illness has introduced, and whether the patient feels a need for help.

3. Ask the patient to draw a self-portrait; note the emphasis put on specific body parts, the patient's ability to reproduce figures on paper, and the representation of any part of the self-portrait. Note the facial features and the feelings portrayed by the picture.

N The patient should demonstrate a realistic awareness and understanding of self.

A Unrealistic perceptions of self.

P Euphoric stages of bipolar affective disorders, endogenous anxiety states, depressed states.

Spatial Perception

Spatial perception is the ability to recognize the relationships of objects in space.

E 1. Ask the patient to copy figures that you have previously drawn, such as a circle, triangle, square, cross, and a three-dimensional cube.

2. Ask the patient to draw the face of a clock, including the numbers around the dial.

3. Ask the patient to identify a familiar sound while keeping the eyes closed, for example, a closing door, running water, or a finger snap.

4. Have the patient identify right from left body parts.

N The patient should be able to draw the objects without difficulty and as closely as possible to the original drawing, and to identify familiar sounds and left and right body parts.

A Agnosia, the inability to recognize the form and nature of objects or persons (visual, auditory, somatosensory).

P Lesions in the non-dominant parietal lobe impair the patient's ability to appreciate self in relation to the environment and to conceive three-dimensional objects. Lesions in the occipital lobe will cause visual agnosia, and temporal lesions will cause auditory agnosia.

A Apraxia, the inability to perform purposeful movements despite the preservation of motor ability and sensation.

P Lesions of the precentral gyrus of the frontal lobe.

Calculation

The patient's ability to perform serial 7s was discussed in the section on attention and is also an assessment of calculation.

Abstract Reasoning

E 1. Ask the patient to describe the meaning of a familiar fable, proverb, or metaphor. Some examples from dominant Canadian culture are:
   • The squeaky wheel gets the grease.
   • A stitch in time saves nine.

2. Note the degree of concreteness versus abstraction in the answers.

N Patients should be able to give the abstract meanings of proverbs, fables, or metaphors within their cultural understanding.

A Conceptual concreteness—the inability to describe in abstractions, to generalize

---

E **Examination**   N **Normal Findings**   A **Abnormal Findings**   P **Pathophysiology**

from specifics, and to apply general principles.

P   Dementia, frontal tumours, schizophrenia, low intelligence.

Thought Process and Content

E   1. Observe the patient's pattern of thought for relevance, consistency, coherence, logic, and organization.
    2. Listen throughout the interview for flaws in content of conversation.

N   Thought processes should be logical, coherent, and goal oriented. Thought content should be based on reality.

A   Unrealistic, illogical thought processes and interruptions of the thinking processes, such as blocking.

P   Schizophrenia.

A   Flight of ideas, demonstrated when the patient changes from subject to subject within a sentence.

P   Manic episode of bipolar affective disorder.

A   Confabulation, the making up of answers unrelated to facts.

P   Memory loss, disorientation, Korsakoff's psychosis, psychopathic disorders.

A   Echolalia, the involuntary repetition of a word or sentence that was uttered by another person.

P   Schizophrenics, dementia.

A   Neologism, a word coined by the patient that is meaningful only to the patient.

P   Patients who are delirious or schizophrenic.

A   Delusions of persecution, grandiose delusions, hallucinations, illusions, obsessive-compulsiveness, and paranoia.

P   Schizophrenia, dementia, drug toxicities.

Suicidal Ideation

E   If the patient has expressed feelings of sadness, hopelessness, despair, worthlessness, or grief, explore his or her feelings further with more specific questions such as:
    1. Have you ever felt so bad that you wanted to hurt yourself?
    2. Do you feel like hurting yourself now?

N   The patient should provide a negative response and be able to verbalize his or her self-worth.

A   Suicidal ideation.

P   Depression, substance abuse, schizophrenia.

Sensory Assessment

Exteroceptive Sensation

For the entire exteroceptive sensation assessment, expose the patient's legs, arms, and abdomen.

Light Touch

E   1. Use a wisp of cotton and apply the stimulus with very light strokes. If the skin is calloused, or for thicker skin on the hands and soles, the stimulus may need to be intensified, although care must be taken not to stimulate subcutaneous tissues.
    2. Begin with distal areas of the patient's limbs and move proximally.
    3. Test the hand, lower arm, abdomen, foot, and leg. Assessment of sensation of the face is discussed in the cranial nerve section.
    4. To prevent the patient from being able to predict the next touch, alter the rate and rhythm of stimulation. Also, vary the sites of stimulation, keeping in mind that the right and left sides must be compared.
    5. Instruct the patient to respond by saying "now" or "yes" when the stimulus is felt, and to identify the

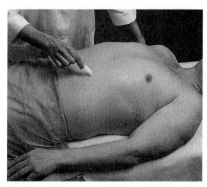

FIGURE 19-4 Assessment of Light Touch.

E **Examination**   N **Normal Findings**   A **Abnormal Findings**   P **Pathophysiology**

area that was stimulated either verbally or by pointing to it.

N/A/P Refer to Temperature.

Superficial Pain

E   1. Use a sharp object: sterile needle or sterile safety pin.
    2. Establish that the patient can identify sharp and dull sensations by touching the patient with each stimulus and asking the patient to describe what is felt. This will help alleviate some of the fears the patient may have about being touched with a sharp object.
    3. Hold the object loosely between the thumb and first finger to allow the sharp point to slide if too much pressure is applied.
    4. Begin peripherally, moving in a distal to proximal direction and following the dermatomal distribution. If impaired sensation is identified move from impaired sensation to normal sensation for comparison. Attempt to define the area of impaired sensation (mapping) by proceeding from the analgesic area to the normal area.
    5. Alternate the sharp point with the dull end to test the patient's accuracy of shear sensation.
    6. Instruct the patient to reply "sharp," "dull," or "I don't know" as quickly as the stimulus is felt and to indicate areas of the skin that perceive differences in pain sensation.
    7. Again, compare the two sides, taking care not to proceed too quickly or to cue the patient with regularity in the stimulus presentation.

N/A/P Refer to Temperature.

Temperature

Assess temperature sensation only if abnormalities in superficial pain sensation are noted.

E   1. Use glass vials containing warm water (40° to 45°C) and cold water (5° to 10°C). Hotter or colder temperatures will stimulate pain receptors.
    2. Touch the warm or cold test tubes on the skin, distal to proximal and following dermatome distribution.
    3. Instruct the patient to respond "hot," "cold," or "I can't tell" and to indicate where the sensation is felt.

N   The patient should be able to perceive light touch, superficial pain, and temperature accurately, and be able to correctly perceive the location of the stimulus.

A   Anesthesia refers to an absence of touch sensation. Hypesthesia is a diminished sense of touch; this may also be called hypoesthesia. Hyperesthesia is marked acuteness to the sensitivity of touch. Paresthesia is numbness, tingling, or pricking sensation. Dysesthesia is an abnormal interpretation of a stimulus such as burning or tingling from a stimulus such as touch or superficial pain.

P   Peripheral nerve lesions may cause anesthesia, hypesthesia, or hyperesthesia. Lesions of the nerve roots produce areas of anesthesia and hypesthesia limited to the segmental distribution of the roots involved. Lesions in the brain stem or spinal cord can cause anesthesia, paresthesia, or dysesthesia.

A   Analgesia refers to insensitivity to pain. Hypalgesia refers to diminished sensitivity to pain. Hyperalgesia is increased sensitivity to pain.

P   Lesions of the thalamus and the peripheral nerves and nerve roots can cause analgesia, hypalgesia, and hyperalgesia.

A   Total unilateral loss of all forms of sensation.

P   Extensive lesion of the thalamus.

A   A "saddle" pattern of sensation loss.

P   Lesion of the cauda equina.

A   The loss of touch sensation in the hands and lower legs (glove and stocking anesthesia).

P   Polyneuritis.

A   Unilateral loss of all exteroceptive sensation.

P   Partial lesion of the thalamus or a lesion laterally situated in the upper brain stem.

E   Examination   **N   Normal Findings**   **A   Abnormal Findings**   **P   Pathophysiology**

Proprioceptive Sensation

Motion and Position

E 1. Grasp the patient's index finger with your thumb and index finger. Hold the finger at the sides (parallel to the plane of movement) in order not to exert upward or downward pressure with your fingers and thus give the patient any clues as to which direction the finger is moving. The patient's fingers should be relaxed.

2. Have the patient shut the eyes and show the patient what "up" and "down" feel like by moving the finger in those directions.

3. Use gentle, slow, and deliberate movements. Begin with larger movements that become smaller and less perceptible.

4. Instruct the patient to respond "up," "down," or "I can't tell" after each time you raise or lower the finger.

5. Repeat this several times. Vary the motion in order not to establish a predictable pattern.

6. Repeat steps 2 through 5 with the finger of the patient's opposite hand, and then with the great toes.

7. If there appears to be a deficit in motion sense, proceed to the proximal joints such as wrists or ankles, and repeat the test.

N The patient should be able to correctly identify the changes of position of the body.

A Inability to perceive direction of movement.

P Peripheral neuropathies, lesion of the posterior column, the sensory cortex, the thalamus, or the connections between them.

Vibration Sense

E 1. Strike the prongs of a low-pitch tuning fork (128 or 256 Hz) against the ulnar surface of your hand or your knuckles, and place the base of the fork firmly on the patient's skin over bony prominences (Figure 19-5). Be sure that your fingers touch only the stem of the fork, not the tines.

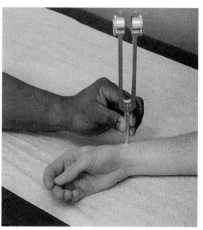

FIGURE 19-5 Assessment of Vibration.

2. Begin with distal prominences such as a toe or finger, testing each extremity by touching the base of the fork against it.

3. Instruct the patient to say "now" when the vibrating tuning fork is felt, and to report immediately when the vibrations are no longer felt.

4. Ensure that the patient is reporting the vibration sense rather than hearing a humming sound or just feeling pressure from the tuning fork.

5. After the patient can no longer feel the vibrations, determine whether the vibrations can, in fact, still be felt by holding the prongs while the tuning fork is left on the patient.

6. If you detect a deficit in vibratory sense in the peripheral bony prominences, progress toward the trunk by testing ankles, knees, wrists, elbows, anterior superior iliac crests, ribs, sternum, and spinous processes of the vertebrae.

N Normally, the patient should be able to perceive vibration over all bony prominences.

A Inability to perceive vibration sense.

P Polyneuropathies (e.g., diabetic) or spinal cord lesions involving the posterior columns.

E **Examination**   N **Normal Findings**   A **Abnormal Findings**   P **Pathophysiology**

Cortical Sensation
Stereognosis
Stereognosis is the ability to identify objects by manipulating and touching them.

E   1. Place a familiar object (coin, button, closed safety pin, key) into the patient's hand.
    2. Ask the patient to manipulate the object, appreciating size and form.
    3. Ask the patient to name the object.
    4. Repeat in the opposite hand with a different object.

N   The patient should be able to identify the objects by holding them.

A   Inability to recognize the nature of objects by touch manipulation, termed astereognosis.

P   Dysfunction of the parietal lobe.

Graphesthesia
The ability to identify numbers, letters, or shapes drawn on the skin is termed graphesthesia.

E   1. Draw a number or letter with a blunt object (such as a closed pen or the stick of a cotton-tipped applicator) on the patient's outstretched palm. Ensure the number or letter is facing the patient's direction.
    2. Ask the patient to identify what has been written.
    3. Repeat on the opposite side.

N   The patient should be able to identify the number or letter written on the palm or other skin surface.

A   Graphanesthesia is the inability to recognize a number or letter drawn on the skin.

P   Parietal lobe dysfunction.

Two-Point Discrimination
Two-point discrimination is tested by simultaneously and closely touching various parts of the body with two identical, sharp objects.

E   1. With two sterile pins, tips of opened paperclips, or broken cotton-tipped applicators, simultaneously touch the tip of the patient's finger, starting with the objects far apart.
    2. Ask the patient whether one or two points are felt.
    3. Continue to move the two points closer together until the patient is unable to distinguish two points. Note the minimum distance between the two points at which the patient reports feeling the objects separately.
    4. Irregularly alternate, using one or two pins throughout the test to verify that the patient is feeling two points.
    5. Repeat steps 1 to 4 with the fingers of the opposite hand.
    6. Other areas of the body that may be tested include the dorsum of the hand, the tongue, the lips, the feet, or the trunk.

N   The patient should be able to identify two points at 5 mm apart on the fingertips. Other parts of the body vary widely in normal distance of discrimination, such as the dorsum of the hand or feet, where a separation of as much as 20 mm may be necessary for discrimination. The patient may be able to detect two points as close as 2 to 3 mm on the tip of the tongue.

A   Distances greater than those described previously that are required to identify two points.

P   Lesions in the parietal lobe.

Extinction
Extinction (sensory inattention) is tested by simultaneously touching opposite sides of the body at the identical site. Use cotton-tipped applicators or your fingers.

E   1. Ask the patient if one or two points are felt and where they are felt.
    2. Remove the stimulus from one side while maintaining the stimulus on the opposite side.
    3. Ask the patient if one or two points are felt and where the sensations are felt.

N   The patient should be able to feel both stimuli.

| E | Examination | N | Normal Findings | A | Abnormal Findings | P | Pathophysiology |

A   Inability to feel the two points simultaneously and to discriminate that one point has been removed.

P   Lesion in parietal lobe.

Cranial Nerves

Refer to Table 19-1 to assist in the review of cranial nerves.

Olfactory Nerve (CN I)

E   1. Ask the patient to close the eyes.
2. Test each side separately by asking the patient to occlude one nostril by pressing against it with a finger.
3. Ask the patient to inhale deeply in order to cause the odour to surround the mucous membranes and adequately stimulate the olfactory nerve.
4. Ask the patient to identify the contents of each vial.
5. Present one odour at a time and alternate them from nostril to nostril.
6. Allow enough time to pass between presentation of vials to prevent confusion of the olfactory system.
7. Record the number of substances tested and the number of times the patient was able to correctly identify the contents.
8. Note whether a difference between the right and the left sides was apparent.

N   The patient should be able to distinguish and identify the odours with each nostril.

A   Anosmia, the loss of the sense of smell.

P   Trauma to the cribriform plate, sinusitis, colds, heavy smoking. Unilateral anosmia may be the result of an intracranial neoplasm.

Optic Nerve (CN II)

Visual acuity, visual fields, and funduscopic examination, ENAP: see Chapter 12.

Oculomotor Nerve (CN III)

Cardinal fields of gaze, eyelid elevation, pupil reactions (direct, consensual, accommodation), ENAP: see Chapter 12.

Trochlear Nerve (CN IV)

Cardinal fields of gaze, ENAP: see Chapter 12.

Trigeminal Nerve (CN V)

Motor Component

E   1. Instruct the patient to clench the jaw.
2. Palpate the contraction of the temporalis (Figure 19-6A) and masseter (Figure 19-6B) muscles on each side of the face by feeling for contraction

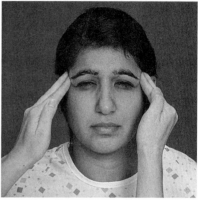

A. Temporalis muscles

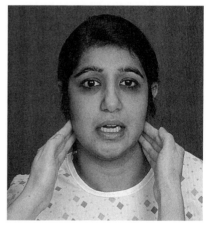

B. Masseter Muscles

FIGURE 19-6 Assessment of the Motor Component of CN V.

E Examination   N Normal Findings   A Abnormal Findings   P Pathophysiology

of the muscles with the finger pads of the first three fingers.

3. Ask the patient to move the jaw from side to side against resistance from your hand. Feel for weakness on one side or the other as the patient pushes against resistance.

4. Test the muscles of mastication by having the patient bite down with the molars on each side of a tongue blade and comparing the depth of the impressions made by the teeth. If you can pull the tongue blade out while the patient is biting on it, there is weakness of the muscles of mastication.

5. Observe for fasciculation and note the bulk, contour, and tone of the muscles of mastication.

Sensory Component

E 1. Instruct the patient to close the eyes.

2. Test light touch by using a cotton wisp to lightly stroke the patient's face in each area of the sensory distribution of the trigeminal nerve (Figure 19-7).

3. Instruct the patient to respond by saying "now" each time the touch of the cotton wisp is felt.

4. Test and compare both sides of the face.

5. To assess superficial pain sensation, use a sterile needle or open paperclip. Before testing, show the patient how the sharpness of the needle or paperclip feels compared to the dullness of the opposite, blunt end. Testing with the blunt end will give some reliability to the assessment.

a. Instruct the patient to respond by saying "sharp" or "dull" when each sensation is felt.

b. Irregularly alternate the sharp and dull ends, and again test each distribution area of the trigeminal nerve on both sides of the face.

6. Test temperature sensation if other abnormalities have been detected. Use vials of hot and cold water.

a. Touch the vials to each dermatomal distribution area, irregularly alternating hot and cold.

b. The patient should respond by saying "hot" or "cold."

7. Because sensation to the cornea is supplied by the trigeminal nerve, test the corneal reflex (the motor component is CN VII). The corneal reflex should not be routinely assessed in conscious patients, unless there is a clinical suspicion of trauma to CN V or CN VII.

a. Ask the patient to open the eyes and look away from you.

b. Approach the patient out of the line of vision to eliminate the blink reflex. You can stabilize the patient's chin with your hand if it is moving.

c. Lightly stroke the cornea with a slightly moistened cotton wisp. Avoid stroking just the sclera or the lashes of the eye. An alternative technique is to instill normal saline eye drops instead of a light stroke of a cotton wisp.

d. Observe for bilateral blinking of the eyes.

e. Repeat on the opposite eye.

N The temporalis and masseter muscles should be equally strong on palpation. The jaw should not deviate and should be equally strong during side-to-side movement against resistance. The volume and

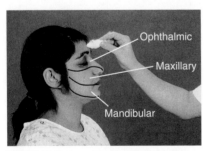

Ophthalmic

Maxillary

Mandibular

FIGURE 19-7 Assessment of the Sensory Component of CN V: Light Touch.

E   Examination   **N   Normal Findings**   **A   Abnormal Findings**   **P   Pathophysiology**

bulk of the muscles should be bilaterally equal. Sensation to light touch, superficial pain, and temperature should be present on the sensory distribution areas of the trigeminal nerve. The corneal reflex should cause bilateral blinking of eyes.

A   Reduced sensory perception or facial pain.

P   Aneurysms of the internal carotid artery, neoplasms, such as meningiomas, pituitary adenomas, and malignant tumours of the nasopharynx, head injuries.

A   Trigeminal neuralgia (tic douloureux), characterized by brief, paroxysmal unilateral facial pain along the distribution of the trigeminal nerve.

P   Multiple sclerosis due to demyelinization of the root of CN V, posterior fossa tumour.

A   Postherpetic neuralgia. The pain is continuous and is described as a constant, burning ache with occasional stabbing pains.

P   Herpes zoster.

A   Tetanus is characterized by tonic spasms interfering with the muscles that open the jaw (trismus).

P   Motor root involvement of the trigeminal nerve.

Abducens Nerve (CN VI)

Cardinal fields of gaze, ENAP: see Chapter 12.

Facial Nerve (CN VII)

Motor Component

E   1. Observe the patient's facial expressions for symmetry and mobility throughout the assessment.

2. Note any asymmetry of the face, such as wrinkles or lack of wrinkles on one side of the face or one-sided blinking.

3. Test muscle contraction by asking the patient to:
   a. Frown
   b. Raise the eyebrows
   c. Wrinkle the forehead while looking up

d. Close the eyes lightly and then keep them closed against your resistance.

e. Smile, show teeth, purse lips, and whistle

f. Puff out the cheeks against the resistance of your hands

4. Observe for symmetry of facial muscles and for weakness during the above manoeuvres.

5. Note any abnormal movements such as tremors, tics, grimaces, or immobility.

N   Normal findings of the motor portion of the facial nerve include symmetry between the right and the left sides of the face as well as the upper and lower portions of the face at rest and while executing facial movements. There should be an absence of abnormal muscle movement.

A   Bell's palsy (idiopathic facial palsy), characterized by complete flaccid paralysis of the facial muscles on the involved side.

P   Damage to the facial nerve.

Sensory Component

E   1. Sensory assessment of the facial nerve is limited to testing taste. The portions of the tongue that are tested are:
   a. The tip of the tongue for sweet and salty tastes
   b. Along the borders and at the tip for sour taste
   c. The back of the tongue and the soft palate for bitter taste

2. Test both sides of the tongue with each solution.

3. The patient's tongue should protrude during the entire assessment of taste, and talking is not allowed. In order for the patient to identify the substance, the words "sweet," "salty," "bitter," and "sour" should be written on a card so the patient can point to what is tasted. Be sure the patient does not see which solution is being tested.

E   **Examination**   N   **Normal Findings**   A   **Abnormal Findings**   P   **Pathophysiology**

4. Cotton swabs may be used as applicators, using a different one for each solution.
5. Dip the cotton swab into the solution being tested and place it on the appropriate part of the tongue.
6. Instruct the patient to point to the word that best describes taste perception.
7. Instruct the patient to rinse the mouth with water before the next solution is tested.
8. Repeat steps 5 to 7 until each solution has been tested on both sides of the tongue.

N Normal sensation would be accurate perceptions of sweet, sour, salty, and bitter tastes.

A Ageusia (loss of taste) and hypogeusia (diminution of taste).

P Age, excessive smoking, extreme dryness of the oral mucosa, colds, medications, lesions of the medulla oblongata, lesions of the parietal lobe.

Acoustic Nerve (CN VIII)

Cochlear Division
Hearing, ENAP: see Chapter 13.
Weber and Rinne tests, ENAP: see Chapter 13.

Vestibular Division
The vestibular division of CN VIII assesses for vertigo.

E 1. During the history, ask the patient if vertigo is experienced.
   2. Note any evidence of equilibrium disturbances. Refer to the section on cerebellar assessment.
   3. Note the presence of nystagmus.

N Vertigo is not normally present.

P Vertigo, an uncomfortable sensation of movement of the environment or the movement of self within a stationary environment.

P Disorder of the labyrinth or the vestibular nerve. Causative factors include migraine headache, tumours of the cerebellopontine angle, head injuries, blockage of the eustachian.

A Ménière's disease, characterized by vertigo that lasts for minutes or hours, low-pitched roaring tinnitus, progressive hearing loss, nausea, and vomiting.

P Distension of the endolymphatic system, with degenerative changes in the organ of Corti.

Glossopharyngeal and Vagus Nerves (CN IX and CN X)
The glossopharyngeal and vagus nerves are tested together because of their overlap in function.

E 1. Examine soft palate and uvula movement and gag reflex as described in Chapter 13.
   2. Assess the patient's quality of speech for a nasal quality or hoarseness. Ask the patient to produce guttural and palatal sounds, such as *k, q, ch, b,* and *d.*
   3. Assess the patient's ability to swallow a small amount of water. Observe for regurgitation of fluids through the nose. If the patient is unable to swallow, observe how oral secretions are handled.
   4. The sensory assessment of the glossopharyngeal and vagus nerves is limited to taste on the posterior one-third of the tongue. This assessment was previously discussed in the section on CN VII.

N Refer to Chapter 13 for normal soft palate and uvula movement and gag reflex findings. The speech is clear, without hoarseness or a nasal quality. The patient is able to swallow water or oral secretions easily. Taste (sweet, salty, sour, and bitter) is intact in the posterior one-third of the tongue.

A Unilateral lowering and flattening of the palatine arch, weakness of the soft palate, deviation of the uvula to the normal side, mild dysphagia, regurgitation of fluids, nasal quality of the voice, loss of taste in the posterior one-third of the tongue, and hemianesthesia of the palate and pharynx.

E Examination   N Normal Findings   A Abnormal Findings   P Pathophysiology

P   Unilateral glossopharyngeal and vagal paralysis, such as with trauma or skull fractures at the base of the skull, bilateral vagus nerve paralysis (lower brain stem cranial nerve dysfunction).

Spinal Accessory Nerve (CN XI)

E   1. Place the patient in a seated or a supine position. Inspect the sterno-cleidomastoid muscles for contour, volume, and fasciculation.

2. Place your right hand on the left side of the patient's face. Instruct the patient to turn the head sideways against the resistance of your hand.

3. Use the other hand to palpate the sternocleidomastoid muscle for strength of contraction. Inspect the muscle for contraction.

4. Repeat steps 2 and 3 in the opposite direction. Compare the strength of the two sides.

5. To assess the function of the trapezius muscle, stand behind the patient and inspect the shoulders and scapula for symmetry of contour. Note any atrophy or fasciculation.

6. Place your hands on top of the patient's shoulders and instruct the patient to raise the shoulders against the downward resistance of your hands. This can be performed in front of or behind the patient.

7. Observe the movements and palpate the contraction of the trapezius muscles. Compare the strength of the two sides.

N   The patient should be able to turn the head against resistance with a smooth, strong, and symmetrical motion. The patient should also demonstrate the ability to shrug the shoulders against resistance with strong, symmetrical movement of the trapezius muscles.

A   Inability to turn the head toward the paralyzed side, and a flat, non-contracting muscle on that side. The contralateral ster-nocleidomastoid muscle may be contracted.

P   Unilateral paralysis of the sternocleido-mastoid muscle due to trauma, tumours, or infection affecting the spinal accessory nerve.

A   Inability of the patient to elevate one shoulder, asymmetrical drooping of the shoulder and scapula, and a depressed outline of the neck.

P   Unilateral paralysis of the trapezius muscle, usually due to trauma, tumours, or infection.

A/P   For information on torticollis, see Chapter 11.

Hypoglossal Nerve (CN XII)

E   1. See Chapter 13 for assessment of tongue movement.

2. Assess lingual sounds by asking the patient to say "la la la."

N   See Chapter 13 for normal tongue movements. Lingual speech is clear.

A   Inability or difficulty in producing lingual sounds.

P   Hypoglossal nerve lesions.

Motor System

For ENAP on muscle size, tone, and strength, and involuntary movements, see Chapter 18.

A   Extrapyramidal rigidity is evident when resistance is present during passive movement of the muscles in all directions.

P   Lesions in the basal ganglia.

A   Decerebrate rigidity (decerebration) (Figure 19-8A).

P   Diencephalic injury, midbrain dysfunction, severe metabolic disorders.

A   Decorticate rigidity (decortication) (Figure 19-8B).

P   Cerebral hemisphere lesions that interfere with the corticospinal tract.

Pronator Drift

E   1. Have the patient extend the arms out in front with palms up for 20 seconds.

2. Observe for downward drifting of an arm.

E **Examination**   N **Normal Findings**   A **Abnormal Findings**   P **Pathophysiology**

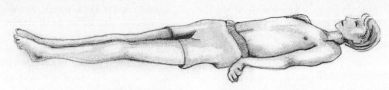

A. Decerebrate Rigidity (Abnormal Extension)

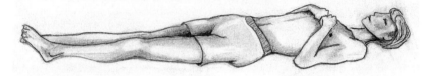

B. Decorticate Rigidity (Abnormal Flexion)

FIGURE 19-8 Motor System Dysfunction.

N   There should be no downward drifting of an arm.

A   Downward drifting of an arm.

P   Hemiparesis, such as in stroke.

Cerebellar Function (Coordination and Gait)

Coordination

E   1. Instruct the patient to sit comfortably facing you, with eyes open and arms outstretched.

2. Ask the patient to first touch the index finger to the nose, then to alternate rapidly with the index finger of the opposite hand.

3. With the patient's eyes closed, have the patient continue to rapidly touch the nose with alternate index fingers.

4. With the patient's eyes open, ask the patient to again touch finger to nose. Next, ask the patient to touch your index finger, which is held about 45 cm away from the patient.

5. Change the position of your finger as the patient rapidly repeats the manoeuvre with one finger.

6. Repeat steps 4 and 5 with the other hand.

7. Observe for intention tremor or overshoot or undershoot of the patient's finger.

8. To assess rapid alternating movements, ask the patient to rapidly alternate patting the knees, first with the palms and then alternating palms with the backs of the hands (rapid supinating and pronating of the hands).

9. Ask the patient to repeatedly touch the thumb to each of the fingers of the hand in rapid succession from index to the fifth finger, and back.

10. Repeat step 9 with the other hand.

11. Observe coordination and the ability of the patient to perform these in rapid sequence.

12. With the patient in a seated or supine position, ask the patient to place the heel just below the knee on the shin of the opposite leg and to slide it down to the foot.

13. Repeat with the opposite foot.

14. Observe coordination of the two legs.

15. Ask the patient to draw a circle or a figure 8 with the foot either on the ground or in the air.

E   Examination   N   Normal Findings   A   Abnormal Findings   P   Pathophysiology

16. Repeat with the other foot.
17. Observe for coordination and regularity of the figure.
18. Test the lower extremities for rapid alternating movement by asking the patient to rapidly extend the ankle ("tap your foot") or to rapidly flex and extend the toes of one foot.
19. Repeat with the opposite foot.
20. Note rate, rhythm, smoothness, and accuracy of the movements.

N The patient is able to rapidly alternate touching finger to nose and moving finger from nose to your finger in a coordinated fashion. The patient is able to perform alternating movements in a purposeful, rapid, coordinated manner.

The patient demonstrates the ability to purposefully and smoothly run heel down shin with equal coordination in both feet and to draw a figure 8 or circles with the foot.

A Dyssynergy, the lack of coordinated action of the muscle groups, movements appear jerky, irregular, and uncoordinated; dysmetria, impaired judgment of distance, range, speed, and force of movement; dysdiadochokinesia, the inability to perform rapid alternating movements.

P Cerebellar disease.

Gait

See Chapter 18 for gait assessment technique.

◄ NURSING CHECKLIST ►

Assessing Reflexes

1. When testing reflexes, the patient should be relaxed and comfortable.
2. Position the patient so the extremities are symmetrical.
3. To elicit true reflexes, distract the patient by talking about another topic.
4. Hold the reflex hammer loosely between the thumb and index finger and strike the tendon with a brisk motion from the wrist. The reflex hammer should make contact with the correct point on the tendon in a quick, direct manner.
5. Observe the degree and speed of response of the muscles after the reflex hammer makes contact. Grading of DTR is as follows:
   0: absent
   + (1+): present but diminished
   ++ (2+): normal
   +++ (3+): mildly increased but not pathological
   ++++ (4+): markedly hyperactive, clonus may be present
6. Compare reflex responses of the right and the left sides. The normal response to taps in the correct area should elicit a brisk (++ or +++) contraction of the muscles involved.
7. When documenting the DTRs, you may use a stick figure.

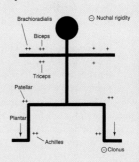

E **Examination**   N **Normal Findings**   A **Abnormal Findings**   P **Pathophysiology**

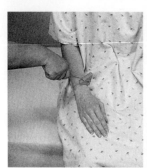

A. Brachioradialis

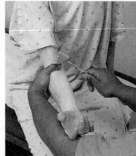

B. Biceps

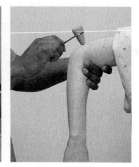

C. Triceps

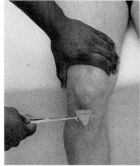

D. Patellar

E. Achilles

FIGURE 19-9 Assessment of Deep Tendon Reflexes.

Reflexes

Deep Tendon Reflexes

Brachioradialis

E 1. Flex the patient's arm to 45°.
   2. Support the patient's relaxed arm either on the lap or semipronated on your forearm.
   3. With the blunt end of the reflex hammer, strike the tendon of the brachioradialis above the styloid process of the radius (a few centimetres above the wrist on the thumb side) (Figure 19-9A).

N   Observe for flexion and supination of the forearm. An exaggerated reflex may also show flexion of the wrist and fingers and adduction of the forearm. Innervation of this reflex is through the radial nerve, with segmental innervation of C5, C6.

A/P   See Achilles.

Biceps

E 1. Flex the patient's arm to between 45° and 90°.
   2. Support the patient's forearm on your forearm.
   3. Place your thumb firmly on the biceps tendon just above the crease of the antecubital fossa (Figure 19-9B).
   4. Wrap your fingers around the patient's arm and rest them on the biceps muscle to feel it contract.
   5. Tap the thumb briskly with the pointed end of the reflex hammer.

N   Observe for contraction of the biceps muscle and flexion of the elbow. Innervation of the biceps reflex is through the musculocutaneous nerve with segmental innervation of C5, C6.

A/P   See Achilles.

| E | **Examination** | N | **Normal Findings** | A | **Abnormal Findings** | P | **Pathophysiology** |

Triceps

E   1. Flex the patient's arm to between 45° and 90°.
    2. Support the patient's arm either on the lap or on your hand as shown in Figure 19-9C.
    3. With the pointed end of the reflex hammer, tap the triceps tendon just above its insertion above the olecranon process (elbow).

N   Observe for contraction of the triceps muscle and extension of the arm. Innervation of the triceps reflex is through the radial nerve, with segmental innervation of C7, C8.

A/P   See Achilles.

Patellar

E   1. Ask the patient to sit in a chair or at the edge of the examination table.
    2. Place your hand over the quadriceps femoris muscle to feel contraction.
    3. With the other hand, tap the patellar tendon just below the patella with the blunt end of the reflex hammer (Figure 19-9D).
    4. If the patient cannot tolerate a sitting position, support the flexed knee with your hand under it so the foot is hanging freely.

N   There should be contraction of the quadriceps muscle and extension of the leg. Innervation of the patellar reflex is through the femoral nerve, with segmental innervation of L2, L3, L4.

A/P   See Achilles.

Achilles

E   1. Ask the patient to sit with the feet dangling.
    2. Slightly dorsiflex the patient's foot.
    3. With the blunt end of the reflex hammer, tap the Achilles tendon just above its insertion in the heel.
    4. If the patient is lying down, flex the leg at the knee and externally rotate the thigh. Place your non-dominant hand under the foot to produce dorsiflexion (Figure 19-9E). Apply the stimulus as described in step 3.

N   The normal response is contraction of the muscles of the calf (gastrocnemius, soleus, and plantaris) and plantar flexion of the foot. Innervation of the Achilles reflex is through the tibial nerve, with segmental innervation of L5, S1, S2.

A   Absent or decreased deep tendon reflexes.

P   Interference in the reflex arc, deep coma, narcosis, deep sedation, hypothyroidism, sedative or hypnotic drugs, infectious diseases, increased intracranial pressure, spinal shock.

A   Hyperactive deep tendon reflexes.

P   Loss of inhibition of the higher centres in the cortex and reticular formation, lesions of the pyramidal system, light coma, tetany, and tetanus.

Superficial Reflexes

Abdominal

E   1. Drape and place the patient in a recumbent position, arms at sides and knees slightly flexed. Stand to the right of the patient.
    2. Use a moderately sharp object to stroke the skin, such as the wooden tip of a cotton-tipped applicator or a split tongue blade.
    3. To elicit the upper abdominal reflex, stimulate the skin of the upper abdominal quadrants. From the tip of the sternum, stroke in a diagonal (downward and inward) fashion.
    4. Repeat step 3 on the opposite side.
    5. To elicit the lower abdominal reflex, stimulate the skin of the lower abdominal quadrants. From the area below the umbilicus, stroke in a diagonal (downward and inward) fashion to the symphysis pubis.
    6. Repeat step 5 on the opposite side.

N   Observe for contraction of the upper abdominal muscles upward and outward with a deviation of the umbilicus toward the stimulus. The upper abdominal reflex is innervated by the intercostal nerves through T7, T8, T9. Observe for contraction of the lower abdominal muscles and contraction of the umbilicus

---

| E Examination | N Normal Findings | A Abnormal Findings | P Pathophysiology |

toward the stimulus. The lower abdominal reflex is innervated by the lower intercostal, iliohypogastric, and ilioinguinal nerves through segments T10, T11, T12.

A/P   See Bulbocavernosus.

Plantar

E   1. With the handle of the reflex hammer, stroke the outer aspect of the sole of the foot from the heel across the ball of the foot to just below the great toe.
    2. Repeat on the opposite foot.

N   Observe for plantar flexion of the toes. The plantar reflex is innervated by the tibial nerve with segmental innervation of L5, S1, S2.

A/P   See Bulbocavernosus.

Cremasteric

E   1. The male patient should be lying down with the thighs exposed and the testicles visible.
    2. Stroke the skin of the inner aspect of the thigh near the groin in a downward movement.
    3. Repeat step 2 on the opposite side.

N   Observe contraction of the cremasteric muscle with corresponding elevation of the ipsilateral testicle. Innervation of the cremasteric reflex is through the ilioinguinal and genitofemoral nerves with segmental innervation of T12, L1, L2.

A/P   See Bulbocavernosus.

Bulbocavernosus

E   1. Pinch the skin of the foreskin or the glans penis.
    2. Observe for a contraction of the bulbocavernosus muscle in the perineum at the base of the penis.

N   Contraction of the bulbocavernosus muscle occurs. The presence of this reflex in a paraplegic patient after acute spinal cord injury indicates that the initial stage of spinal shock is past. The bulbocavernosus reflex is innervated by segments S3 and S4.

A   Decreased or absent superficial reflexes.

P   Dysfunction of the reflex arc, lesions in the pyramidal tracts, deep sleep, coma.

Pathological Reflexes

All the reflexes described following are abnormal findings in adults and are not usually assessed unless the patient's clinical presentation warrants it.

Glabellar

E   1. With your finger, tap the patient on the forehead between the eyebrows.
    2. Observe for a hyperactive blinking response.

A   The presence of this reflex is abnormal.

P   Lesions of the corticobulbar pathways from the cortex to the pons, Parkinson's disease, glioblastoma of the corpus callosum.

Clonus

E   1. Have the patient assume a recumbent position. Stand to the side.
    2. Support the patient's knee in a slightly flexed position.
    3. Quickly dorsiflex the foot and maintain it in that position.
    4. Assess for clonus (a rhythmic oscillation of involuntary muscle contraction).

A   Sustained clonus.

P   Sustained clonus, in combination with muscle spasticity and hyperreflexia, indicates upper motor neuron disease; women with preeclampsia and eclampsia.

Babinski

E   With the handle of the reflex hammer, stroke the patient's sole as you did for the plantar reflex. Use a slow and deliberate motion.

N   A Babinski reflex is normal in infants and toddlers until 15 to 18 months of age.

A   A positive Babinski's reflex is noted when the patient's toes abduct (fan) and the great toe dorsiflexes.

P   Lesions in the pyramidal system, stroke, trauma.

E **Examination**   N **Normal Findings**   A **Abnormal Findings**   P **Pathophysiology**

REFERENCES

[1]Canadian Heart and Stroke Foundation. *Stroke risk factors*. Retrieved November 3, 2006, from http://ww2.heartandstroke.ca/Page. asp?PageID=33&ArticleID=438&Src=stroke &From=SubCategory

20

Female Genitalia

ANATOMY AND PHYSIOLOGY

The components of the external female genitalia are collectively referred to as the vulva. They consist of the mons pubis, labia majora, labia minora, clitoris, vulval vestibule and its glands, urethral meatus, and vaginal introitus (Figure 20-1).

The vestibule is the area between the two skin folds of the labia minora that contains the urethral meatus, openings of the Skene's glands, hymen, openings of the Bartholin's glands, and vaginal introitus.

The perineum is located between the fourchette and the anus. Its composition of muscle, elastic fibres, fascia, and connective tissue gives it an exceptional capacity for stretching during childbirth. The anal orifice is located at the seam of the gluteal folds, and it serves as the exit to the gastrointestinal tract.

The components of the internal female genitalia are the vagina, uterus, fallopian tubes, and ovaries (Figure 20-2).

The vagina is a pink, hollow, muscular tube extending from the cervix to the vulva.

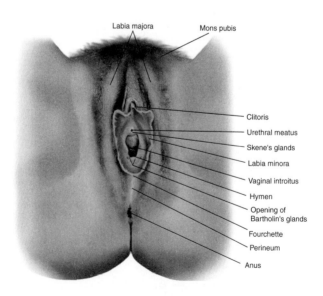

Labia majora
Mons pubis
Clitoris
Urethral meatus
Skene's glands
Labia minora
Vaginal introitus
Hymen
Opening of
Bartholin's glands
Fourchette
Perineum
Anus

FIGURE 20-1 External Female Genitalia.

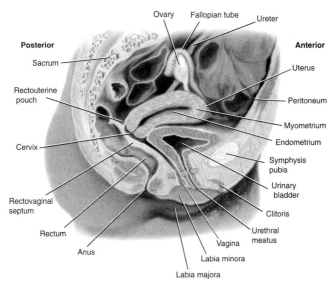

FIGURE 20-2 Left-Sided Sagittal Section at Midline of Internal Pelvic Organs.

HEALTH HISTORY

Medical History	See Table 20-1
Surgical History	Hysterectomy, myomectomy, salpingectomy, oophorectomy, dilatation and curettage, laparoscopy, vulvectomy, tubal ligation, colpotomy, cesarean section, colposcopy, cryotherapy, uterine cryoablation
Communicable Diseases	STI: gonorrhea, syphilis, herpes, HIV/AIDS, hepatitis, chlamydia, human papillomavirus (HPV), hepatitis B and C, trichomoniasis, chancroid, molluscum contagiosum
Injuries and Accidents	Abdominal trauma, rape, sexual abuse, vaginal trauma or injuries, pelvic fractures, lumbar spine, sacrococcygeal injuries
Childhood Illnesses	Fetal diethylstilbestrol (DES) exposure
Family Health History	Cancers of the reproductive organs, mother received DES while pregnant with patient, transfer of STIs during delivery, placental transfer of hepatitis B and hepatitis C, HIV/AIDS, multiple pregnancies, congenital anomalies

The uterus is an inverted pear-shaped, hollow, muscular organ in which an impregnated ovum develops into a fetus. The inferior aspect is the cervix; the superior aspect is the fundus.

The adnexa of the uterus consists of the fallopian tubes, the ovaries, and their supporting ligaments. The fallopian tubes extend from the cornu of the uterus to the ovaries and are

TABLE 20-1	**Female Reproductive Health History**

MENSTRUAL HISTORY

Age of menarche, last menstrual period (LMP), length of cycle, regularity of cycle, duration of menses, amenorrhea, menorrhagia, presence of clots or vaginal pooling, number and type of tampons or pads used during menses, dysmenorrhea, spotting between menses, missed menses.

PREMENSTRUAL SYNDROME (PMS)

Symptoms occur from 3 to 7 days before the onset of menses with cessation of symptoms after second day of cycle. Symptoms include: breast tenderness, bloating, moodiness, cravings for salt, sugar, or chocolate, fatigue, weight gain, headaches, joint pain, nausea and vomiting.

OBSTETRIC HISTORY

See Chapter 23.

MENOPAUSE HISTORY

Menopause (cessation of menstruation), spotting, associated symptoms of menopause (such as hot flashes, palpitations, numbness, tingling, drenching sweats, mood swings, vaginal dryness, itching), treatment for symptoms (including estrogen replacement therapy), feelings about menopause.

VAGINAL DISCHARGE

Colour, consistency, odour, pruritus (itching), amount.

HISTORY OF UTERINE BLEEDING

Consistency, colour, number of pads or tampons used in 24 hours, duration, frequency of flow, pain, clots.

SEXUAL FUNCTIONING

Sexual preference, number of partners, interest, satisfaction, dyspareunia, inorgasmia.

REPRODUCTIVE MEDICAL HISTORY

Vaginal infections, yeast infections, salpingitis, endometritis, endometriosis, cervicitis, fibroids, ovarian cysts, cancer of the reproductive organs, infertility, Pap smear records.

METHOD OF BIRTH CONTROL

Type, frequency of use, methods to prevent STIs, any associated problems with birth control or STI prevention methods, such as a reaction to the spermicides used with vaginal sponges, diaphragms, and condoms.

supported by the broad ligaments. The ovaries are a pair of almond-shaped glands in the upper pelvic cavity.

The female reproductive cycle consists of two interrelated cycles called the ovarian and the menstrual cycles. The ovarian cycle consists of two phases: the follicular phase and the luteal phase. During the follicular phase, the actions of the follicle-stimulating hormone (FSH) and the luteinizing hormone (LH) stimulate the ripening of one ovarian follicle. During the luteal phase, LH stimulates the development of the corpus luteum.

The menstrual cycle begins if implantation does not occur. The menstrual flow lasts from two to seven days and the cycles continue every 25 to 34 days, with the average being 28 days.

If conception and implantation of the fertilized ovum occur, the corpus luteum is maintained by the presence of human chorionic gonadotropin (HCG), which is secreted by the

◄ NURSING CHECKLIST ►

General Approach to Female Genitalia Assessment

Prior to the assessment:

1. Ensure that the patient will not be menstruating at the time of the examination for optimal cytological specimen collection.
2. Instruct the patient not to use vaginal sprays, to douche, or to have coitus 24 to 48 hours before the scheduled physical assessment. The products of coitus and commercial sprays and douches may affect the Pap smear and other vaginal cultures.
3. Encourage the patient to express any anxieties and concerns about the physical assessment. Reassure the patient by acknowledging anxieties and validating concerns. Virgins need reassurance that the pelvic assessment should not affect the hymen.
4. Show the speculum and other equipment to the patient and allow her to touch and explore any items that do not have to remain sterile.
5. Inform the patient that the assessment should not be painful but may be uncomfortable at times, and tell her to inform you if she is experiencing any pain.
6. Instruct the patient to empty her bladder and then to undress from the waist to the ankles.
7. Ensure that the room is warm enough to prevent chilling, and provide additional draping material as necessary.
8. Place drapes or sheep skin over the stirrups to increase patient comfort.
9. Warm your hands with warm water prior to gloving.
10. Ensure that privacy will be maintained during the assessment. Provide screens and a closed door.
11. Warm the speculum with warm water or a warming device before insertion.

During the assessment:

1. Inform the patient of what you are going to do before you do it. Tell her she may feel pressure when the speculum is opened and a pinching sensation when the Pap smear is done.
2. Adopt a non-judgmental and supportive attitude.
3. Maintain eye contact with the patient as much as possible to reinforce a caring relationship.
4. Use a mirror to show the patient what you are doing and to educate her about her body. Help her with positioning the mirror during the examination so she will feel comfortable using this technique at home to assess her genitalia.
5. Offer the patient the opportunity to ask questions about her body and sexuality.
6. Encourage the patient to use relaxation techniques such as deep breathing or guided imagery to prevent muscle tension during the assessment.

After the assessment:

1. Assess whether the patient needs assistance in dressing.
2. Offer tissues with which to wipe excess lubrication.
3. After the patient is dressed, discuss the experience with her, invite questions and comments, listen carefully, and provide her with information regarding the assessment and any laboratory information that is available.
4. Tell the patient she may experience a small amount of spotting following the Pap smear.

implanting blastocyst. HCG is the hormone tested in at-home pregnancy kits.

EQUIPMENT

- Examination table with stirrups
- Stool, preferably mounted on wheels
- Large hand mirror
- Gooseneck lamp
- Clean gloves
- Linens for draping
- Vaginal specula:
  – Graves' bivalve specula, sizes medium and large, useful for most adult sexually active women
  – Pederson bivalve specula, sizes small and medium, useful for non–sexually active women, children, menopausal women
- Cytological materials:
  – Wood spatulas i.e., Ayre
  – Cervical broom
  – Cytobrushes
  – Cotton-tipped applicators
  – Liquid-based preparation vials
  – Microscope slides, cover slips, culture plates labelled with the patient's name, identification number, and date specimen was collected
  – Cytology fixative spray
  – Reagents: normal saline solution, potassium hydroxide (KOH), acetic acid (white vinegar)
- Warm water

ASSESSMENT OF THE FEMALE GENITALIA

Inspection of the External Genitalia

1. With the patient seated, place a drape over the patient's torso and thighs until positioning is completed.
2. Instruct the patient to first sit on the examination table between the stirrups, facing the foot of the table.
3. Assist the patient in assuming a dorsal recumbent or lithotomy position on the examination table. Assist the patient in placing her heels in the stirrups, thus abducting her legs and flexing her hips.
4. Don clean gloves.

5. Assist the patient as she moves her buttocks down to the lower end of the examination table so that the buttocks are flush with the edge of the table. If the patient desires, raise the head of the examination table slightly to elevate her head and shoulders. This position allows you to maintain eye contact with the patient and prevents abdominal muscle tension.
6. Readjust the drape to cover the abdomen, thighs, and knees; adjust the stirrups as necessary for patient comfort. Push the drape down between the patient's knees so you can see the patient's face.
7. Sit on a stool at the foot of the examination table facing the patient's external genitalia.
8. Adjust your lighting source and provide the patient with a mirror. Instruct her on how to hold the mirror in order to view the examination prior to touching the patient's genitalia.
9. Finally, remember to inform the patient of each step of the assessment process before it is performed, and be gentle.

Pubic Hair

E 1. Observe the pattern of pubic hair distribution.
   2. Note the presence of nits or lice.

N The distribution of the female pubic hair should be shaped like an inverse triangle. There may be some growth on the abdomen and upper inner thighs. A diamond-shaped pattern from the umbilicus may be due to cultural or familial differences. There are no nits or lice.

A Extensive hair extending beyond the pubic hair triangle to the abdomen and upper inner thighs.

P Hirsutism, indicative of an endocrine disorder.

A Hair distribution is sparse or hair is absent at the genitalia area.

P Alopecia from genetic factors, aging, systemic disease, and obesity.

A Nits or lice.

P Pubic lice (pediculosis pubis) is the infestation of the hairy regions of the body, usually the pubic area.

E **Examination** N **Normal Findings** A **Abnormal Findings** P **Pathophysiology**

Skin Colour and Condition
Mons Pubis and Vulva

E   1. Observe the skin coloration and condition of the mons pubis and vulva.
2. Inform the patient that you will touch the inside of her thigh before you touch her genitals.
3. With gloved hands, separate the labia majora using the thumb and index finger of the dominant hand.
4. Observe both the labia majora and the labia minora for coloration, lesions, or trauma.

N   The skin over the mons pubis should be clear except for nevi and normal hair distribution. The labia majora and minora should appear symmetrical with a smooth to somewhat wrinkled, unbroken, slightly pigmented skin surface. There should be no ecchymosis, excoriation, nodules, swelling, rash, or lesions. An occasional sebaceous cyst is within normal limits. These cysts are non-tender, yellow nodules that are less than 1 cm in diameter.

A   Ecchymosis.
P   Trauma from an accident or abuse.
A   Edema or swelling of the labia.
P   Hematoma formation, Bartholin's cyst, obstruction of the lymphatic system.
A   Broken areas on the skin surface.
P   Ulcerations or abrasions secondary to infection or trauma.
A   Rash over the mons pubis and labia.
P   Contact dermatitis, infestations.
A   Non-tender, reddish, round ulcer with a depressed centre, and raised, indurated edges (chancre).
P   Primary stages of syphilis.
A   Flat or raised, round, wartlike papules that have moist surfaces covered by grey exudate (condyloma latum).
P   Secondary stage of syphilis.
A   White, dry, cauliflower-like growths that have narrow bases are suggestive of condyloma acuminatum.
P   Human papillomavirus.

A   Small, swollen, red vesicles that fuse together to form a large, burning ulcer that may be painful and itch.
P   Herpes simplex virus.
A   A painless mass that may be accompanied by pruritus or a mass that develops into a cauliflower-like growth.
P   Suggestive of malignancy.
A   Venous prominences of the labia.
P   Varicose veins due to a congenital predisposition, prolonged standing, pregnancy, aging.

Clitoris

E   1. Using the dominant thumb and index finger, separate the labia minora laterally to expose the prepuce of the clitoris.
2. Observe the clitoris for size and condition.

N   The clitoris is approximately 2.0 cm in length and 0.5 cm in diameter and without lesions.

A   Hypertrophy.
P   Female pseudohermaphroditism due to androgen excess.
A   A reddish, round ulcer with a depressed centre and raised, indurated edges (chancre).
P   The primary lesion of syphilis.

Urethral Meatus

E   1. Using the dominant thumb and index finger, separate the labia minora laterally to expose the urethral meatus. Do not touch the urethral meatus; this may cause pain and urethral spasm.
2. Observe the shape, colour, and size of the urethral meatus.

N   The urethral opening is slit-like in appearance and midline; it is free of discharge, swelling, or redness and is about the size of a pea.

A   Discharge of any colour from the meatus.
P   Urinary tract infection.
A   Swelling or redness around the urethral meatus.

E **Examination**   N **Normal Findings**   A **Abnormal Findings**   P **Pathophysiology**

P   Infection of the Skene's glands, urethral caruncle (small, red growth that protrudes from the meatus), urethral carcinoma, prolapse of the urethral mucosa.

Vaginal Introitus

E   1. Keep the labia minora retracted laterally to inspect the vaginal introitus.
    2. Ask the patient to bear down.
    3. Observe for patency and bulging.

N   The introitus mucosa should be pink and moist. Normal vaginal discharge is clear to white and free of foul odour; some white clumps may be seen that are mass numbers of epithelial cells. The introitus should be patent and without bulging.

A   Pale colour and dryness.

P   Atrophy from topical steroids, the aging process, and estrogen deficiency.

A   Malodorous white, yellow, green, or grey discharge.

P   Gonorrhea, *chlamydia*, *Candida* vaginosis, *Trichomonas* vaginitis, bacterial vaginosis, atrophic vaginitis, or cervicitis are possible infectious processes or vectors (Table 20-2).

A   An external tear or impatency of the vaginal introitus.

P   Trauma, fissure of the introitus.

A   Bulging of the anterior vaginal wall indicates a cystocele.

P   Weakened supporting tissues and ligaments.

A   Bulging of the anterior vaginal wall, bladder, and urethra into the vaginal introitus indicates a cystourethrocele.

P   Weakening of the entire anterior vaginal wall, fissure.

A   Bulging of the posterior vaginal wall with a portion of the rectum indicates a rectocele.

P   Weakening of the entire posterior vaginal wall.

Perineum and Anus

E   1. Observe for colour and shape of the anus.
    2. Observe texture and colour of the perineum.

N   The perineum should be smooth and slightly darkened. A well-healed episiotomy scar is normal after vaginal delivery. The anus should be dark pink to brown and puckered. Skin tags are not uncommon around the anal area.

A   A fissure or tear of the perineum.

P   Trauma, abscess, unhealed episiotomy.

A   Venous prominences of the anal area indicate external hemorrhoids.

P   Varicose dilatation of a vein of the inferior hemorrhoidal plexus.

Palpation of the External Genitalia
Labia

E   1. Palpate each labium between the thumb and the index finger of your dominant hand.
    2. Observe for swelling, induration, pain, or discharge from a Bartholin's gland duct.

N   The labium should feel soft and uniform in structure with no swelling, pain, induration, or purulent discharge.

A   Swelling, redness, induration, or purulent discharge from the labial folds with hot, tender areas.

P   Bartholin's gland infection. Causative organisms include gonococci, *chlamydia trachomatis*, syphilis.

Urethral Meatus and Skene's Glands

E   1. Insert your dominant index finger into the vagina.
    2. Apply pressure to the anterior aspect of the vaginal wall and milk the urethra (Figure 20-3).

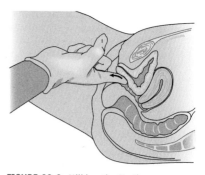

FIGURE 20-3 Milking the Urethra.

E **Examination**   N **Normal Findings**   A **Abnormal Findings**   P **Pathophysiology**

TABLE 20-2	Vaginal Discharge—Diagnostic Features and Laboratory Diagnosis		
	BACTERIAL VAGINOSIS	**CANDIDIASIS**	**TRICHOMONIASIS**
Sexual transmission	• Not usually considered sexually transmitted	• Not usually considered sexually transmitted	• Sexually transmitted
Predisposing factors	• Often absent • More common if sexually active • New sexual partner • IUD use	• Often absent • More common if sexually active • Current or recent antibiotic use • Pregnancy • Corticosteroids • Poorly controlled diabetes • Immunocompromised	• Multiple partners
Symptoms	• Vaginal discharge • Fishy odour • 50% asymptomatic	• Vaginal discharge • Itch • External dysuria • Superficial dyspareunia • Up to 20% asymptomatic	• Vaginal discharge • Itch • Dysuria • 10–50% asymptomatic
Signs	• White or grey, thin, copious discharge	• White, clumpy, curdy discharge • Erythema and edema of vagina and vulva	• Off-white or yellow, frothy discharge • Erythema of vulva and cervix ("strawberry cervix")
Vaginal pH	• >4.5	• <4.5	• >4.5
Wet mount	• PMNs • Clue cells*	• Budding yeast • Pseudohyphae	• Motile flagellated protozoa (38–82% sensitivity)
Gram stain	• Clue cells • Decreased normal flora • Predominant Gram-negative curved bacilli and coccobacilli	• PMNs • Budding yeast • Pseudohyphae	• PMNs • Trichomonads
Whiff test	• Positive	• Negative	• Negative
Preferred treatment	• Metronidazole • Clindamycin	• Antifungals	• Metronidazole • Treat partner

IUD = intrauterine device   PMN = polymorphonuclear leukocytes   *Clue cells are vaginal epithelial cells covered with numerous coccobacilli.
†Culture is more sensitive than microscopy for T vaginalis.

Source: Compiled from information on the Health Canada website.

3. Observe for discharge and patient discomfort.

N   Milking the urethra should not cause pain or result in any urethral discharge.

A   Pain on contact and discharge from the urethra.

P   Skene's gland infection, urinary tract infection.

Vaginal Introitus

E   1. While your finger remains in the vagina, ask the patient to squeeze the vaginal muscles around your finger.
    2. Evaluate muscle strength and tone.

N   Vaginal muscle tone in a nulliparous woman should be tight and strong; in a parous woman, it will be diminished.

A   Significantly diminished or absent vaginal muscle tone, bulging of vaginal or pelvic contents.

P   Weakened muscle tone from injury, age, childbirth, or medication.

Perineum

E   1. Withdraw your finger from the introitus until you can place only your dominant index finger posterior to the perineum and place the dominant thumb anterior to the perineum.
    2. Assess the perineum between the dominant thumb and index finger for muscular tone and texture.

N   The perineum should be smooth, firm, and homogenous in the nulliparous woman, and thinner in the parous woman. A well-healed episiotomy scar is also within normal limits for a parous woman.

A   A thin, tissue-like perineum, fissures, or tears.

P   Atrophy, trauma, unhealed episiotomy.

Speculum Examination of the Internal Genitalia

Cervix

E   1. Select the appropriate-sized speculum. This selection should be based on the patient's history, size of vaginal introitus, and vaginal muscle tone.

2. Lubricate and warm the speculum by rinsing it under warm water. Do not use other lubricants because they may interfere with the accuracy of cytological samples and cultures.

3. Hold the speculum in your dominant hand with the closed blades between the index and middle fingers. The index finger should rest at the proximal end of the superior blade. Wrap the other fingers around the handle, with the thumbscrew over the thumb.

4. Insert your non-dominant index and middle fingers, ventral sides down, just inside the vagina and apply pressure to the posterior vaginal wall. Encourage the patient to bear down. This will help to relax the perineal muscles.

5. Encourage the patient to relax by taking deep breaths. Be careful not to pull on pubic hair or pinch the labia.

6. When you feel the muscles relax, insert the speculum at an oblique angle on a plane parallel to the examination table until the speculum reaches the end of the fingers that are in the vagina (Figure 20-4A).

7. Withdraw the fingers of your non-dominant hand.

8. Gently rotate the speculum blades to a horizontal angle and advance the speculum at a 45° downward angle against the posterior vaginal wall until it reaches the end of the vagina.

9. Using your dominant thumb, depress the lever to open the blades and visualize the cervix (Figure 20-4B).

10. If the cervix is not visualized, close the blades and withdraw the speculum 2 to 3 cm and reinsert it at a slightly different angle to ensure that the speculum is inserted far enough into the vagina.

11. Once the cervix is fully visualized, lock the speculum blades into place.

E **Examination**   N **Normal Findings**   A **Abnormal Findings**   P **Pathophysiology**

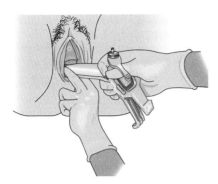

A. Opening of the Vaginal Introitus

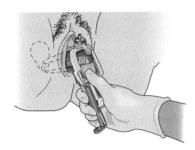

B. Opening the Speculum Blades

FIGURE 20-4 Speculum Examination.

This procedure varies based on the type of speculum being used.

12. Adjust your light source so that it shines through the speculum.
13. If any discharge obstructs the visualization of the cervix, clean it away with a cotton-tipped applicator.
14. Inspect the cervix and the os for colour, position, size, surface characteristics such as polyps or lesions, discharge, and shape.

Colour

N   The normal cervix is a glistening pink; it may be pale after menopause or blue (Chadwick's sign) during pregnancy.
A   Redness or a friable appearance.
P   Infection and inflammation, such as *chlamydia* or gonorrhea.

Position

N   The cervix is located midline in the vagina with an anterior or posterior position relative to the vaginal vault and projecting approximately 2.5 cm into the vagina.
A   Lateral positioning of the cervix.
P   Tumour, adhesions.
A   Projection of the cervix into the vaginal vault greater than normal limits.
P   Uterine prolapse.

Size

N   Normal size is 2.5 cm.
A   Cervical size greater than 4 cm is indicative of hypertrophy.
P   Inflammation, tumour, multiparous.

Surface Characteristics

N   The cervix is covered by the glistening pink squamous epithelium, which is similar to the vaginal epithelium, and the deep pink to red columnar epithelium, which is a continuation of the endocervical lining.
A   A reddish circle around the os.
P   Ectropion or eversion occurs when the squamocolumnar junction appears on the ectocervix. It results from lacerations during childbirth or possibly from congenital variation.
A   Small, cystic, yellow lesions on the cervical surface indicate nabothian cysts.
P   Obstruction of cervical glands.
A   Bright-red, soft protrusion through the cervical os indicates a cervical polyp.
P   Polyps originate from the endocervical canal; they are usually benign but tend to bleed if abraded.
A   Hemorrhages dispersed over the surface and known as strawberry spots.
P   Trichomonal infections.
A   Mucopurulent discharge, erythema, and friability of the cervix.
P   *Chlamydia trachomatis*.
A   Irregularities of the cervical surface that may look cauliflower-like.

E   **Examination**   N   **Normal Findings**   A   **Abnormal Findings**   P   **Pathophysiology**

P   Carcinoma of the cervix.
A   Columnar epithelium covering most of the cervix and extending to the vaginal wall (vaginal adenosis), and a collar-type ridge between the cervix and the vagina.
P   Exposure to DES.

Discharge
E/A/P See Table 20-2.

Shape of the Cervical Os
N   In the nulliparous woman, the os is small and either round or oval. In the parous woman who has had a vaginal delivery, the os is a horizontal slit.
A   A unilateral transverse, bilateral transverse, stellate, or irregular cervical os (Figure 20-5).
P   Rapid second-stage childbirth delivery, forceps delivery, trauma.

Collecting Specimens for Cytological Smears and Cultures
Collect the Pap smear first, followed by the gonococcal and any other vaginal smears.

Nursing Alert

Risk Factors for Female Genitalia Cancer

Cervical Cancer
- Early age at first intercourse (before 17 or 18 years of age)
- Multiple sex partners or male partners who have had multiple partners
- Prior history of human papillomavirus, herpes simplex virus
- Current or prior human papillomavirus or condylomata, or both
- Family history
- Tobacco use
- Drug use
- HIV
- Immunosuppressed
- History of STIs, cervical dysplasia or cervical cancer, endometrial, vaginal, or vulvar cancer
- Women of lower socioeconomic state

Endometrial Cancer
- Early or late menarche (before age 11 or after age 16)
- History of infertility
- Failure to ovulate
- Unopposed estrogen therapy
- Use of tamoxifen
- Obesity
- Family history

Ovarian Cancer*
- Advancing age
- Nulliparity
- History of breast cancer
- Family history of ovarian cancer
- Infertility treatment

Vaginal Cancer
- Daughters of women who ingested DES during pregnancy
- Prior human papillomavirus

***Ovarian Cancer Signs and Symptoms**
Changes in bowel function (constipation, diarrhea); abdominal bloating, distention or discomfort; nausea, indigestion, flatulence; urinary frequency/nocturia; menstrual irregularities; back pain; pelvic discomfort, heaviness; weight gain or loss; fatigue/sleep changes.

Normal

Nulliparous   Parous

Lacerations

Unilateral transverse   Bilateral transverse   Stellate

FIGURE 20-5 Speculum Examination.

E Examination   N Normal Findings   A Abnormal Findings   P Pathophysiology

Papanicolaou (Pap) Smear

The Pap smear is a collection of three specimens that are obtained from three sites: the endocervix (covered by columnar epithelium), cervix (or transformative zone—covered by metaplastic epithelium), and the vaginal pool (also called the exocervix or posterior fornix—covered by squamous epithelium). The purpose of the Pap smear is to evaluate cervicovaginal cells for pathology that may indicate carcinoma.

Endocervical Smear

E 1. Using your dominant hand, insert the Cytobrush or cervical broom through the speculum into the cervical os approximately 1 cm. Many patients find that this procedure causes a cramping sensation, so forewarn your patient that she may feel discomfort during this element of the assessment.

2. Rotate the Cytobrush between your index finger and thumb 90° clockwise, then counterclockwise. Keep the Cytobrush in contact with the cervical tissue. *Note:* If you have to use a cotton-tipped applicator instead of a Cytobrush, leave the applicator in the cervical os for 30 seconds to ensure saturation. If you use the cervical broom, rotate the broom six times clockwise and place the broom in the liquid-based preparation container.

3. Remove the Cytobrush and, using a rolling motion, spread the cells on the section of the slide marked *E*, if a sectional slide is being used. Do not press down hard or wipe the Cytobrush back and forth because doing so will destroy the cells.

4. Discard the brush.

N/A/P Refer to Vaginal Pool Smear.

Cervical (Transformative Zone) Smear

E 1. Insert the bifurcated end of the wooden spatula through the speculum base. Place the longer projection of the bifurcation into the cervical os. The shorter projec-

tion should be snug against the ectocervix.

2. Rotate the spatula 360° one time only. Make sure the transformation zone is well sampled.

3. Remove the spatula and gently spread the specimen on the section of the slide labelled *C*, if a sectional slide is being used.

N/A/P Refer to Vaginal Pool Smear.

Vaginal Pool (Exocervical) Smear

E 1. Reverse the spatula and insert the rounded end into the posterior vaginal fornix and gently scrape the area. *Note:* a cotton-tipped applicator can also be used to obtain the smear. The cotton-tipped applicator may be the preferred vehicle for obtaining the specimen if vaginal secretions are viscous or dry. By moistening the cotton-tipped applicator with normal saline solution, viscous secretions can be removed with less trauma to the surrounding membranes.

2. Remove the spatula and gently spread the specimen on the section of the slide marked *V*, if a sectional slide is being used.

3. Dispose of the spatula or cotton-tipped applicator.

4. Spray the entire slide or the slides with cytological fixative.

5. Submit the specimens to the appropriate laboratory following your institution's guidelines for cytology specimens.

N Normal classifications for cervicovaginal cytology (meaning no pathogenesis) include "within normal limits (WNL)" (using Bethesda System); or "no abnormal cells" or "metaplasia noted" (using CIN/Modified Walton System).

A Report finding of benign cellular changes.

P Fungal, bacterial, protozoan, or viral infections.

A A report finding of "atypical squamous cells of undetermined significance."

| E **Examination** | N **Normal Findings** | A **Abnormal Findings** | P **Pathophysiology** |

P Inflammatory or infectious processes, a preliminary lesion, unknown phenomenon.

A A report finding of epithelial cell abnormalities.

P Squamous intraepithelial lesion, which may or may not be transient; squamous cell carcinoma; glandular cell abnormalities.

Chlamydia Culture Specimen

E 1. Insert a sterile cotton swab applicator 1 cm into the cervical os.
   2. Hold the applicator in place for 20 seconds.
   3. Remove the swab.
   4. Place the swab in a viral, *chlamydia*, or mycoplasma culture transport tube.
   5. Dispose of the cotton swab applicator.
   6. Submit the specimens to the appropriate laboratory following your institution's guidelines for culture specimens.

N Cervicovaginal tissues are normally free of *Candida albicans*. There should be no odour.

A *Trachomatis*, serotypes D through K, or obligate, intracellular bacteria in cervicovaginal secretions.

P *Trachomatis* may invade the cervix or fallopian tubes, but is often asymptomatic in women.

Gonococcal Culture Specimen

E 1. Insert a sterile cotton swab applicator 1 cm into the cervical os.
   2. Hold the applicator in place for 20 to 30 seconds.

3. Remove the swab.
4. Roll the swab in a large Z pattern over the culture plate. Simultaneously rotate the swab as you roll it to ensure that all of the specimen is used.
5. Dispose of the swab.
6. Submit the specimens to the appropriate laboratory following your institution's guidelines for culture specimens.

N Cervicovaginal tissues are normally free of *Neisseria gonorrhoeae*.

A Large number of Gram-negative diplococci present in cervicovaginal secretions.

P *N. gonorrhoeae* are Gram-negative diplococci organisms that invade columnar and stratified epithelium.

Saline Mount or Wet Mount

This test is performed for the rapid evaluation of white blood cells and protozoa.

E 1. Spread a sample of the cervical or vaginal pool specimen onto a microscope slide, add one drop of normal saline (0.9%) solution, and apply a cover slip.
   2. Examine under a microscope.

N The sample should have fewer than ten white blood cells (WBCs) per field.

A A sample with more than ten WBCs per field, protozoa, bacteria-filled epithelial cells (clue cells).

P A large number of WBCs can be indicative of an inflammatory response, *chlamydia trachomatis*, or a bacterial infection. Protozoa are indicative of *trichomoniasis*.

Reflective Thinking

Examining the Patient with an STI

Your patient has told you that she has noticed an odourless greenish discharge from her vagina during the past two weeks. She has been married for 37 years and has not had any sexual partners other than her husband during that time. You observe that her vulva is erythematous, and there is pus in her cervical os. How would you further assess this patient? What additional questions would you ask? What anticipatory guidance would you provide?

E **Examination**   N **Normal Findings**   A **Abnormal Findings**   P **Pathophysiology**

Whiff Test or KOH Prep

This test is performed for the rapid evaluation of *Candida*.

E 1. Spread a sample of the cervical or vaginal pool specimen onto a microscope slide, add one drop of 10% KOH (potassium hydroxide), and apply a cover slip.
   2. Note any odour.
   3. Examine under a microscope.

N Cervicovaginal tissues are normally free of *Candida albicans* except in a small percentage of women. There should be no odour.

A The presence of yeast and pseudohyphae forms (chains of budding yeast).

P Overgrowth of *Candida*.

A Odour.

P An amine (fishy odour) indicates bacterial vaginosis.

Five Percent Acetic Acid Wash

E After completing all other vaginal specimens, swab the cervix with a cotton-tipped applicator that has been soaked in 5% acetic acid.

N The normal response is no change in the appearance of the cervix.

A A rapid acetowhitening or blanching with jagged borders.

P Human papillomavirus (causative agent of genital warts).

Anal Culture

E 1. Insert a sterile cotton swab applicator 1 cm into the anal canal.
   2. Hold the applicator in place for 20 to 30 seconds.
   3. Remove the swab. If fecal material is collected, discard the applicator and start again.
   4. Roll and rotate the swab in a large Z pattern over a culture plate.
   5. Dispose of the swab.

N Anal tissues are normally free of *Neisseria gonorrhoeae*.

A Large number of Gram-negative diplococci.

P *N. gonorrhoeae*.

Inspection of the Vaginal Wall

E 1. Disengage the locking device of the speculum.
   2. Slowly withdraw the speculum but do not close the blades.
   3. Rotate the speculum into an oblique position as you retract it to allow full inspection of the vaginal walls. Observe vaginal wall colour and texture.

N The vaginal walls should be pink, moist, deeply rugated, and without lesions or redness.

A Spots that appear as white paint on the walls.

P Leukoplakia from *Candida albicans*, HIV infection.

A Pallor of the vaginal walls.

P Anemia, menopause.

A Redness of the vaginal walls.

P Inflammation, hyperemia, trauma from tampon insertion or removal.

A Vaginal lesions or masses.

P Carcinoma, tumours, DES exposure.

Bimanual Examination

E 1. Observe the patient's face for signs of discomfort during the assessment process.
   2. Inform the patient of the steps of the bimanual assessment, and warn her that the lubricant gel may be cold.
   3. Squeeze water-soluble lubricant onto the fingertips of your dominant hand.
   4. Stand between the legs of the patient as she remains in the lithotomy position, and place your

---

Nursing Alert

Reporting of STIs

Reporting of STIs to public health officials and partners is important to meet legal and ethical obligations.

E Examination **N** Normal Findings **A** Abnormal Findings **P** Pathophysiology

non-dominant hand on her abdomen and below the umbilicus.

5. Insert your dominant index and middle fingers 1 cm into the vagina. The fingers should be extended with the palmar side up. Exert gentle posterior pressure.

6. Inform the patient that pressure from palpation may be uncomfortable. Instruct the patient to relax the abdominal muscles by taking deep breaths.

7. When you feel the patient's muscles relax, insert your fingers to their full length into the vagina. Insert your fingers slowly so that you can simultaneously palpate the vaginal walls.

8. Remember to keep your thumb widely abducted and away from the urethral meatus and clitoris throughout the palpation in order to prevent pain or spasm.

Vagina

E Complete steps 1–8 from bimanual examination. Rotate the wrist so that the fingers are able to palpate all surface aspects of the vagina.

N The vaginal wall is non-tender and has a smooth or rugated surface with no lesions, masses, or cysts.

A Lesions, masses, scarring, cysts.

P Benign lesions (inclusion cysts, myomas, fibromas), malignant lesions.

Cervix

E
1. Position the dominant hand so that the palmar surface faces upward.
2. Place the non-dominant hand on the abdomen approximately one-third of the way down between the umbilicus and the symphysis pubis.
3. Use the palmar surfaces of the dominant hand's finger pads, which are in the vagina, to assess the cervix for consistency, position, shape, and tenderness.
4. Grasp the cervix between the fingertips and move the cervix from side to side to assess mobility (Figure 20-6).

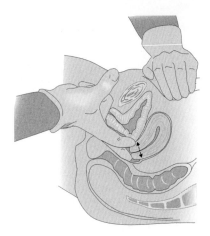

FIGURE 20-6 Assessment of Cervical Mobility.

N The normal cervix is mobile without pain, smooth and firm, symmetrically rounded, and midline.

A The presence of pain on palpation or the assessment of mobility is a positive Chandelier's sign.

P Pelvic inflammatory disease, ectopic pregnancy.

A Softening of the cervix (Goodell's sign).

P Fifth to sixth week of pregnancy.

A Irregular surface, immobility, or nodular surface.

P Malignancy, fibroids, nabothian cysts, polyps.

Fornices

E
1. With the fingertips and palmar surfaces of the fingers, palpate around the fornices.
2. Note nodules or irregularities.

N The walls should be smooth and without nodules.

A Nodules or irregularities.

P Malignancy, polyps, herniations (if the walls of the fornices are impatent).

Uterus

E
1. With the dominant hand, which is in the vagina, push the pelvic organs out of the pelvic cavity and provide stabi-

---

E Examination   N Normal Findings   A Abnormal Findings   P Pathophysiology

lization while the non-dominant hand, which is on the abdomen, performs the palpation (Figure 20-7).

2. Press the hand that is on the abdomen inward and downward toward the vagina, and try to grasp the uterus between your hands.

3. Evaluate the uterus for size, shape, consistency, mobility, tenderness, masses, and position.

4. Place the fingers of the intravaginal hand into the anterior fornix and palpate the uterine surface.

N The size of the uterus varies based on parity; it should be pear-shaped in the non-gravid patient and more rounded in the parous patient. The uterus should be smooth, firm, mobile, non-tender, and without masses. A uterus may be non-palpable if it is retroverted or retroflexed. The uterus in these positions can be assessed only via rectovaginal examination. A non-palpable uterus in the older woman may be a normal finding secondary to uterine atrophy.

A Significant exterior enlargement and changes in the shape of the uterus.

P Uterine enlargement indicates possible intrauterine pregnancy or tumour.

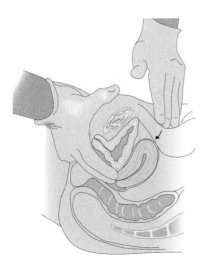

FIGURE 20-7 Uterine Palpation.

A Nodules or irregularities.

P Leiomyomas are tumours containing muscle tissue.

A Inability to assess the uterus.

P Hysterectomy, retroverted and retroflexed uterus.

Adnexa

Fallopian tubes are rarely palpable, and palpation of the ovaries depends on patient age and size. Many times, the ovaries are not palpable, and this procedure can be painful to the patient during the luteal phase of the menstrual cycle (postovulation) or due to normal visceral tenderness.

E 1. Move the intravaginal hand to the right lateral fornix, and the hand on the abdomen to the right lower quadrant just inside the anterior iliac spine. Press deeply inward and upward toward the abdominal hand.

2. Push inward and downward with the abdominal hand and try to catch the ovary between your fingertips.

3. Palpate for size, shape, consistency, and mobility of the adnexa.

4. Repeat the above manoeuvres on the left side (Figure 20-9).

N The ovaries are normally almond shaped, firm, smooth, and mobile without tenderness.

A Enlarged ovaries that are irregular, nodular, painful, with decreased mobility, or pulsatile.

P Ectopic pregnancy, ovarian cyst, pelvic inflammatory disease, malignancy.

Rectovaginal Examination

E 1. Withdraw your dominant hand from the vagina and change gloves. Apply additional lubricant to the fingertips of your dominant hand.

2. Tell the patient you will be inserting one finger into her vagina and one finger into her rectum. Remind her that the lubricant jelly will feel cold

E Examination   **N** Normal Findings   **A** Abnormal Findings   **P** Pathophysiology

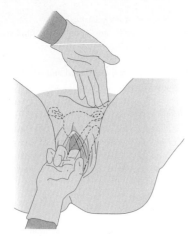

FIGURE 20-8 Palpation of the Left Adnexa.

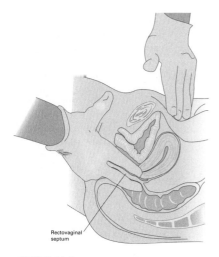

Rectovaginal
septum

FIGURE 20-9 Rectovaginal Examination.

and that the rectal examination will be uncomfortable.

3. Insert the dominant index finger back into the vagina.

4. Ask the patient to strain down as if she is having a bowel movement in order to relax the anal sphincter. Assess anal sphincter tone.

5. Insert the middle finger of the dominant hand into the patient's rectum

as she strains down (Figure 20-10). If the rectum is full of stool, carefully remove the stool digitally from the rectum.

6. Advance the rectal finger forward while using the non-dominant hand to depress the abdomen. Assess the rectovaginal septum for patency, the cervix and uterus for anomalies such as posterior lesions, and the rectouterine pouch for contour lesions.

7. On completion of the assessment, withdraw the fingers from the vagina and rectum, and if any stool is present on the glove, test for occult blood.

8. Clean the patient's genitalia and anal area with a tissue and assist her back to a sitting position.

N   The rectal walls are normally smooth and free of lesions. The rectal pouch is rugated and free of masses. Anal sphincter tone is strong. The cervix and uterus, if palpable, are smooth. The rectovaginal septum is smooth and intact. Refer to Chapter 22 for further information on the complete rectal examination.

A   Masses or lesions.

P   Malignancy, internal hemorrhoids.

A   Lax sphincter tone.

P   Perineal trauma from childbirth or anal intercourse, neurological disorders.

E **Examination**   N **Normal Findings**   A **Abnormal Findings**   P **Pathophysiology**

21

Male Genitalia

ANATOMY AND PHYSIOLOGY

The male reproductive system includes essential and accessory organs, ducts, and supporting structures (Figure 21-1). The essential organs are the testes, or male gonads. The accessory organs include the seminal vesicles and bulbourethral glands. There are also several ducts, including the epididymis, ductus (vas) deferens, ejaculatory ducts, and urethra. The supporting structures include the scrotum, penis, and spermatic cords. The prostate is discussed in Chapter 22.

The testes, or testicles, are two oval glands located in the scrotum. The seminal vesicles are two pouches located posteriorly to and at the base of the bladder. They contribute about 60% of the volume of semen.

The bulbourethral glands, or Cowper's glands, are pea-sized glands located just below the prostate. The bulbourethral glands secrete an alkaline substance that protects sperm by neutralizing the acidic environment of the vagina.

The epididymis is a comma-shaped, tightly coiled tube that is located on the top and behind the testis and inside the scrotum. Sperm mature and develop the power of motility as they pass through the epididymis. The ductus

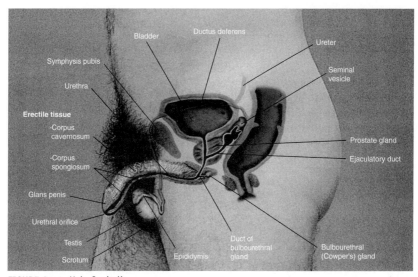

FIGURE 21-1 Male Genitalia.

HEALTH HISTORY

Medical History	Prior history of STI, prostatitis, urinary tract infection, nephrolithiasis, cryptorchidism, trauma, cancer, benign prostatic hypertrophy (BPH), congenital or acquired deformity (epispadias, hypospadias), premature ejaculation, impotence, infertility
Surgical History	Prostatectomy, transurethral prostatectomy (TURP), circumcision, orchiectomy, correction of malposition of testes, vasectomy, lesion or nodule removal, epispadias repair, hypospadias repair, hernia repair
Medications	Antibiotics, hormone replacements, 5-alpha-reductase inhibitors, antihypertensives, psychotropic agents
Communicable Diseases	HSV, HPV, molluscum contagiosum, condyloma acuminata, syphilis, penile lesion, *chlamydia*, gonorrhea, ureaplasma
Injuries and Accidents	Trauma, testicular torsion
Childhood Illnesses	Mumps: orchitis, infertility
Family Health History	Varicocele, testicular cancer, hypospadias, infertility, mother's use of hormones (diethylstilbestrol [DES]) during pregnancy
Drug Use	Cocaine: priapism with chronic abuse, impotence, increased sexual excitability
	Barbiturates: impotence
	Amphetamines: increased libido and delayed orgasm in moderate users, impotence in chronic users
Sexual Practice	Multiple partners, partner with multiple partners, new sexual partner, condom use (frequency and accuracy of use), sexual orientation, anal or oral intercourse

(vas) deferens is an extension of the tail of the epididymis. The ejaculatory ducts are two short tubes posterior to the bladder. The urethra is the terminal duct of the seminal fluid passageway. It measures about 20 cm in length, passes through the prostate gland and penis, and terminates at the external urethral orifice.

The scrotum is a pouchlike supporting structure for the testes and consists of rugated, deeply pigmented, loose skin. The penis, or male organ of copulation and urination, is hairless, slightly pigmented, and cylindrical in shape. The penis contains the urethra, a slitlike opening on the tip of the glans. The urethra terminates at the urethral meatus and is the passageway for urine.

The spermatic cord is made up of testicular arteries, autonomic nerves, veins that drain the testicles, lymphatic vessels, and the cremaster muscle. The testicles are suspended by the spermatic cord. The left side of the spermatic cord is longer than the right side, causing the left testicle to be lower in the scrotal sac.

The primary function of the male reproductive system is to produce sperm to fertilize eggs. The male sexual act consists of four stages: erection, lubrication, emission, and ejaculation.

EQUIPMENT

- Non-sterile gloves
- Penlight
- Stethoscope
- Culturette tube
- Sterile cotton swabs
- Absorbent underpad
- Culture plate
- 10 × power magnifying lens

◄ NURSING CHECKLIST ►

General Approach to Male Genitalia Assessment

1. Greet the patient and explain the assessment techniques that you will be using.
2. Ensure that the examination room is at a warm, comfortable room temperature to prevent patient chilling and shivering.
3. Use a quiet room that will be free from interruptions.
4. Ensure that the light in the room provides sufficient brightness to adequately observe the patient.
5. Assess the patient's apprehension level about the assessment and address this with him, reassuring him that this is normal.
6. Instruct the patient to remove his pants and underpants.
7. Place the patient on the examination table in the supine position with the legs spread slightly, and cover with a drape sheet. Stand to the patient's right side or
7a. Have the patient stand in front of you while you are sitting.
8. Don clean gloves.
9. Expose the entire genital and groin area.

ASSESSMENT OF THE MALE GENITALIA

Inspection

Sexual Maturity Rating (SMR)

E 1. Assess the developmental stage of the pubic hair, penis, and scrotum.
   2. Determine the SMR.

N Males usually begin puberty between the ages of $9\frac{1}{2}$ and $13\frac{1}{2}$. The average male proceeds through puberty in about three years, with a possible range of two to five years.

A SMR less than expected for a male's age.

P Familial, chronic illnesses.

A A normally formed but diminutive penis is abnormal. There is a discrepancy between the penile size and the age of the individual.

Hair Distribution

E 1. Note hair distribution pattern.
   2. Note the presence of nits or lice.

N Pubic hair is distributed in a triangular form. It is sparsely distributed on the scrotum and inner thigh and absent on the penis. Genital hair is more coarse than scalp hair. There are no nits or lice.

A Hair distribution is sparse or hair is absent at the genitalia area. This is called alopecia.

P Genetic factors, aging, or local or systemic disease.

A Nits or lice.

P Pediculosis.

Penis

E 1. Inspect the glans, foreskin, and shaft for lesions, swelling, and inflammation. If the patient is uncircumcised, ask him to retract the foreskin so that the underlying area can be inspected. Ensure the foreskin is replaced after the assessment.
   2. Inspect the anterior surface of the penis first. Then lift the penis to check the posterior surface.
   3. Note the shape of the penis.

N Skin is free of lesions and inflammation. The shaft skin appears loose and wrinkled in the male without an erection. The glans is smooth and without lesions, swelling, and inflammation. The foreskin retracts easily and there is no discharge.

E **Examination**   N **Normal Findings**   A **Abnormal Findings**   P **Pathophysiology**

Nursing Alert

Signs and symptoms of STI in men

- Urethral discharge, bloody or purulent
- Scrotal or testicular pain
- Burning or pain during urination
- Penile lesion, rashes

There may be a small amount of smegma, a white, cottage cheese–like substance, present. The dorsal vein is sometimes visible. The penis is cylindrical in shape. The glans penis varies in size and shape and may appear rounded or broad.

P Inflammation of the glans penis.

A Balanitis, bacterial infection.

A Small papular lesion that enlarges and undergoes superficial necrosis to produce a sharply marginated ulcer on a clean base.

P The chancre is the lesion of primary syphilis.

A Tender, painful, ulcerated, exudative, papular lesion with an erythematous halo, surrounding edema, and a friable base.

P Chancroid is caused by inoculation of *Haemophilus ducreyi*.

A Penile lesion from subtle induration to a small papule.

P Penile carcinoma.

A Pinhead papules to cauliflower-like groupings of filiform, skin-coloured, pink, or red lesions.

P Condyloma acuminatum (genital warts).

A Multifocal maculopapular lesions that are tan, brown, pink, violet, or white.

P Intraepithelial neoplasia.

A Erythematous, painful ulcers developing into vesicular lesions that may become pustular are abnormal.

P Herpes simplex virus infection.

A Multiple, discrete, flat pustules with slight scaling and surrounding edema.

P *Candida* is a superficial mycotic infection of moist cutaneous sites.

A Erythematous plaques with scaling, papular lesions with sharp margins, and occasionally clear centres, and pustules.

P Tinea cruris, a fungal infection, usually caused by *Epidermophyton floccosum* or *Trichophyton rubrum*.

A An unusually narrow foreskin or one that cannot be retracted over the glans penis.

P Phimosis. Inability to retract the foreskin is normal in infancy. In later years, an acquired constricting circumferential scar may follow healing of a split foreskin.

A Retracted foreskin develops a fixed constriction proximal to the glans.

P If the foreskin is retracted and not returned to its original position, paraphimosis can ensue.

A A continuous and pathological erection of the penis.

P Priapism associated with leukemia, metastatic carcinoma, sickle cell anemia, intracavernous injection, alcohol abuse, genital trauma, and neurologic disorders, antihypertensives, antipsychotics, and antidepressants.

A Penile curvature, or chordee, is either a ventral or a dorsal curvature of the penis.

P Congenitally caused by a fibrous band along the usual course of the corpus spongiosum, Peyronie's disease.

Scrotum

E 1. Displace the penis to one side in order to inspect the scrotal skin.
  2. Lift up the scrotum to inspect the posterior side.
  3. Observe for lesions, inflammation, swelling, and nodules.
  4. Note size and shape.
  5. The patient should then stand with legs slightly spread apart.
  6. Have the patient perform the Valsalva manoeuvre.
  7. Observe for a mass of dilated testicular veins in the spermatic cord above and behind the testes.

N Scrotal skin appears rugated and thin and appears more deeply pigmented than body colour. The skin should hug the testicles firmly in the young male and become elongated and flaccid in the elderly male. All skin areas should be free of

---

E **Examination**   N **Normal Findings**   A **Abnormal Findings**   P **Pathophysiology**

any lesions, nodules, swelling, or inflammation. Scrotal size and shape vary greatly from one individual to another. The left scrotal sac is lower than the right. There should be no dilated testicular veins.

A Condyloma acuminatum, tinea cruris, and *Candida*.

A Enlargement of or masses within the scrotum.

P Benign or malignant conditions. Scrotal swelling is seen with inguinal hernia, hydrocele, varicocele, spermatocele, tumour, edema.

A Large, pear-sized mass in the scrotum.

P Hydrocele created by the accumulation of fluid between the two layers of the tunica vaginalis.

A A well-defined cystic mass on the superior testis or in the epididymis.

P Spermatocele: sperm-filled cysts at the top of the testis or in the epididymis.

A In light-skinned individuals, a scrotal mass with a bluish discoloration.

P Dilated veins in the pampiniform plexus of the spermatic cord cause varicocele.

A Round, firm, cystic nodule confined within the scrotal skin.

P Sebaceous cyst contains sebum, an oily, fatty matter secreted by the sebaceous glands.

Urethral Meatus

E 1. Note the location of the urethral meatus.
   2. Observe for discharge.
   3. Obtain a culture of any discharge.
   4. If the patient complains of penile discharge but none is present, ask the patient to milk the penis from the shaft to the glans.

N The urethral meatus is located centrally. It is pink and without discharge.

A Erythema and swelling at the urethral meatus.

P Urethritis, a localized tissue inflammation resulting from bacterial, viral, or fungal infection, urethral trauma.

A Urethral meatus displaced dorsally.

P Epispadias is a congenital abnormality caused by a complete or partial dorsal fusion defect of the urethra.

A Urethral meatus open on the ventral aspect of the glans penis.

P Hypospadias is a congenital abnormality, usually associated with chordee.

Inguinal Area

E 1. If the patient is supine, ask the patient to stand.
   2. Stand facing the patient.
   3. Observe for swelling or bulges.
   4. Ask the patient to bear down.
   5. Observe for swelling or bulges.

N The inguinal area is free of any swelling or bulges.

A Bulge in the inguinal area.

P Hernia.

Palpation

Penis

E 1. Stand in front of the patient's genital area.
   2. Don clean gloves.
   3. Between the thumb and the first two fingers, palpate the entire length of the penis.
   4. Note any pulsations, tenderness, masses, or plaques.

N Pulsations are present on the dorsal sides of the penis. The penis is non-tender. No masses or firm plaques are palpated.

A Fibrotic plaques or ridges along the dorsal shaft.

P Perivascular inflammation between the tunica albuginea and the underlying spongy erectile tissue.

A Vascular insufficiency is evidenced by diminished or absent palpable pulse or pulsations.

P Systemic disease, localized trauma, localized disease.

A Generalized penile swelling.

P Fluid accumulation in the loose tissue of the penile integument, trauma.

| E **Examination** | N **Normal Findings** | A **Abnormal Findings** | P **Pathophysiology** |

Urethral Meatus

E **1.** Stand in front of the patient's genital area.

    2. Between the thumb and forefinger, grasp the glans and gently squeeze to expose the meatus (Figure 21-2).

    3. If discharge is seen, or if the patient complains of a urethral discharge, a culture should be taken.

N The urethral meatus is free of discharge and drainage.

A Urethral discharge of pus.

P Bacterial infection.

Scrotum

E **1.** Between the thumb and the first two fingers, gently palpate the left testicle (Figure 21-3).

    2. Note the size, shape, consistency, and presence of masses.

    3. Palpate the epididymis.

    4. Note the consistency and presence of tenderness or masses.

    5. Between the thumb and the first two fingers, palpate the spermatic cord from the epididymis to the external ring.

    6. Note the consistency and presence of tenderness or masses.

    7. Repeat on the left side.

N The scrotum contains on each side a testicle and an epididymis. The testicles should be firm (but not hard), ovoid, smooth, and equal in size bilaterally. They should be sensitive to pressure but not tender. The epididymis is comma-shaped and should be distinguishable from the testicle. The epididymis should be insensitive to pressure. The spermatic cord should feel smooth and round.

A A unilateral mass palpated within or about the testicle.

P Intratesticular masses should be considered malignant until proven otherwise.

A/P Refer to the section on scrotal inspection for a description of hydrocele.

A A soft testis.

P Hypogonadism.

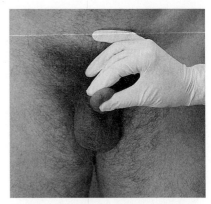

FIGURE 21-2 Palpation of the Urethral Meatus.

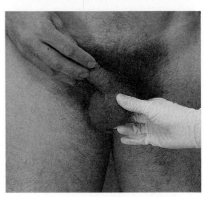

FIGURE 21-3 Palpation of the Testicle.

Nursing Alert

Risk Factors of Testicular Cancer

- Caucasian race, especially Scandinavian background
- Higher socioeconomic status
- Unmarried
- Rural resident
- History of cryptorchidism (even if previously repaired)

E **Examination**   N **Normal Findings**   A **Abnormal Findings**   P **Pathophysiology**

Nursing Tip

Teaching Testicular Self-Examination

Testicular self-examination (TSE) should be taught to the patient during the scrotal examination.

- Ask the patient if monthly testicular self-examination is performed.
- Explain the rationale for the examination. Monthly testicular examination will allow for earlier detection of testicular cancer.
- Tell the patient to pick a date to perform the exam every month. The best time to perform the examination is after a warm shower when both hands and the scrotum are warm.
- Instruct the patient to gently feel each testicle using the thumb and first two fingers (Figure 21-4A).
- Remind the patient that the testicles are ovoid and movable, and that they feel firm and rubbery. The epididymis is located on top and behind the testis, is softer, and feels ropelike.
- Instruct the patient to report any changes from these findings, including any lumps and nodules, especially if they are non-mobile.
- Instruct the patient to squeeze the tip of the penis and check for any discharge (Figure 21-4B).

A   Palpation of a scrotal mass superior to the testis.

P   Varicocele.

A   Testicle enlarged, retracted, in a lateral position, and/or extremely sensitive.

P   Twisting or torsion of the testis causes venous obstruction, secondary edema, and eventual arterial obstruction.

A   Indurated, swollen, tender epididymis.

P   Bacterial pathogens such as *chlamydia trachomatis* and *Neisseria gonorrhoeae*.

A   One or both testes undescended.

P   Cryptorchidism related to testicular failure, deficient gonadotrophic stimulation, mechanical obstruction, gubernacular defects.

A   An acute, painful onset of swelling of the testicle along with warm scrotal skin.

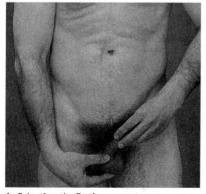

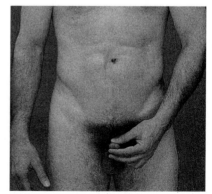

A. Palpating the Testis

B. Assessing for Penile Discharge

FIGURE 21-4 Testicular Self-examination.

| E **Examination** | N **Normal Findings** | A **Abnormal Findings** | P **Pathophysiology** |

P   Orchitis can be caused by mumps, cox-sackievirus B, infectious mononucleosis, varicella.

A   In light-skinned individuals, it is abnormal for the scrotum to be enlarged, taut with pitting edema, and reddened.

P   Scrotal edema associated with the lower half of the body, such as in congestive heart failure (CHF), renal failure, portal vein obstruction.

A   Acute, painful, scrotal swelling.

P   Trauma, testicular rupture.

Inguinal Area

E   1. With the index and middle fingers of the right hand, palpate the skin overlying the inguinal and femoral areas for lymph nodes.

2. Note size, consistency, tenderness, and mobility.

3. Ask the patient to bear down while you palpate the inguinal area.

4. Place the right index finger in the patient's right scrotal sac above the right testicle and invaginate the scrotal skin. Follow the spermatic cord until you reach a triangular, slitlike opening (the external inguinal ring).

5. The finger is placed with the nail facing inward and the finger pad outward (Figure 21-5).

6. If the inguinal ring is large enough, continue to advance the finger along the inguinal canal and ask the patient to turn his head and cough.

7. Note any masses felt against the finger.

8. Repeat on the left side using the left hand to perform the palpation.

9. Palpate the femoral canal. Ask the patient to bear down.

N   It is normal for there to be small (1 cm), freely mobile lymph nodes present in the inguinal area. There should not be any bulges present in the inguinal area. There should not be any palpable masses in the inguinal canal. No portions of the bowel should enter the scrotum. There should be no palpable mass at the femoral canal.

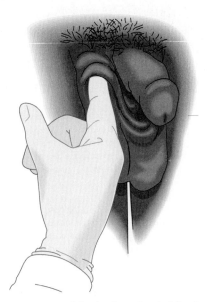

FIGURE 21-5 Palpation for an Inguinal Hernia.

A   Unilateral enlargement of the lymph nodes with erythematous overlying skin.

P   Lymphogranuloma venereum (LV).

A   Unilateral or bilateral enlargement of the inguinal lymph nodes.

P   Bacterial infections, trauma, carcinoma.

A/P Table 21-1 compares the different types of hernias. Refer to Figures 21-6, 21-7, and 21-8.

Auscultation

Auscultation is performed if a scrotal mass is found on inspection or palpation.

Scrotum

E   1. Place the patient in a supine position.

2. Stand at the patient's right side at the genitalia area.

3. Place your stethoscope over the scrotal mass.

4. Listen for the presence of bowel sounds.

N   No bowel sounds are present in the scrotum.

E **Examination**   N **Normal Findings**   A **Abnormal Findings**   P **Pathophysiology**

TABLE 21-1 Comparison of Inguinal and Femoral Hernias

FEATURE	INDIRECT INGUINAL HERNIA	DIRECT INGUINAL HERNIA	FEMORAL HERNIA
Occurrence	More common in infants <1 year and males 16 to 25 years of age.	Middle-aged and elderly men.	More frequent in women.
Origin of Swelling	Above inguinal ligament. Hernia sac enters canal at internal ring and exits at external ring. Can be found in the scrotum.	Above inguinal ligament. Directly behind and through external ring.	Below inguinal ligament.
Cause	Congenital or acquired.	Acquired weakness brought on by heavy lifting, obesity, COPD.	Acquired, due to increased abdominal pressure and muscle weakness.
Signs and Symptoms	Lump or fullness in the groin that may be associated with a cough or crying.	Lump or fullness in the groin area. It may cause an aching or dragging sensation	Firm a rubbery lump in the groin. Plain may be severe.

A   An indirect inguinal hernia is present if bowel sounds are present in the enlarged scrotum.

P   Loops of bowel extending into the scrotum via an indirect hernia.

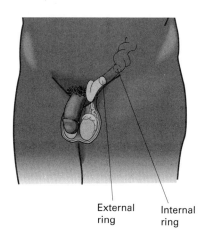

FIGURE 21-6 Indirect Inguinal Hernia.

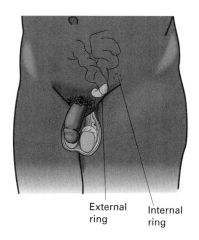

FIGURE 21-7 Direct Inguinal Hernia.

E **Examination**   N **Normal Findings**   A **Abnormal Findings**   P **Pathophysiology**

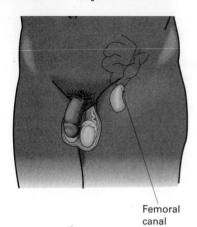

Femoral
canal

FIGURE 21-8 Femoral Hernia.

22

Anus, Rectum, and Prostate

ANATOMY AND PHYSIOLOGY

Rectum

The large intestine is composed of the cecum, colon, rectum, and anal canal. The cecum and colon are discussed in Chapter 17. The sigmoid colon begins at the pelvic brim. Beyond the sigmoid colon, the large intestine passes downward in front of the sacrum. This portion is called the rectum (Figure 22-1). The rectum contains three transverse folds, or valves of Houston. These valves work to retain fecal material so it is not passed along with flatus.

Anus

The terminal 3 to 4 cm of the large intestine is called the anal canal. The anal canal fuses with the rectum at the anorectal junction, or the dentate line, and together these structures form the anorectum.

In the superior half of the anal canal are anal columns, which are longitudinal folds of mucosa (also called columns of Morgagni). The anal valves are formed by inferior joining anal columns. There are pockets located superior to the valves and are called the anal sinuses. These sinuses secrete mucus when they are compressed

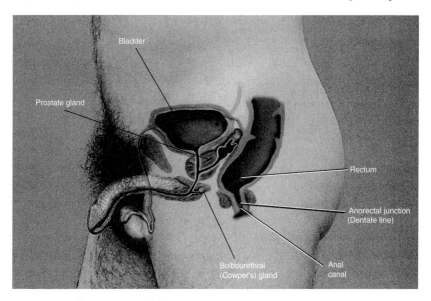

FIGURE 22-1 The Anorectum and Prostate.

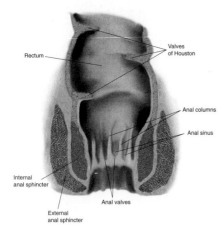

FIGURE 22-2 Anal Canal.

by feces, providing lubrication that eases fecal passage during defecation (Figure 22-2).

The anal canal opens to the exterior through the anus. Internal and external anal sphincter muscles surround the anus. Smooth muscle, which is under involuntary control, forms the internal sphincter. Skeletal muscle forms the external sphincter and is under voluntary control, allowing a person to control bowel movements.

Prostate

Contiguous with part of the anterior rectal wall in the male is the prostate gland. The prostate is an accessory male sex organ the size and shape of a chestnut, approximately 3.5 cm long by 3 cm wide. It consists of glandular tissue and muscle, and its small ducts drain into the urethra.

HEALTH HISTORY

Medical History	Trauma, inflammatory bowel disease, prior history of STIs, polyps, rectal cancer, hemorrhoids, pruritus ani, constipation, diarrhea, incontinence
	Prostate cancer, prostatitis, benign prostatic hypertrophy
Surgical History	Sigmoidoscopy, colonoscopy, rubber band ligation, injection sclerotherapy, hemorrhoidectomy, drainage of fistula or abscess
	Prostatectomy, transurethral resection of the prostate (TURP)
Medications	Laxatives, constipating agents, alpha blockers, 5-alpha-reductase inhibitors, antifungals, astringent ointments, suppositories
Communicable Diseases	HIV, *Neisseria gonorrhoeae, Treponema pallidum* (syphilis), *chlamydia trachomatis*, human papillomavirus (HPV), herpes simplex virus (HSV)
Family Health History	Rectal polyps, rectal cancer, pilonidal cyst, prostate cancer
Sexual History	Rectal penetration increases the risk for anal carcinoma and anorectal STIs.
	Use of foreign objects in the rectum can lead to anal valve incompetence.
Diet	Increased amounts of dietary fats, cured and smoked meats, and charcoal-broiled foods, and decreased amounts of fibre, fruits, and vegetables are associated with prostate and rectal cancers; excessive intake of milk, coffee, tea, cola, and spices is associated with pruritus ani. Vitamins A, C, E, and folate may protect against developing rectal cancer.

The prostate has five lobes: anterior, posterior, median, and two lateral. The median sulcus is the groove between the lateral lobes. The right and left lateral lobes are accessible to examination.

EQUIPMENT

- Non-sterile gloves
- Water-soluble lubricant
- Hemoccult cards
- Gooseneck lamp

ASSESSMENT OF THE ANUS, RECTUM, AND PROSTATE

Inspection

Perineum and Sacrococcygeal Area

E   Inspect the buttocks and sacral region for lesions, swelling, inflammation, and tenderness.

N   This area should be smooth and free of lesions, swelling, inflammation, and

---

◄ NURSING CHECKLIST ►

General Approach to Anus, Rectum, and Prostate Assessment

1. Greet the patient and explain the assessment techniques that you will be using.
2. Ensure that the examination room is at a warm, comfortable temperature to prevent patient chilling and shivering.
3. Use a quiet room that will be free from interruptions.
4. Ensure that the light in the room provides sufficient brightness to adequately observe the patient. It may be helpful to have a gooseneck lamp available for additional lighting when lesions are observed.
5. Instruct the patient to void prior to the assessment.
6. Instruct the patient to remove pants and underpants and to cover up with a drape sheet.
7. Assess the patient's apprehension level about the assessment and reassure the patient that apprehension is normal.
8. For inspection, place the patient in the left lateral decubitus position and visualize the perianal skin (Figure 22-3A). This position can also be used for palpation.
9. For palpation, have the patient stand at the side or end of the examination table, bending over the table resting the elbows on the table and spreading the legs slightly apart (Figure 22-3B).
   9a. For the patient who cannot stand, have the patient assume the knee-chest position (Figure 22-3C).
   9b. For the female who is undergoing a rectovaginal examination, have her assume the lithotomy position. See Chapter 20.
10. Don non-sterile gloves.
11. Use a systematic approach every time the assessment is performed. Proceed from the anus to the rectum in the female patient. Proceed from the anus to the prostate in the male patient.

| E **Examination** | N **Normal Findings** | A **Abnormal Findings** | P **Pathophysiology** |

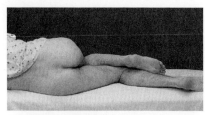

A. Left Lateral Decubitus

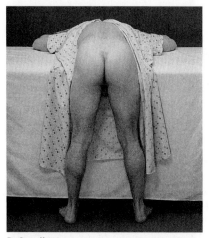

B. Standing

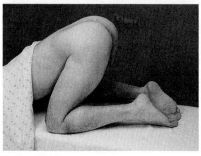

C. Knee-Chest

FIGURE 22-3 Patient Positions for the Anus, Rectum, and Prostate Examination.

tenderness. There should be no evidence of feces or mucus on the perianal skin.

A One or several tiny openings in the midline over the sacral region, often with hair protruding.

P Pilonidal disease.

A Hyperpigmentation, coupled with excoriation and thickened skin.

P Pruritus ani caused by pinworms in children, fungal infections in adults.

A Well-demarcated, erythematous, sometimes itchy, exudative patches of varying size and shape and rimmed with small, red-based pustules.

P *Candida albicans.*

Anal Mucosa

E 1. Spread the patient's buttocks apart with both hands, exposing the anus.
   2. Instruct the patient to bear down as though moving the bowels.
   3. Examine the anus for colour, appearance, lesions, inflammation, rash, and masses.

N The anal mucosa is deeply pigmented, coarse, moist, and hairless. It should be free of lesions, inflammation, rash, masses, or additional openings. The anal opening should be closed. There should not be any leakage of feces or mucus from the anus with straining and there should not be any tissue protrusion.

A A spherical, bluish lump that appears suddenly at the anus, and that ranges in size from a few millimetres to several centimetres in diameter. The overlying anal skin may be tense and edematous. Pain and pruritus may be present.

P Hemorrhoids from dilatation of the superior and inferior hemorrhoidal veins.

A Excess anal or perianal tissue of varying sizes that is soft, pliable, and covered by normal skin.

P Anal skin tags (residual resolved thrombosed external hemorrhoids).

A Linear tears in the epidermis of the anal canal beginning below the dentate line and extending distally to the anal orifice. Extreme pain, pruritus, and bleeding may accompany these findings.

P Anal fissures are the result of trauma, such as the forced passage of a large, hard stool, and anal intercourse, especially forced.

E Examination   N Normal Findings   A Abnormal Findings   P Pathophysiology

A   Undrained collections of perianal pus of the tissue spaces in and adjacent to the anorectum.

P   Anorectal abscess is infection of the anal glands, usually located posteriorly and situated between the internal and the external sphincters.

A   An inflamed, red, raised area with purulent or serosanguinous discharge on the perianal skin (Figure 22-4).

P   Anorectal fistula, fibrous tract lined by granulation tissue and having an opening inside the anal canal or rectum and one or more orifices in the perianal skin. Usually the result of incomplete healing of drained anorectal abscesses.

A   Soiling of the skin with stool and gaping of the anus.

P   Anal incontinence caused by neurological diseases, traumatic injuries, or surgical damage to the puborectalis or sphincter muscles.

A   Protrusion of the rectal mucosa (pinkish red doughnut with radiating folds) through the anal orifice (see Figure 22-5).

P   Rectal prolapse: chronic straining at stool, fecal incontinence, neurological disease or traumatic damage to the pelvis.

A   Erythematous plaques that develop into vesicular lesions that may become pustules and ulcerate.

P   HSV.

A   Warts or lesions that are beefy red, flesh coloured, irregular, and pedunculated.

P   Condylomata acuminatum caused by HPV.

A   Mucoid or creamy exudate, possibly blood, from the rectum.

P   Gonococcal proctitis.

A   Perianal fissures and edematous skin tags of varying degrees.

P   Perianal disease.

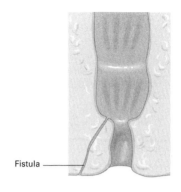

Fistula

Skin
surface
opening

FIGURE 22-4 Anorectal Fistula.

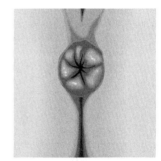

FIGURE 22-5 Rectal Prolapse.

Palpation

Anus and Rectum

To perform anal and rectal wall palpation:

E   1. Have the patient assume one of the positions described in Figure 22-3.

2. Reassure the patient that sensations of urination and defecation are common during the rectal assessment.

3. Lubricate a gloved index finger.

4. Place your finger by the anal orifice and instruct the patient to bear down (Valsalva manoeuvre) as you gently insert the flexed tip of your gloved finger into the anal sphincter, with the tip of the finger

---

E Examination   N Normal Findings   A Abnormal Findings   P Pathophysiology

toward the anterior rectal wall (pointed toward the umbilicus) (Figure 22-6). The anus should never be approached at a right angle (with the index finger extended).

4a. If the patient tightens the sphincter, remove your finger, reassure the patient, and try again, using a relaxation technique such as deep breathing.

5. Feel the sphincter relax. Insert finger as far as it will go (Figure 22-7). Note anal sphincter tone.

6. Palpate the lateral, posterior, and anterior walls of the rectum in a sequenced manner. The lateral walls are felt by rotating the finger along the sides of the rectum. Palpate for nodules, irregularity, masses, and tenderness.

6a. Ask the patient to bear down again (which may help to palpate masses).

7. Slowly withdraw the finger; inspect any fecal matter on your glove and test it for occult blood. Table 22-1 lists common stool findings and etiologies. Table 22-2 lists the common causes of rectal bleeding.

8. Offer the patient tissues to wipe off any remaining lubricant.

N   The rectum should accommodate the index finger. There should be good sphincter tone at rest and with bearing

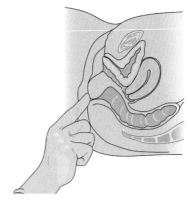

FIGURE 22-6 Position of the Index Finger for Anorectal Palpation.

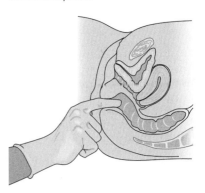

FIGURE 22-7 Position of the Index Finger in the Anorectum.

TABLE 22-1   Common Stool Findings and Etiologies

STOOL FINDING	ETIOLOGY
Black, tarry (melena)	Upper gastrointestinal bleeding
Bright red	Rectal bleeding
Black	Iron or bismuth ingestion
Gray, tan	Obstructive jaundice
Pale yellow, greasy, fatty (steatorrhea)	Malabsorption syndromes (e.g., celiac disease), cystic fibrosis
Mucus with blood and pus	Ulcerative colitis, acute diverticulitis
Maroon or bright red	Diverticulosis

E   **Examination**   N   **Normal Findings**   A   **Abnormal Findings**   P   **Pathophysiology**

TABLE 22-2	Common Causes of Rectal Bleeding

- Cancer of the colon
- Benign polyps of the colon
- Hemorrhoids
- Anal fissure
- Inflammatory bowel disease
- Forced or vigorous anal intercourse
- Traumatic sexual practices

down. There should be no excessive pain, tenderness, induration, irregularities, or nodules in the rectum or rectal wall.

A   Anal canal tight (making insertion of the index finger very difficult and painful or impossible).

P   Anal stenosis can occur congenitally, or is acquired (anorectal operations, diarrheal disease, inflammatory conditions, and the habitual use of laxatives).

A   Internal masses of vascular tissue in the anal canal.

P   Internal hemorrhoids.

A   A soft nodule in the rectum.

P   Rectal polyps: pedunculated (attached to a stalk) or sessile (adhering to the rectal mucosal wall).

A   Tender, indurated mass in the anorectum.

P   Anorectal abscess.

A   An indurated cord palpated in the anorectum.

P   Anorectal fistula tracts (may be palpated from the secondary orifice toward the anus).

A   A small, symmetrical projection 2 to 4 cm long.

P   Rectal prolapse: anal sphincter is lax.

A   Foreign bodies palpated in the rectum.

P   Thermometers, enema catheters, vibrators, bottles, phallic objects.

A   A hard mass in the anal canal.

P   Anal carcinoma.

A   A firm, sometimes rocklike but often rubbery, puttylike mass.

P   Fecal impaction.

Prostate

E   To perform prostatic palpation:

1. Position the patient as tolerated (the standing position is preferred).
2. Reassure the patient that sensations of urination and defecation are common during the prostatic assessment.
3. Use a well-lubricated, gloved index finger.
4. Insert the gloved index finger and proceed as described in steps 4 and 5 on pages 317 and 318.
5. Perform bidigital examination of the bulbourethral gland by pressing

---

Nursing Alert

Risk Factors for Colorectal Cancer[1]

- Over 50 years of age (most of those diagnosed are 70 years or older)
- Family history of colorectal cancer
- Personal history of adenomatous polyps and/or chronic inflammatory bowel disease (ulcerative colitis, Crohn's disease)
- Personal history of endometrial, ovarian, or breast cancer
- Diet high in red meat and low in fruits and vegetables; high-fat diet
- Obesity
- Lack of physical activity
- Alcohol consumption, especially beer
- Smoking

E **Examination**	N **Normal Findings**	A **Abnormal Findings**	P **Pathophysiology**

your gloved thumb into the perianal tissue while pressing your gloved index finger toward it (Figure 22-8). Assess for tenderness, masses, or swelling.

6. Release pressure of the thumb and index finger. Remove thumb from the perianal tissue and advance your index finger.

7. Palpate the posterior surface of the prostate gland (Figure 22-9). Note the size, shape, consistency, sensitivity, and mobility of the prostate. Note whether the median sulcus is palpable.

8. Attempt to palpate the seminal vesicles by extending your index finger above the prostate gland. Assess for tenderness and masses.

9. Slowly withdraw the finger; inspect any fecal matter on your glove and test it for occult blood (if not previously performed).

N   The prostate gland should be small, smooth, mobile, and non-tender. The median sulcus should be palpable.

A   A soft, tender, enlarged prostate gland.

P   Benign prostatic hypertrophy (BPH) is related to aging and the presence of testosterone, which converts to dihydrotestosterone and leads to prostatic cell growth.

A   A firm, tender, or fluctuant mass on the prostate.

P   Prostatic abscesses are caused mainly by *Escherichia coli*.

A   Firm, hard, or indurated nodules on the prostate.

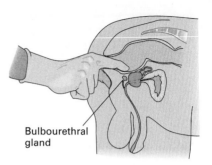

FIGURE 22-8 Bidigital Palpation of the Bulbourethral Gland.

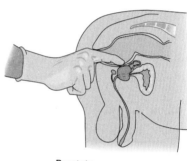

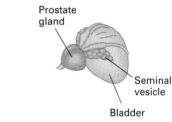

FIGURE 22-9 Prostatic Palpation.

Nursing Alert

Risk Factors for Prostate Cancer[2]

- Family history of prostate cancer
- Age (particularly after 65; uncommon in men under 50)
- Ethnicity—African ancestry

Research is ongoing into other potential risk factors including dietary factors; sexual factors including sexually transmitted infections; occupational exposures; and hormonal factors.

E   Examination   N   Normal Findings   A   Abnormal Finding   P   Pathophysiology

P   Prostate cancer.
A   An exquisitely tender and warm prostate.
P   Bacterial prostatitis usually caused by
     Escherichia coli.

REFERENCES

[1]Health Canada, 2005. Screening for colorectal
     cancer. Retrieved November 9, 2006, from
     http://www.hc-sc.gc.ca/ iyh-vsv/diseases-
     maladies/colorectal_e.html
[2]Centre for Chronic Disease Prevention and
     Control (2005). Prostate Cancer. Retrieved
     November 17, 2006, from http://www.phac-
     aspc.gc.ca/ccdpc-cpcmc/topics/cancer_
     prost_e.html#desc

E Examination	N Normal Findings	A Abnormal Findings	P Pathophysiology

Unit 4

Special Populations

23

Pregnant Patient

ANATOMY AND PHYSIOLOGY

Pregnancy brings about many physiological, hormonal, and psychological changes in a woman during the 280 days, or approximately 40 weeks, of gestation. The pregnancy is subdivided into trimesters of a little more than 13 weeks each, and various symptoms and problems can be specific to each trimester. Physiological changes during pregnancy affect every system in the body.

Skin and Hair

Increased subdermal fat deposit; thickening of the skin; acne may develop or improve; increase in sweat and sebaceous gland production; pigmentation increases in the nipples, areolae, external genitalia, and anal region; the face may develop melasma or chloasma; linea nigra or darkening of the linea alba on the abdomen; skin tags, molluscum fibrosum gravidarum may develop; striae gravidarum (stretch marks) on the abdomen, breasts, and upper thighs; development or enlargement of spider angiomas, hemangiomas, varicosities, palmar erythema; facial hair may increase.

Head and Neck

The thyroid gland may increase in size after approximately 12 weeks of gestation.

Eyes, Ears, Nose, Mouth, and Throat

Corneal thickening and edema; nasal stuffiness, snoring, congestion and epistaxis; impaired hearing or fullness in the ears; decreased sense of smell; soft, edematous, and bleeding gums; ptyalism (excessive secretion of saliva).

Breasts

Enlargement, tingling, and tenderness; Montgomery's tubercles enlarge; lactiferous ducts proliferate; areolae and nipples may become darker; colostrum (thick, yellow discharge) may be secreted.

Thorax and Lungs

Diaphragm elevates approximately 4 cm and the movement of the diaphragm increases; the thoracic cage relaxes and expands by 5 to 7 cm; tidal volume increases 30% to 40%; increased respiratory rate, hyperventilation, or shortness of breath on exertion.

Heart and Peripheral Vasculature

Blood volume increases by 30% to 50%; heart lies more horizontally and shifts upward and to the left; heart rate increases by 10 to 15 beats per minute, a split first heart and S_3 sound may be heard, physiological systolic murmurs of grade 2/6 may be heard; blood pressure varies according to position and trimester; supine hypotension; diastolic pressure may lower by 5 mm Hg; dependent edema.

Abdomen

Decreased tone and motility, decreased bowel sounds, increased emptying time for the stomach and intestines; increased flatulence and constipation; hemorrhoids; indigestion (heartburn); nausea and vomiting; separation of the rectus muscle (diastasis recti).

Urinary System

Glomerular filtration rate (GFR) increases by approximately 50%; urinary frequency; glycosuria (glucose in the urine); proteinuria; nocturia.

Musculoskeletal System

Widening (and, occasionally, a separation) of the symphysis pubis at approximately 28 to 32 weeks; increased pelvic mobility to accommodate vaginal delivery; unsteady gait known as the "waddle of pregnancy"; upper back or rib pain; lordosis of the lumbar spine; sciatic nerve pain; muscle cramps, particularly in the calves, thighs, and buttocks.

Neurological System

Headaches; numbness, and tingling; seizure activity with no prior history (may indicate eclampsia or pregnancy-induced hypertension); dizziness and lightheadedness.

Female Genitalia

Amenorrhea; uterus begins as a pelvic organ, becoming palpably enlarged at six to seven weeks (Figure 23-1), and to an abdominal organ at approximately 12 weeks of gestation; at 16 weeks the fundus of the uterus is midway between the symphysis pubis and the umbilicus; at 20 weeks it is typically at the umbilicus; between weeks 18 and 32, the height of the uterine fundus above the symphysis pubis is measured in centimetres and is used to confirm the gestational age in weeks; round and broad ligaments elongate to accommodate the growing fetus; lightening (a decrease in fundal height) occurs approximately three weeks prior to the onset of labour in a nulliparous woman; Braxton Hicks contractions (irregular and usually painless) begin as early as the first trimester; the cervix experiences increased vascularity and increased friability (susceptibility to bleeding); mucus production occurs to form an endocervical protective plug (referred to as the mucous plug); the vaginal mucosa thickens secondary to hormonal changes; vaginal discharge increases

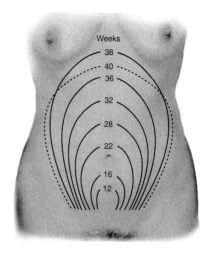

FIGURE 23-1 Uterine and Abdominal Enlargement of Pregnancy.

and is typically of a white, milky consistency; from 36 weeks on, vaginal discharge may become thicker and clumps may be present when the mucous plug is expelled; increased risk of yeast infection.

Anus and Rectum

Decreased gastrointestinal tract tone and motility produce a sense of fullness, indigestion, constipation, bloating, and flatulence. Development of hemorrhoids is common. As the uterus enlarges, mechanical pressure may aggravate constipation and hemorrhoids. Vitamin and iron supplementation may darken the stool.

Hematological System

Increased white blood cell count (WBC), increased total red blood cell (RBC) volume; increased plasma volume; decreased number and increased size of platelets; increased fibrinogen and clotting factors VII through X; physiological anemia of pregnancy.

Endocrine System

The basal metabolic rate (BMR) increases by 15% to 25%; increasing resistance to insulin develops; glycosuria may be noted; less resistant to infection.

HEALTH HISTORY

Medical History	Table 23-1 illustrates a typical obstetric history. Asthma, diabetes mellitus, cardiac disease, renal disease, seizure disorder, autoimmune disorders
Surgical History	Uterine surgery, cone or excisional biopsy of the cervix, abdominal surgery leading to internal or external scarring or adhesions
Communicable Diseases	TORCH diseases (toxoplasmosis, rubella, cytomegalovirus, herpes), measles, varicella, mumps, human parvovirus B19, HIV, hepatitis B. A rubella titer, VDRL, and hepatitis B surface antigen are routinely drawn on pregnant patients. HIV testing is recommended, if the patient agrees to it. Rubella (German measles), especially in the first trimester, and syphilis during pregnancy can cause anomalies and complications. Other infectious diseases may affect the pregnancy depending on their severity and the gestational age at which the disease is contracted; e.g., varicella may present a problem to the fetus if active at the time of delivery. Other infectious diseases to review include tuberculosis and sexually transmitted illnesses (STIs).
Family Health History	*Pregnancy-related conditions and diseases that are familial are listed.*
	Preterm labour or delivery; hypertensive disorders of pregnancy; diethylstilbestrol (DES) exposure; multiple births in female relatives of patient's mother; chromosome abnormalities such as Down syndrome; genetic disorders such as Tay-Sachs or Gaucher's diseases or sickle cell disease; inheritable diseases, such as Huntington's chorea; congenital anomalies such as cleft lip or palate; neural tube defects; cardiac deformities; blood disorders; diabetes (gestational, Type 1 or 2 diabetes mellitus); neuromuscular diseases; psychiatric disorders; any history of abuse, neglect, or substance abuse
	Family history of baby's father: genetic, hereditary, or chromosomal disorders, abuse or neglect, substance abuse
Social History **Alcohol Use**	Alcohol is a teratogen that can lead to fetal alcohol syndrome (FAS) or fetal alcohol effects (FAE). The absolute safe level of alcohol consumption is unknown. Problems have been documented with an average of 1–2 drinks of alcohol per day and with binge drinking.
Drug Use	Drug effects on the fetus vary according to the drug(s) used and the gestational age at time of use. The most common complications are spontaneous abortion, preterm delivery, congenital anomalies, and stillbirth.
Tobacco Use	Smoking can lead to a small-for-gestational-age (SGA) infant, preterm labour, spontaneous abortions, and lower Apgar scores (refer to Chapter 24).

TABLE 23-1 Obstetric History

PRESENT OBSTETRIC HISTORY

Last menstrual period (LMP)

History since LMP (e.g., fever, rashes, disease exposures, abnormal bleeding, nausea and vomiting, medication use, toxic exposures)

Signs and symptoms of pregnancy

Use of fertility drugs

Estimated date of delivery (EDD) or estimated date of confinement (EDC)*

Genetic predispositions

PAST OBSTETRIC HISTORY

Gravidity/gravida (number of pregnancies)

Parity/para (number of births 20 weeks or greater) usually listed as term (37–42 weeks gestational age), preterm (20–37 weeks gestational age), or postterm (>42 weeks gestational age)

Spontaneous abortion

Therapeutic abortion

Ectopic pregnancy

Multiples or multiple births (more than one fetus or baby)

Number of living children

Pregnancy history (Table 23-2 for high-risk factors):
- Complications during pregnancy
- Duration of gestation
- Date of delivery
- Type of delivery
  (vaginal versus cesarean)
  (if cesarean, reason)
  (forceps or vacuum extraction)
  (episiotomy or laceration, and degree)
- Length of labour
- Medications and anesthesia used
- Complications during labour and delivery
- Postpartum complications

Infant weight and sex, Apgar score

Type of feeding (breastfeeding versus bottle feeding)

Breastfeeding: difficulties

Use Naegele's rule to determine EDD: subtract 3 months from the first day of the LMP, then add 7 days. This is based on a 28-day cycle and may have to be adjusted for shorter or longer cycles. For example, if the LMP is September 1, 9/1 – 3 months = 6/1
$$6/1 + 7 \text{ days} = 6/8$$
The EDD for this patient is June 8.
A pregnancy wheel may also be used.

TABLE 23-2   Risk Factors for Pregnancy

There are many risk factor tools and scoring systems available with varying degress of sensitivity and specificity. Some prenatal forms include a risk screen in the history.

MATERNAL

Age less than 18 or older than 40

Single

Abusive relationship and other violence or family relationship stresses

Low socioeconomic status, poverty, or low educational level

Long work hours, long commute or long tiring trip; excessive fatigue

Stress or unusual anxiety, or both, per patient perception

Unplanned pregnancy or conflict about pregnancy, or both

Height less than 1.5 metres.

Weight less than 45 kgs.

Inadequate diet

Habits: smoking, excessive caffeine (greater than 400 mg caffeine per day – 4 to 5 cups of coffee), alcohol consumption, drug addiction

REPRODUCTIVE HISTORY

More than one prior abortion (some risk tools differentiate first and second trimester)

Uterine anomaly

Molar pregnancy/hydatidiform mole

Myomas (leiomyomas)

Sexually transmitted infections or diseases

Perinatal death

Preterm delivery or premature labour, or both

Delivery of infant less than 2500 g

Delivery of infant greater than 4000 g

Delivery of infant with congenital or perinatal disease

Delivery of infant with isoimmunization or ABO incompatibility

Gestational diabetes

Operative delivery

Cervical incompetence

Prior cerclage

MEDICAL PROBLEMS

Hypertension

Renal disease, pyelonephritis, asymptomatic bacteriuria

Diabetes mellitus

Heart disease

Sickle cell disease

Anemia

Pulmonary disease

Endocrine disorder

Neurological disorder

Autoimmune disorder

Hematological disorder

PRESENT PREGNANCY

Late, inadequate, or no prenatal care

Abdominal surgery

Bleeding

Placenta previa

Premature rupture of membranes

Anemia

Hypertension

Preeclampsia or eclampsia

Hydramnios

Multiple pregnancy

Abnormal glucose screen

Low or excessive weight gain

Rh-negative sensitization

Teratogenic exposure

Viral infections (especially fever-rash with first trimester)

Sexually transmitted infection(s) or disease(s)

Bacterial infections (bacterial vaginosis and group B streptococcus, in particular)

Protozoal infections

Abnormal presentation (i.e., breech, transverse) at approximately 36 weeks

Postdates

Nursing Tip

Obstetric Abbreviations

You can classify pregnant patients according to their prior obstetric outcomes by using the following abbreviations. During the initial visit it is important to note all of the categories. In subsequent visits, every category may not be documented, just the number of pregnancies (gravida) and deliveries (para).

G = gravida
P = para
T = term
P = preterm
VP = very preterm
A = abortion (either therapeutic or
    spontaneous; may be listed separately)
E = ectopic pregnancy
LC = living children

Examples:
G 4, P 2, T 2, P 0, VP 0, A 1, E 1, LC 2 = 4 pregnancies, 2 births, 2 term births, 0 preterm or very preterm births, 1 abortion, 1 ectopic pregnancy, 2 living children

EQUIPMENT

- Stethoscope
- Doppler or fetoscope
- Centimetre tape measure
- Watch with a second hand
- Non-sterile gloves
- Speculum
- Genital culture supplies
- Pap smear supplies (see Chapter 20)
- Sphygmomanometer
- Urine cup
- Urine dipsticks

ASSESSMENT OF THE PREGNANT PATIENT

Assessment of the pregnant woman includes a complete initial assessment as well as subsequent specific follow-up prenatal visits. The initial assessment is done when the woman first seeks care. Optimally, a health assessment should be conducted prior to conception. Generally, the schedule for prenatal visits is as follows: every four weeks for weeks 6–28 of gestation, every two weeks for weeks 28–36 of gestation, and weekly from 36 weeks until delivery. Women who go beyond the 40th week of gestation (postdates) require additional evaluations.

General Assessment, Vital Signs, and Weight

E   1. Conduct a general assessment, including obtaining vital signs.
    2. Obtain the patient's weight.

N   See Chapter 9 for normal general assessment and page 324 for blood pressure changes that occur in pregnancy. See Chapter 7 for the recommended weight gain in pregnancy.

A   Hypertension at any time in pregnancy (systolic pressure greater than 140 and a diastolic pressure greater than 90 or a systolic pressure increase of 30 mm Hg and a diastolic pressure increase of 15 mm Hg above pre-pregnancy pressures).

P   PIH.

A   Weight gain that is more than the recommended amount.

P   Increased caloric intake, multiple pregnancies, polyhydramnios, edema secondary to PIH.

A   Weight gain that is less than the recommended amount.

P   Hyperemesis gravidarum, decreased caloric intake, malabsorption syndromes.

Skin and Hair

E   Examine the skin and hair.
N   See Chapter 10.
A   Prurigo of pregnancy; highly pruritic; excoriated papules, usually distributed on the hands and feet.
P   Etiology poorly understood.
A   Papular dermatitis: erythematous, pruritic, widespread, soft papules.
P   Poorly understood.

E Examination   N Normal Findings   A Abnormal Findings   P Pathophysiology

◄ NURSING CHECKLIST ►

General Approach to Assessment of the Pregnant Patient

1. Greet the patient and explain how the assessment will proceed.
2. Ensure that the examination room is ready and supplies are at hand.
3. Use a quiet room that will be free from interruptions.
4. Ensure that there is adequate lighting, including a light that is appropriate for the pelvic assessment.
5. Prior to the physical assessment, complete the health history and the nutritional and psychosocial assessments. (This is usually done in an office before proceeding to the examination room.)
6. Ask the patient to void prior to the examination, both for patient comfort and to facilitate uterine and adnexal evaluation (which can be impeded by a full bladder). The urine should be saved and checked for glucose and acetone.
7. For the physical assessment, instruct the patient to remove all street clothes, don an examination gown, and cover her lap with a sheet.
8. Perform the initial assessment in a head-to-toe manner. Try to minimize the patient's time in the supine position. Assist the patient in assuming the lithotomy position via verbal guidance and by assisting in placing her feet in the foot or leg stirrups. Always inform the patient before touching her of what you will be doing and what to expect. Special sensitivity should be given to adolescents and the patient who is having her first pelvic examination. The patient may be dizzy upon sitting up or upon standing. It may be beneficial to assist her to a sitting position or to brace her arm. She should be cautioned not to stand or sit up abruptly.

A   Erythematous plaques that develop into vesicular lesions that may become pustular.

A   Primary herpes contracted in the first trimester places the fetus at risk for abnormalities.

Head and Neck

E/N   See Chapter 11.

A   Hyperthyroidism and hypothyroidism.

P   Neoplastic disorders such as choriocarcinoma, ovarian teratoma, hydatidiform mole; single active thyroid nodule or multinodular goiter.

Eyes, Ears, Nose, Mouth, and Throat

E/N   See Chapters 12 and 13.

A   Arterial constriction of retinal vessels.

P   PIH.

A   Any growth in the mouth.

P   Benign tumours secondary to hormonal changes.

Breasts

E   1. Examine the breasts as described in Chapter 14.
    2. Don gloves.
    3. Assess the shape of each nipple by putting your thumb and index finger on the areola and pressing inward to express any discharge. Note whether the nipple protracts (becomes erect) or retracts (inverts).

N   Refer to Chapter 14. Nipples normally protract when stimulated.

A/P   See Chapter 14 for additional information.

| E   Examination | N   Normal Findings | A   Abnormal Findings | P   Pathophysiology |

Thorax and Lungs

E See Chapter 15.

N See Chapter 15.

A/P Pathology noted in Chapter 15 would also be considered abnormal for the pregnant patient.

Heart and Peripheral Vasculature

E Assess the patient as described in Chapter 16.

N See Chapter 16.

A Generalized edema, in contrast to the dependent edema of pregnancy.

P PIH, kidney disease, cardiovascular disease.

Abdomen

E Assess the patient as described in Chapter 17.

N See Chapter 17.

A Severe nausea and vomiting (hyperemesis gravidarum).

P Unknown etiology.

A Epigastric pain.

P Liver inflammation or necrosis from PIH.

Urinary System

E 1. Obtain a complete urinalysis at the initial prenatal visit.
   2. Obtain a urine culture if indicated by urinalysis or patient history.
   3. It is common to assess urine for protein, glucose, leukocytes, and nitrates at each subsequent prenatal visit.

N The urine may turn a brighter yellow as a result of prenatal vitamins. Trace amounts of protein may be noted. Glycosuria may be noted without pathology, but concern for diabetes mellitus cannot be ignored. Leukocytes and nitrates are normally absent.

A Nitrates or large amounts of leukocytes.

P Urinary tract infection.

A Dysuria (difficulty in initiating urinary flow, increased urinary frequency, a feeling of being unable to empty the bladder).

P Bacterial infection, inflammation of the bladder (cystitis), urinary tract infection.

A Pain in the flank area (costovertebral angle tenderness).

P Pyelonephritis.

A Proteinuria greater than trace as shown on a urine dipstick.

P PIH; collagen disorders; kidney diseases.

Musculoskeletal System

E Assess the patient as described in Chapter 18.

N See Chapter 18.

A/P Abnormalities and pathology described in Chapter 18 are also considered abnormal for the pregnant patient.

Neurological System

E Assess the patient as described in Chapter 19.

N See Chapter 19.

A Seizures.

P Eclampsia, stroke, tumours, epilepsy.

A Hyperreflexia and clonus.

P PIH can cause these findings.

Female Genitalia

E 1. For the initial prenatal visit, perform the assessment as described in Chapter 20.
   2. Perform cultures as indicated (see Chapter 20).
   3. Postdate pregnancies and pregnancies complicated by preterm labour symptoms or preterm labour risk factors may require a cervical assessment at each visit.

N See Chapter 20 for normal findings of the female genitalia assessment. The multiparous vulva and vagina may appear more relaxed in tone, with a shorter perineum. There is often a visible, white, milky discharge during pregnancy, and the cervix may show more ectropion (also called eversion and friability). Ectropion is the condition where the columnar epithelium extends from the os past the normal squamocolumnar junction, often

E Examination	**N** Normal Findings	**A** Abnormal Findings	**P** Pathophysiology

producing a red, possibly inflamed appearance. Manual assessment should show uterine size appropriate for gestational age, and the uterus may be slightly more tender than in a non-pregnant woman. The retroverted and retroflexed uterus may be more difficult to assess. Palpation of the adnexa may demonstrate a slight tenderness and enlargement of the ovulatory ovary secondary to the corpus luteum of pregnancy.

A Persistent abdominal pain or tenderness.

P PIH, abruptio placenta.

A Painful adnexal masses.

P Ectopic pregnancy (pregnancy other than intrauterine, such as in the abdomen or fallopian tube), infection, cancerous growth.

Uterine Size
Fundal Height by Centimetres

E 1. Place the patient in a supine position.
   2. Place the zero centimetre mark of the tape measure at the symphysis pubis in the midline of the abdomen.
   3. Palpate the top of the fundus and pull tape measure to the top.
   4. Note the centimetre mark.

N A 16-week uterus is between the symphysis pubis and umbilicus, a 20-week uterus is at the umbilicus, and from 18 to 32 weeks the size is equal to the centimetre height of the uterine fundus. After 32 weeks, although still used, this measurement is less accurate.

A Uterine size larger than expected given LMP.

P Hydatidiform mole or molar pregnancy (especially in the absence of fetal heart tones), multiple gestation, inaccurate dating, uterine pathology (fibroid), polyhydramnios, or, in later pregnancy, macrosomia (newborn weighing greater than 4000 gm).

A Uterine size smaller than expected given LMP.

P Non-viable pregnancy, inaccurate dating, or, later in pregnancy, intrauterine growth restriction (IUGR) or transverse lie of the fetus.

Fetal Heart Rate

E 1. Place the patient in the supine position.
   2. Place Doppler or fetoscope on abdomen and move it around until fetal heart tones (FHTs) are heard.
   3. Count the FHR for sufficient time to determine rate and absence of an irregularity (optimally one minute).

N During early gestation, the fetal heart is generally heard in the midline area between the symphysis pubis and the umbilicus. It can be heard via Doppler by approximately 12 weeks (and maybe as early as nine weeks). Use Doppler to auscultate FHT prior to 20 weeks; a fetoscope can be used after 20 weeks. Doppler is commonly used throughout pregnancy, as it is more convenient and also allows the patient to hear FHTs. The normal rate is 110 to 160 bpm. If the FHT seems low, check the mother's pulse rate to verify it is the FHT that you are listening to and not the mother's heart rate. Near-term FHTs are generally heard at maximum intensity in the left or right lower quadrant. If FHTs are best heard above the umbilicus, one should suspect a breech presentation or placenta previa. The fetal heart is best heard through the fetal back, which can be located by performing Leopold's manoeuvre as described later.

A FHR below 110 bpm indicates bradycardia.

P Fetal distress, drug use.

A Absence of fetal heart activity.

P Ectopic pregnancy, a blighted ovum, fetal demise, molar pregnancy.

A FHR above 160 bpm indicates tachycardia.

P Cardiac dysrhythmia, maternal fever, drug use.

Leopold's Manoeuvre

Beginning at 36 weeks, determine fetal presentation using Leopold's manoeuvre (Figure 23-2).

First Manoeuvre

E 1. Place the patient in a supine position with the knees bent.

E **Examination**   N **Normal Findings**   A **Abnormal Findings**   P **Pathophysiology**

2. Stand to the patient's right side facing her head.
3. Keeping the fingers of your hand together, palpate the uterine fundus.
4. Determine which fetal part presents at the fundus.

Second Manoeuvre

E
1. Move each of your hands to a side of the uterus.
2. Keep your left hand steady and palpate the patient's abdomen with the right hand.

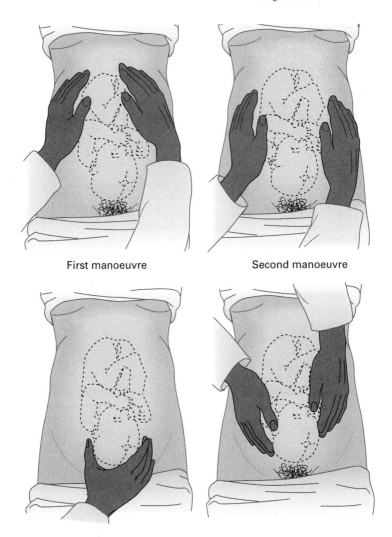

First manoeuvre

Second manoeuvre

Third manoeuvre

Fourth manoeuvre

FIGURE 23-2 Leopold's Manoeuvre.

| E Examination | N Normal Findings | A Abnormal Findings | P Pathophysiology |

3. Determine the positions of the fetus's back and small parts.
4. Keep your right hand steady and palpate the patient's abdomen with your left hand.

Third Manoeuvre

E   Place your right hand above the symphysis pubis with your thumb on one side of the fetus's presenting part and your fingers on the other side.
   1. Gently palpate the fetus's presenting part.
   2. Determine if the buttocks or the head is the presenting part in the pelvis. (This should confirm the findings of the first manoeuvre.)

Fourth Manoeuvre

E   1. Change your position so you are facing the patient's feet.
   2. Place your hands on each side of the uterus above the symphysis pubis and attempt to palpate the cephalic prominence (forehead). This will assist you in determining the fetal lie (long axis of fetus in relationship to long axis of mother) and attitude (head flexed or extended).
N   The fetus's head is usually the presenting part. It feels firm, round, and smooth. The head can move freely when palpated. If the baby is in a breech position, the buttocks feel soft and irregular. With palpation, the fetus's whole body seems to move but not with as much ease as the head. The fetus's back is firm, smooth, and continuous. The limbs are bumpy and irregular. The long axis is vertical, and the fetal head is flexed. A fetus not in a vertex presentation can affect the type of delivery; e.g., a fetus in a persistent transverse or oblique lie will need to be delivered by cesarean. A breech fetus may be delivered vaginally or by cesarean, depending on the health care provider's comfort and experience in doing a vaginal breech delivery. Breech presentation, if uncorrected (i.e., by external version [the manual turning of the fetus by the health care provider]), is associated with an increased rate of perinatal morbidity and mortality, prolapsed umbilical cord, placenta previa, fetal anomalies and abnormalities (which may not manifest immediately after birth), and uterine anomalies.
A   Inability to determine fetal outline.
P   Polyhydramnios and maternal obesity.

Hematological System
See Table 23-3.

Endocrine System
See Table 23-3 and Table 23-4.

Nutritional Assessment
See Chapter 7.

Special Antepartum Tests and Evaluations
Table 23-4 lists special antepartum tests and evaluations that can be performed in pregnant women.

Psychosocial Assessment and Learning Needs
The meaning of the pregnancy to the woman and her family; the planned versus unplanned nature of the pregnancy, reason for becoming pregnant; response of family and friends; previous experience with pregnancy (personal or vicarious), socioeconomic status, presence of difficult symptoms of pregnancy, body image changes, presence of co-morbidities, and usual mood changes of pregnancy can all play a role in how the woman copes with the trajectory of pregnancy.

E   Examination   N   Normal Findings   A   Abnormal Findings   P   Pathophysiology

TABLE 23-3 Laboratory Tests and Values in Pregnancy

TEST	REFERENCE RANGE (UNITS)*	TIMING
Prenatal Panel includes		
ABO and Rh (D) blood group antibody screening	A, B, O, AB, Rh(D) positive or negative	Initial visit; repeat antibody screening between 24 and 49 weeks if mother is Rh(D) negative; repeat if spontaneous or induced abortion, amniocentesis, CVS, or obstetrical complications. Repeat antibody screening within 72 hours of delivery of a Rh(D) positive baby.[1]
VDRL (Venereal disease research laboratory)	Negative for Treponema pallidum	Initial visit; may repeat at 36 weeks
Rubella (Canada has a very low incidence of rubella and congenital rubella syndrome [0–0.6/100,000 births] as a result of effective immunization programs. Immigrant women who have not had access to immunization programs are at higher risk)	Immune (non-immune patients should be cautioned to avoid contact with any possible exposure during the first trimester and will require a postpartum immunization)	Initial visit
Hepatitis B surface antigen	Negative	Initial visit; may repeat at 36 weeks
HIV (offered)	Negative	Initial visit; repeat based on history or exposure
Varicella	Immune	Initial visit if uncertain history
Human parvovirus B19 (fifth disease) IgG and IgM status	Positive IgG and negative IgM means immunity; negative IgG and IgM means precautions must be taken to avoid exposure; positive or negative IgG and positive IgM indicates possible recent infection.[2]	May be done on initial visit or as indicated by exposure
Hepatitis C antibody	Negative	Initial visit if indicated by history

continued

TABLE 23-3 Laboratory Tests and Values in Pregnancy *continued*

TEST	REFERENCE RANGE (UNITS)*	TIMING
Prenatal Panel includes		
CBC to include:		
HGB	100–140 g/L	Initial visit; repeat at 26–28 weeks and 36 weeks
HCT	0.32–0.42	
MCV	80–100 fL	
Platelets	150–450 × 109	
Maternal serum alpha fetal protein (MSAFP) or triple marker screen	Both are maternal blood screening tests. MSAFP screens for neural tube defects and ventral wall defects, an elevation being a positive screen. As a screening test, there are false negatives (misses 20% of actual defects) and false positives, which may result from inaccurate dates, multiple fetus pregnancy, or bleeding with pregnancy. The MSAFP incidentally picks up 20% of Down-affected infants, as the alpha fetal protein will be diminished. Poorly understood is the association of an increased MSAFP with a normal fetus, but increased pregnancy complications such as preterm labour or delivery or PIH. The triple screen adds estradiol and HCG to the test and thus increases the detection of Down to approximately 60%.	15–20 weeks; 16–18 weeks is optimal
Cystic fibrosis screening	Non-carrier. Inherited as an autosomal recessive pattern and may not manifest with symptoms until later in childhood. Carried by 1 in 25 of Canadian Caucasians with 94–98.4% cases in Canada being in Caucasians.[3]	Ideally, prior to pregnancy, if not; at initial prenatal visit

continued

TABLE 23-3 Laboratory Tests and Values in Pregnancy *continued*

TEST	REFERENCE RANGE (UNITS)*	TIMING
Genital Cultures or Probes		
Chlamydia and gonorrhea by DNA probe or culture	Negative	Initial visit; may repeat at 36 weeks
Genital bacterial/group beta Streptococcus (GBS)	Normal flora or negative for pathogens	Initial visit; screening for GBS at 35–37 weeks gestation.[4] Intrapartum chemoprophylaxis of colonized women reduces colonization in neonate.
Urinalysis	Same as non-pregnant; glycosuria is a normal variant	Initial visit; as needed per symptoms and history
Urine culture	No notable pathogens	Screening once by culture method for asymptomatic bacteriuria at 12–16 weeks of pregnancy;[5] as needed per symptoms and history
Toxoplasma IgG	Negative; antibodies indicate past or current infection	As indicated by any history of exposures and symptoms
Glucose screen* for gestational diabetes mellitus (GDM): 1 hour post 50 gram glucose challenge test[6]	1 hour: < 7.8 mmol; if ≥ 10.3 then gestational diabetes mellitus is diagnosed with no further testing	24–28 weeks for all pregnant women and an early test, preferably with initial prenatal panel, for a woman with a family history of diabetes or a prior macrosomic baby, or who is 34 years or older or obese
Oral glucose tolerance test (100 grams)	1 hour: < 10 mmol/L 2 hour: < 8.6 mmol/L 3 hour: < 7.8 mmol/L	If indicated by elevated screening glucose or with history of failure with screening in prior pregnancies

* A small but significant number of Canadian obstetricians and hospital centres have a "no screen" policy for GDM unless risk factors other than pregnancy as they believe there are insufficient RTCs to indicate benefit.

TABLE 23-4	Special Antepartum Tests and Evaluations

TEST	DESCRIPTION
Ultrasound	At any time for pregnancy dating, although more accurate for dates early in pregnancy. Confirm or rule out placenta previa, multiple pregnancy; confirm presenting fetal part. Evaluate amniotic fluid volume or fetal growth (especially to rule out intrauterine growth restriction or discordant growth with a multiple pregnancy). Evaluate for ectopic pregnancy or fetal demise.
Genetic testing: chorionic villi sampling (CVS), amniocentesis, chromosome studies	• CVS for chromosome studies is usually performed between 10 and 13 weeks. There may be an approximately 1% increased risk of limb deformities associated with CVS, as well as a 1% increased risk of spontaneous abortion. • Amniocentesis is performed at mid-trimester between 15 to 16 weeks and has a 0.5–1% increased risk of spontaneous abortion. Early amniocentesis, performed between 11 to 12 weeks, carries increased risks. • Blood or tissue chromosome studies can be done at any time and are best done with a known family history prior to conception.
Non-stress test (NST) or contraction stress test (CST) (not common in Canada) for fetal well-being, e.g., with decreased fetal movement, known decreased fluid volume, history of certain maternal diseases (insulin dependent diabetes, collagen vascular disease) or obstetric complications, such as IUGR, postdates, pre-eclampsia, discordant twin, or multiples	For a non-stress test, an electrical fetal monitor is applied to the woman's abdomen, with a tocodynamometer to monitor and record uterine activity and fetal movement, and a Doppler to monitor and record FHR, looking at fetal heart response to fetal movement (and any spontaneous uterine contractions). Timing is typically 1 or 2 times per week, and may start as early as 32 weeks depending on the risk factor. With a contraction stress test, uterine activity is induced by timed breast nipple stimulation (which induces uterine contractions); failing adequate uterine stimulation from nipple stimulation, pitocin intravenously via a pump is used to induce uterine activity. (Relative contraindications for contraction stress test include any risk for uterine rupture, e.g., previous vertical cesarean section; premature delivery risk; any bleeding risk such as known placenta previa; or any unexplained vaginal bleeding.) Timing is typically once per week after 36 weeks.
Amniotic fluid volume (AFV), which may be described as amniotic fluid index (AFI), most commonly ordered with postdates pregnancies	Ultrasound measurement of AFV using an index to determine normal, increased, or decreased fluid levels.
Biophysical profile	A composite test that includes amniotic fluid volume, non-stress test, fetal breathing movements, fetal limb movements, and fetal tone; each rated on 0–2 score. This study is done most commonly for the same reasons as an NST or CST.

continued

TABLE 23-4	Special Antepartum Tests and Evaluations *continued*

TEST	DESCRIPTION
Fetal movement count	Can be done by all pregnant women, requires no equipment, and incurs no direct cost. There are many methods of doing fetal movement or kick counts, e.g., number of movements during the day, or at certain times of the day.
	Cardiff technique: starting at 09:00 women lie or sit and count how long it takes to experience 10 movements; if <10 have been felt by 10:00 then consultation should occur.
	Sadovsky technique: Women lie down for one hour after meals; if 4 movements have not been felt within 1 hour then monitoring continues for 1 more after which consultation should occur if 4 movements have not been felt.

Nursing Alert

Danger Signs of Pregnancy

Vaginal bleeding*

Leaking or gush of watery fluid*

Abdominal or pelvic pain or cramping*

Severe headache or blurring of vision

Persistent chills or fever greater than 38.5°C

Persistent vomiting

Decreased fetal movement or lack of fetal movement

Change in vaginal discharge or pelvic pressure before 36 to 37 weeks*

Frequent (more than 4 per hour) uterine contractions or painless tightening between 20 and 37 weeks*

Associated with preterm labour

REFERENCES

[1]Beaulieu M.D. (1994). Screening for D (Rh) sensitization in pregnancy. Canadian Task Force on the Periodic Health Examination—Canadian Guide to Clinical Preventive Health Care. Ottawa: Health Canada, 1994; 116–24.

[2]Crane, J. for the Maternal-Fetal Medicine Committee and Infectious Diseases Committee (2002). Parvovirus B19 infection in pregnancy: SOGC Clinical Practice Guidelines. *Journal of Obstetrics and Gynaecology Canada (JOGC), 119*, 1–8.

[3]Canadian Cystic Fibrosis Foundation (2002). *Report of the Canadian cystic fibrosis patient data registry*. Toronto, Ontario.

[4]Canadian Task Force on Preventive Health Care (2002). Prevention of group B streptococcal infection in newborns. *Canadian Medical Association Journal, 166* (7), 928–930.

[5]Nicolle L. E. (1994). Screening for asymptomatic bacteriuria in pregnancy. *Canadian Guide to Clinical Preventive Health Care*. Ottawa: Health Canada, 100–106.

[6]Berger, H., Crane, J., & Farine, D. for the Maternal-Fetal Medicine Committee (2002). Screening for gestational diabetes mellitus: SOGC clinical practice guidelines. *Journal of Obstetrics and Gynaecology Canada JOGN, 121*, 1–10.

24

Pediatric Patient

PHYSICAL GROWTH

Physical growth parameters are required for pediatric health assessment. The parameters of weight, length or height, and head circumference (dependent on age) are essential in serial physical growth measurements. Chest circumference is of less importance.

For infants the average birth weight is 3.5 kg, length is 48 to 53 cm, and head circumference is 33 to 35.5 cm. Infants should double birth weight at six months and triple birth weight by one year of age. An infant's height increases about 2.5 cm per month for the first six months, and then slows to 1.3 cm per month until 12 months. Growth in the toddler period (12–24 months) begins to slow. The birth weight usually quadruples by 2.5 years of age, with an average weight gain during the toddler period of 1.8 to 2.7 kg per year. The toddler usually grows 7.6 cm.

Preschoolers (2–6 years) gain an average of 2.3 kg per year. Height increases 6.4 to 7.6 cm per year. The preschooler's birth length usually is doubled by four years of age. In contrast, the school-age child (6–12 years) grows 2.5 to 5 cm per year and gains 1.3 to 2.7 kg annually.

Infancy and adolescence (13–18 years) are two periods of rapid growth in children. Females commonly experience this between ages 10 and 14, whereas in males it occurs somewhat later, between 12 and 16 years of age.

ANATOMY AND PHYSIOLOGY

Structural and Physiological Variations

Vital Signs

- Infants aged six months and younger are unable to shiver in the face of lower ambient temperature. The absence of this important protective mechanism puts infants at risk for hypothermia, bradycardia, and acidosis.
- By age 4, temperature parameters are comparable to those seen in adults.
- Both pulse and respiratory rates in children tend to decline with advancing age and reach levels comparable to those found in adulthood by adolescence.
- In children one year of age and older, an easy rule of thumb for determining normal systolic blood pressure is:

$$\text{normal systolic BP (mm Hg)} = 80 + (2 \times \text{age in years}).$$

- Normal diastolic blood pressure is generally two-thirds of systolic blood pressure.

Skin and Hair

- Lanugo, a fine, downy hair may be present in the newborn over the temples of the forehead and on the upper arms, shoulders, back, and pinna of the ears.
- Vernix caseosa, a thick, cheesy, protective, integumentary deposit that consists of sebum and shed epithelial cells, is present on the newborn's skin.

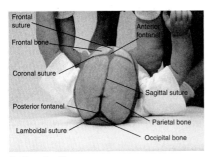

A. Superior View

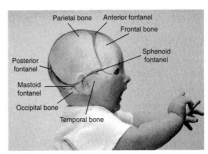

B. Lateral View

FIGURE 24-1 Infant Head Structures.

- Relative to an adult, a child has a higher ratio of body surface area to body surface mass.

Head
- Suture ridges are palpable until approximately six months of age.
- The posterior fontanel usually closes by three months of age (Figure 24-1).
- The anterior fontanel should close by 19 months of age.

Eyes, Ears, Nose, Mouth, and Throat
- At birth, visual acuity is approximately 20/200. The child's visual acuity is usually 20/20 at 6–8 years.
- Newborns do not produce tears until their lacrimal ducts open, at around two to three months of age.
- The external auditory canal of a child is shorter and positioned upward.
- The eustachian tube is more horizontal, wider, and shorter.
- Only the ethmoid and maxillary sinuses are present at birth. At approximately seven years of age, the frontal sinuses develop. The sphenoid sinuses do not develop until after puberty.
- Figure 24-2 summarizes deciduous and permanent teeth eruption.
- Salivation starts at about three months, and the infant drools until the swallowing reflex is more coordinated.

Breasts
- Breast tissue in the female starts to develop between eight and ten years of age. Mature

adult breast tissue is achieved between 14 and 17 years of age.

Thorax and Lungs
- A newborn's chest is circular because the anteroposterior and transverse diameters are approximately equal (Figure 24-5). By six years of age, the ratio of anteroposterior to lateral diameters reaches adult values.
- Ribs are displaced horizontally in infants.
- The trachea is short in the newborn. By 18 months of age, it has grown from the newborn length of 5 cm to 7.6 cm. Toward the latter part of adolescence, the trachea has grown to the adult size.
- Until three to four months of age, infants are obligate nose breathers.

Heart and Peripheral Vasculature
- The infant's, toddler's, and preschooler's heart lies more horizontally than an adult's heart; thus the apex is higher at about the left fourth intercostal space.
- The three fetal shunts (ductus venosus, foramen ovale, and ductus arteriosus) close at birth or shortly thereafter.

Abdomen
- At birth, the neonate's umbilical cord contains two arteries and one vein.
- The infant's liver is proportionately larger in the abdominal cavity than is the liver of an adult.

Musculoskeletal System
- Bone growth ends at age 20, when the epiphyses close.

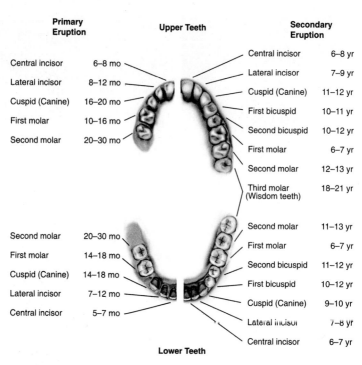

Primary Eruption		Upper Teeth	Secondary Eruption	
Central incisor	6–8 mo		Central incisor	6–8 yr
Lateral incisor	8–12 mo		Lateral incisor	7–9 yr
Cuspid (Canine)	16–20 mo		Cuspid (Canine)	11–12 yr
First molar	10–16 mo		First bicuspid	10–11 yr
Second molar	20–30 mo		Second bicuspid	10–12 yr
			First molar	6–7 yr
			Second molar	12–13 yr
			Third molar (Wisdom teeth)	18–21 yr
			Second molar	11–13 yr
Second molar	20–30 mo		First molar	6–7 yr
First molar	14–18 mo		Second bicuspid	11–12 yr
Cuspid (Canine)	14–18 mo		First bicuspid	10–12 yr
Lateral incisor	7–12 mo		Cuspid (Canine)	9–10 yr
Central incisor	5–7 mo		Lateral incisor	7–8 yr
			Central incisor	6–7 yr

Lower Teeth

FIGURE 24-2 Deciduous and Permanent Teeth.

HEALTH HISTORY

Prenatal

The nature of the prenatal experience and care are important to assess intrauterine health and risks for any subsequent health issues that may arise from such situations as an unplanned pregnancy; use of alcohol, caffeine, or other drugs during pregnancy; smoking status of the mother during pregnancy; or physical abuse toward the mother. Other aspects of maternal health during the pregnancy that are important include any history of pregnancy-induced hypertension, preterm labour, gestational diabetes, group B streptococcus (GBS), TORCH infection (toxoplasmosis, rubella, cytomegalovirus, and herpes), or an abnormal finding on a prenatal ultrasound.

Labour and Delivery

Labour—length of the labour; spontaneous or induced; analgesia or anaesthetic agents used, including mode of delivery (e.g., epidural) are relevant to assess.

Delivery—gestational age of the neonate at delivery; vaginal versus cesarean section delivery; if cesarean, why? Was the baby held or placed at the breast immediately after delivery? What were the baby's Apgar scores at one and five minutes? What were the birth weight and length of the baby? Who was present at the birth, where did it take place (e.g., home, birthing centre, hospital)?

Postnatal	When were mother and baby discharged home? (Indicates overall health as extended stay generally indicates complications.) Did the baby have any breathing or feeding problems during the first week or require any medications or require special attention during the first weeks? Was there any jaundice? Were there any concerns about either maternal or neonatal health? Was the baby circumcised? What is the nature of feeding and were there any problems with the choice of feeding method?
Medical History	Inquire about the circumstances and outcomes of any hospitalizations or emergency department visits.
Injuries and Accidents	Determine if the child has a pattern of frequent injuries or accidents. Repeat trauma may indicate abuse.
Childhood Illnesses	Document any past and current illness experiences the child may have had including any recent exposure to viral or bacterial infections.
Immunizations	See Table 3-1 for the routine immunization schedule of infants, children, and youth.
Family Health History	Sudden infant death syndrome (SIDS), attention deficit hyperactivity disorder (ADHD), congenital disorders or defects, or any situations of delayed cognitive, physical, or social growth in the family.

Neurological System

- The neurological system of the infant is incompletely developed. The autonomic nervous system helps maintain homeostasis as the cerebral cortex develops.
- In the first year, the neurons become myelinated, and primitive motor reflexes are replaced by purposeful movement. The myelinization occurs in a cephalocaudal and proximodistal manner (head and neck, trunk, and extremities).

Urinary System

In infancy, the urinary bladder is between the symphysis pubis and umbilicus.

Female Genitalia

- Development of pubic hair in girls begins at puberty, between 8 and 12 years of age. Within about one year, the pubic hair becomes dark, coarse, and curly but is not considered fully developed. Axillary hair follows six months later. After about age 13–15, pubic hair distribution approaches adult quantity and consistency.

Male Genitalia

- The testes usually descend by the age of one year.
- Puberty usually starts between the ages of $9^1/2$ and $13^1/2$ and can last two to five years. Testicular enlargement is usually the first area of sexual development to occur. Within about one year, the pubic hair becomes dark, coarse, and curly but is not fully developed. Axillary hair follows six months later. Facial hair follows approximately six months after the emergence of axillary hair.

EQUIPMENT

- Equipment listed in Chapters 10–22
- Scale (infant or stand-up)
- Appropriate-sized blood pressure cuff
- Snellen E and Tumbling E charts
- Allen cards
- Ophthalmoscope
- Otoscope, speculum (2.5 to 4 mm), pneumatic attachment
- Pediatric stethoscope
- Growth chart, BMI chart
- Small bell
- Brightly coloured object

◄ NURSING CHECKLIST ►

General Approach to Pediatric Physical Assessment

1. Assess the patient in a warm, quiet room. To prevent hypothermia, always keep infants under the age of six months warm during the examination.

2. Use natural lighting, if available, during the assessment. Fluorescent lighting makes assessing varying degrees of cyanosis and jaundice difficult.

3. To help reduce anxiety and uncooperativeness (especially when assessing young children), have a familiar caregiver present during the assessment.

4. Talk to the child in a soothing voice; even an infant who cannot understand your words will take comfort in a calm and supportive approach.

5. Explain all procedures and allow older infants, toddlers, preschoolers, and younger school-age patients to touch or manipulate medical equipment

6. To promote the child's feeling of security, allow the infant who cannot sit up and the younger child to sit on the caregiver's lap for as much of the examination as possible.

7. Until the infant or toddler is comfortable, maintain eye contact with the caregiver while the assessment is taking place. Maintaining eye contact with the child who experiences anxiety in the presence of strangers can interfere with completing the examination. Maintain eye contact with caregiver if other means of alleviating the fears are not successful.

8. Interview the older school-age child or adolescent separately, without the caregiver. Talking to the individual without the caregiver present may yield important information not gained during a group interview (e.g., that the patient is using drugs).

9. Respect the patient's modesty.

10. Warm equipment (e.g., stethoscope).

11. Avoid making abrupt movements, which may startle a child.

12. If the child is sleeping, perform simple procedures (length, head circumference) and system assessments that require a quiet room (such as the cardiac and respiratory assessments) first.

13. Perform all invasive or uncomfortable procedures (ear inspection, hip palpation) last because they may cause discomfort, crying, fear, and increased heart rate.

14. Always provide comfort measures following pain. It is especially helpful to allow the caregiver the opportunity to provide supportive measures. This shows the child that you are genuinely concerned about his or her feelings.

15. To prevent falls, always keep one hand on any infant who is placed on the examination table.

16. Prior to completing the examination, ask the caregiver and patient if they have questions.

- Clean gloves
- Disposable centimetre tape measure

Growth and Development

Refer to Chapter 4 for a summary of normal cognitive, social, motor, language, and sensory development in children from infancy through adolescence.

PHYSICAL ASSESSMENT

Many assessment techniques for the child are similar to those for the adult. Refer to the specific system chapters for detailed explanations of assessment techniques.

Vital Signs

See Chapter 9.

Temperature
Axillary

E   1. When measuring axillary temperature, have the child sit or lie on the caregiver's lap to free your hands for other observations or to prepare for the next area of assessment.

2. Explain to the child that this type of temperature measurement does not hurt. To pass time, ask the caregiver to read the child a story.

N/A/P See Chapter 9.

Rectal

E   1. Children dislike having rectal temperature taken, so the approach to explanation should be matter of fact: "I need to measure your temperature in your bottom. You need to hold very still while I do this. Your mommy (or other appropriate person) will be right here with you."

2. Place the patient in either a side-lying or a prone position on the caregiver's lap or place the patient on the back on the examination table and firmly grasp the feet with your non-dominant hand.

3. After lubricating the stub-tipped thermometer, insert it gently into the patient's rectum: 1.25 cm for newborns, 1.9 cm for infants, and 2.5 cm for preschoolers and older patients. Hold the thermometer firmly between your fingers to avoid accidentally inserting it too far.

N/A/P See Chapter 9.

Tympanic Thermometry

E   1. The child may feel that a physical boundary has been crossed when the probe is inserted into the ear. To help the child remain calm, the parent can hold the child on the lap or help the child lie comfortably in bed.

2. If the patient is under three years old, pull the pinna down, aiming the probe toward the opposite eye. If the patient is over three years old, grasp the pinna and pull gently up and back, aiming the probe toward the opposite ear.

N/A/P See Chapter 9.

Temporal Artery Thermometry

E   1. This method is not invasive but still requires the child to remain still so the sensor will maintain contact.

2. See Chapter 9.

N/A/P See Chapter 9.

Respiratory Rate

E   1. Try to obtain the rate early in the assessment, when the patient is most cooperative and not crying.

2. See Chapter 9 for full instructions.

N/A/P See Chapter 9.

Physical Growth
Weight

Use the same scale at each visit, if possible, to prevent variations in serial weight checks.

E   1. If using an infant scale, cover it with a paper protector.

2. Balance or zero the scale.

E Examination   N Normal Findings   A Abnormal Findings   P Pathophysiology

3. Place infants and young toddlers nude on the scale. Always keep one hand on the child to prevent falls and lift your hand slightly when obtaining the actual weight reading.

4. Preschoolers and young school-age children can wear street clothes to be weighed. Have the older child undress, don a paper or cloth gown, and step on the standard platform scale.

5. Note and record weight.

N   Usually, neonates lose approximately 10% of birth weight by the third or fourth day after birth, then regain it by two weeks of age. This expected change in weight is called physiological weight loss, and it is due to a loss of extracellular fluid and meconium, a dark-green, sticky, stool-like substance excreted from the rectum within the first 24 hours after birth.

A   A newborn weight less than the tenth gestational age percentile.

P   Small for gestational age (SGA). Potential causes include tobacco, alcohol, or drug abuse, or certain genetic syndromes.

A   A newborn weight greater than the 90th gestational age percentile.

P   A diabetic mother or genetic predisposition may be responsible for producing a large for gestational age (LGA) newborn.

A   A weight below the 3rd percentile.

P   Organic or non-organic failure to thrive, congenital or cyanotic heart disease, cystic fibrosis (CF), fetal alcohol syndrome, malabsorption diseases.

Length and Height

Recumbent length is measured for children less than two years old.

E   1. Position the measuring board flat on the examination table.

2. Place the child's head at the top of the board and the child's heels at the foot of the board, ensuring that the legs are fully extended.

3. Measure and record the length.

4. If a board is not available, place the child in a supine position and mark lines on the paper at the tip of the head and at the heel ensuring that the legs are fully extended.

5. Measure between the lines and record.

Height for all other age groups can be measured in the same fashion as for an adult.

N   Refer to standard growth charts.

A   A height below the 3rd or above the 97th percentiles, a patient who falls two standard deviations below his or her own established curve.

P   Possible causes include organic or non-organic failure to thrive, congenital or cyanotic heart disease, CF, fetal alcohol syndrome, malabsorption diseases.

Head Circumference

Head circumference is measured in all children less than two years of age or serially in patients with known or suspected hydrocephalus. Measuring head circumference is an invaluable tool in the infant with suspected cessation of brain growth.

E   1. Place the patient in a sitting or supine position.

2. Using a tape measure, measure anteriorly from above the eyebrows and around posteriorly to the occipital protuberance.

N   Normal average head growth is 1 to 1.5 cm per month during the first year. Premature infants often have small head circumferences.

A   Microcephaly, a condition characterized by a small brain with a resultant small head.

P   Intrauterine infections, drug or alcohol ingestion (fetal alcohol syndrome) during pregnancy, genetic defects.

A   Hydrocephalus (enlarged head) when an infant's or young child's head circumference is above the 97th percentile and crossing over the patient's established percentile lines from one serial measurement to the next.

E   **Examination**   N   **Normal Findings**   A   **Abnormal Findings**   P   **Pathophysiology**

P Imbalance in cerebrospinal fluid (CSF) production and reabsorption.

Chest Circumference

Chest circumference is measured up to one year of age. It is a measurement that by itself provides little information but is compared to head circumference to evaluate the child's overall growth.

E 1. Stand in front of the supine patient.
  2. Measure the chest circumference by placing the tape measure around the chest at the nipple line.
  3. Measure during exhalation.

N From birth to about one year, the head circumference is greater than the chest circumference. After age one, the chest circumference is greater than the head circumference.

A A measured chest circumference below normal limits.

P Prematurity.

Apgar Scoring

The Apgar score system provides a quick method to assess the need for newborn resuscitation in the delivery room. An Apgar score is given to a newborn at one and five minutes after birth. Perform steps 1 through 5 at one minute following birth; add the score in each category for the total. Repeat at five minutes following birth.

E 1. Auscultate the heart rate for one full minute.
  2. Measure the degree of respiratory effort.
  3. Evaluate muscle tone by attempting to straighten each extremity individually.
  4. Evaluate the newborn's reflex irritability. Use a flicking motion of two fingers against the newborn's sole to rate reflex irritability.
  5. Inspect the newborn's colour.

N A score of 8 to 10 demonstrates that the newborn is in good condition. Table 24-1 outlines the scoring system for each of the five areas assessed.

A A moderately depressed newborn earns a score of 4 to 7. A score of 0 to 3 indicates that the newborn is severely depressed and needs immediate resuscitation.

P Prematurity, central nervous system depression, blood or meconium in the trachea, maternal history of drug abuse, certain drugs that are given to the mother in preparation for delivery and that cross over and cause fetal depression, congenital complete heart block, congenital heart disease.

Skin
Inspection
Colour

E Observe the colour of the body, especially at the tip of the nose, the external ear, the lips, the hands, and the feet. These areas are prominent locations for detecting cyanosis or jaundice.

N The skin of a newborn is reddish in colour for the first 24 hours, then changes to varying shades of pale pink to pink to

TABLE 24-1	Apgar Scoring				
HEART RATE	**RESPIRATORY RATE**	**TONE**	**REFLEX IRRITABILITY**	**COLOUR**	
Absent = 0	Apnea = 0	Flaccid = 0	No response = 0	Cyanosis = 0	
< 100 = 1	Slow, irregular rate = 1	Some degree of flexion = 1	Grimace = 1	Body pink, extremities acrocyanotic = 1	
> 100 = 2	Crying vigorously = 2	Full flexion = 2	Crying = 2	Completely pink = 2	

E Examination	**N** Normal Findings	**A** Abnormal Findings	**P** Pathophysiology

brown or black, depending on the child's race. It is normal for dark-skinned newborns to have a ruddy appearance and for light-skinned newborns to exhibit a bluish-purple colour of the hands and feet while the rest of the body remains pink. This is called acrocyanosis. It may disappear with warming. Mongolian spots, deep-blue pigmentation over the lumbar and sacral areas of the spine, over the buttocks, and sometimes over the upper back or shoulders in newborns of African, Latin American, or Asian descent, are extremely common and not to be confused with ecchymosis or signs of child abuse.

A   A blue hue.

P   Cyanosis associated with a congenital heart defect, decreasing levels of oxygen saturation.

A   A yellowing of the skin or sclera.

P   Physiological jaundice of the newborn occurs on the second or third day of life.

P   Pathological jaundice of the newborn occurs within the first 24 hours of life; Rh/ABO incompatibility, maternal infections (rubella, herpes, syphilis, toxoplasmosis).

A   It is abnormal when the newborn lies on a side and the dependent half becomes red or ruddy.

P   Harlequin colour change is a benign condition due to poor vasomotor control.

A   Erythema of the palms or soles, edema of the hands or feet, or periungal desquamation.

P   Kawasaki disease.

Lesions

E/N   See Chapter 10.

A   Lesions that are asymmetrical, scaly, erythematous patches or plaques with possible exudation and crusting.

A   Eczema, or atopic dermatitis due to pollens, moulds, dust mites, or food allergens.

A   Small, maculopapular lesions on an erythematous base, wheals, and vesicles that erupt on the newborn.

P   Erythema toxicum.

A   Flat, deep, irregular, localized, pink areas in light-skinned children and deeper-red areas in dark-skinned children.

P   Telangiectatic nevi (stork bites) due to capillary dilatation.

A   Diffuse redness, papules, vesicles, edema, scaling, and ulcerations on the area covered by a baby's diaper.

P   Possible causes of diaper dermatitis include fecal enzymes, irritated skin, stool consistency and frequency, *Candida*, cleansing agents, sensitive skin, and poor nutrition.

A   Vesicles located on the palms of hands, soles of feet, and in the mouth; a papular erythematous rash may also be on the buttocks.

P   Hand–foot–mouth disease.

A   A dark–black tuft of hair or a dimple over the lumbosacral area.

P   The neural tube fails to fuse at about the fourth week of gestation and causes a vertebral defect known as spina bifida occulta.

Palpation

Texture

E   1. Use the finger pads to palpate the skin.

    2. The technique of palpating the skin of a younger child can be accomplished by playing games. For example, use the finger pads to walk up the abdomen and touch the nose.

N   Skin of the pediatric patient normally is smooth and soft. Milia, plugged sebaceous glands, present as small, white papules in the newborn. Milia occur mainly on the head, especially the cheeks and nose. Preterm infants have vernix caseosa.

A/P   See Chapter 10.

Hair

Inspection

Lesions

E/N   See Chapter 10.

A   Yellow, greasy-appearing scales on the scalp of a light-skinned infant; in dark-skinned infants, the scaling is light grey.

P   Seborrheic dermatitis (cradle cap) related to increased epidermal tissue growth.

Head

Inspection

Shape and Symmetry

E   With the patient sitting upright either in the caregiver's arms or on the examination table, observe the symmetry of the frontal, parietal, and occipital prominences.

N   The shape of a child's head is symmetrical without depressions or protrusions. The anterior fontanel normally may pulsate with every heartbeat. The Asian infant generally has a flattened occiput, more so than infants of other races.

A   A flattened occipital bone with resultant hair loss over the same area.

P   Prolonged supine position.

Head Control

E   1. Assess head control while the patient is in the position used for assessing shape and symmetry.
    2. With the head unsupported, observe the patient's ability to hold the head erect.

N   At three months of age, the infant is able to hold the head steady without lag.

A   Lack of head control is evidenced by the infant who is unable to hold the head steady while in a sitting position; head lag beyond four to six months of age.

P   Prematurity, hydrocephalus, developmental delays.

Palpation

Fontanel

E   1. Place the child in an upright position.
    2. Using the second or third finger pad, palpate the anterior fontanel at the junction of the sagittal, coronal, and frontal sutures.

3. Palpate the posterior fontanel at the junction of the sagittal and lambdoidal sutures.
4. Assess for bulging, pulsations, and size. To obtain accurate measurements, the patient should not be crying. Crying will produce a distorted, full, bulging appearance.

N   The anterior fontanel is soft and flat. Size ranges from 4 to 6 cm at birth. The fontanel gradually closes between 9 and 19 months of age. The posterior fontanel is also soft and flat. The size ranges from 0.5 to 1.5 centimetres at birth. The posterior fontanel gradually closes between one and three months of age. It is normal to feel pulsations related to the peripheral pulse.

A   Palpation reveals a bulging, tense fontanel.
P   Increased intracranial pressure (meningitis, increased CSF).
A   A sunken, depressed fontanel.
P   Dehydration.
A   A wide anterior fontanel in a child older than 2½.
P   Rickets, hypothyroidism, Down syndrome, hydrocephalus.

Suture Lines

E   1. With the finger pads, palpate the sagittal suture line. This runs from the anterior to the posterior portion of the skull in a midline position.
    2. Palpate the coronal suture line. This runs along both sides of the head, starting at the anterior fontanel.
    3. Palpate the lambdoidal suture. The lambdoidal suture runs along both sides of the head, starting at the posterior fontanel.
    4. Ascertain if these suture lines are open, united, or overlapping.

N   Grooves or ridges between sections of the skull are normally palpated up to six months of age.

A   Suture lines that overlap or override one another.

P   Craniosynostosis (premature ossification of suture lines) caused by metabolic disorders or microcephaly.

E **Examination**   N **Normal Findings**   A **Abnormal Findings**   P **Pathophysiology**

Surface Characteristics

E **1.** With the finger pads, palpate the skull in the same manner as the fontanels and suture lines.

2. Note surface edema and contour of the cranium.

N The skin covering the cranium is flush against the skull and without edema.

A A softening of the outer layer of the cranial bones behind and above the ears combined with a ping-pong ball sensation as the area is pressed in gently with the fingers is indicative of craniotabes.

P Rickets, syphilis, hydrocephaly, hypervitaminosis A.

A A localized, subcutaneous swelling over one of the cranial bones of a newborn.

P Cephalhematoma.

A Swelling over the occipitoparietal region of the skull.

P Caput succedaneum from prolonged delivery.

A Moulding.

P The parietal bone overrides the frontal bone as a result of induced pressure during delivery.

Eyes

General Approach

1. From infancy through about eight to ten years, assess the eyes toward the end of the assessment, with the exception of testing vision, which should be done first. Remember that the child's attention span is short, and attentiveness decreases the longer you evaluate. Children generally are not cooperative for eyes, ears, and throat assessments.

2. Place the young infant, preschooler, school-age, or adolescent patient on the examination table. The older infant or the toddler can be held by the caregiver.

3. Become proficient at performing fundoscopic assessments on adults prior to assessing the pediatric patient.

Vision Screening

General Approach

1. The adult Snellen chart can be used on children as young as six years, provided they are able to read the alphabet. The E chart is used for a patient over three years of age or any child who cannot read the alphabet.

2. Newborn to three months and six to 12 months: complete eye exam including red reflex and corneal light reflex; three to five years: complete eye exam including E acuity card or Allen chart. Test every two years until ten; every three years thereafter.

3. If the child resists wearing a cover patch over the eye, make a game out of wearing the patch. For example, the young child could pretend to be a pirate exploring new territory. Use your imagination to think of a fantasy situation.

4. The Allen test (a series of seven pictures on different cards) can be used with children as young as two years of age.

Tumbling E Chart

E **1.** Ask the child to point an arm in the direction the E is pointing.

2. Observe for squinting.

N Vision is 20/40 from two to approximately six years of age, when it approaches the normal 20/20 acuity. Refer the patient to an ophthalmologist if results are greater than 20/40 in a child two to six years of age or 20/30 or greater in a child six years or older, or if results vary by two or more lines between eyes even if in the passing range.

A/P Chapter 12.

Allen Test

E **1.** With the child's eyes both open, show each card to the child and elicit a name for each picture. Do not use any pictures with which the child is not familiar. Usually, the only pictures children have difficulty with are the 1940s vintage telephone and the Christmas tree if they do not celebrate this holiday.

2. Place the 2- to 3-year-old child 4.5 m (15 feet) from where you will be standing. Place the 3- to 4-year-old child 6 m (20 feet) from you.
3. Ask the caregiver to help cover one of the child's eyes.
4. With the child's eye covered and the child standing at the appropriate distance listed, show the pictures one at a time, eliciting a response after each showing.
5. Show the same pictures in different sequence for the other eye.
6. To record findings, the denominator is always constant at 30, because a child with normal vision should see the picture on the card (target) at 9 m (30 feet). To document the numerator, determine the greatest distance at which three of the pictures are recognized by each eye, for example, right eye = 15/30, left eye = 20/30.

N   The child should correctly identify three of the cards in three trials. Two- to three-year-old children should have 15/30 vision. Three- to four-year-old children should be able to achieve a score of 15/30 to 20/30. Each eye should have the same score.

A/P If the scores for the patient's right and left eyes differ by 1.5 m (5 feet) or more or either or both eyes score less than 15/30.

Strabismus Screening

The Hirschberg test and the cover-uncover test screen for strabismus. The latter is the more definitive test.

Hirschberg Test

E/N See Chapter 12.
A   It is abnormal for the light reflection to be displaced to the outer margin of the cornea as the eye deviates inward.
P   Esotropia is thought to be congenital.

A   It is abnormal for the light reflection to be displaced to the inner margin of the cornea as the eye deviates outward.
P   Exotropia can result from eye muscle fatigue or can be congenital.

Cover/Uncover Test

E   See Chapter 12.
N   Neither eye moves when the occluder is being removed. Infants less than six months of age display strabismus due to poor neuromuscular control of eye muscles.
A   It is abnormal for one or both eyes to move to focus on the penlight during assessment. Assume strabismus is present.
P   Strabismus after six months of age is abnormal and indicates eye muscle weakness.

Inspection

Eyelids

E   1. Sit at the patient's eye level.
     2. Observe for symmetrical palpebral fissures and position of eyelids in relation to the iris.
N   The palpebral fissures of both eyes are positioned symmetrically. The upper eyelid normally covers a small portion of the iris, and the lower lid meets the iris. Epicanthal folds are normally present in children of Asian descent.
A   Portion of the sclera is seen above the iris.
P   Hydrocephalus.
A   A fold of skin covering the inner canthus and lacrimal caruncle.
P   Down syndrome; fetal alcohol syndrome.

Lacrimal Apparatus

E/N See Chapter 12.
A   Unable to produce tears.
P   Dacryocystitis when the distal end of the membranous lacrimal duct fails to open or a blockage occurs.

E **Examination**   N **Normal Findings**   A **Abnormal Findings**   P **Pathophysiology**

Anterior Segment Structures

Sclera

E See Chapter 12.

N The newborn exhibits a bluish-tinged sclera. The sclera is white in light-skinned children and a slightly darker colour in some dark-skinned children.

A/P See Chapter 12.

Iris

E Conduct the examination in the same manner as for an adult.

N Up to about six months of age, the colour of the iris is blue or slate grey in light-skinned infants and brownish in dark-skinned infants. Between six and 12 months of age, complete transition of iris colour has occurred.

A Small white flecks, called Brushfield's spots, noted around the perimeter of the iris.

P Down syndrome.

Pupils

E See Chapter 12.

N When the pupils' reaction to light is assessed, a newborn will normally blink and flex the head closer to the body. This is called the optical blink reflex.

A/P See Chapter 12.

Posterior Segment Structures

General Approach

1. Observe the red reflex, retina, and optic disc.
2. The assessment is easier to accomplish if the infant or toddler is lying supine on an examination table. The assistance of another individual, such as the caregiver, to hold the patient in position is essential. The older patient may be allowed to sit, if cooperative.

Inspection

Red Reflex

E/N See Chapter 12.

A Absent red reflex.

P Chromosomal disorders, intrauterine infections, ocular trauma.

A Yellowish or white light reflex.

P Retinoblastoma.

Retina

E/N See Chapter 12.

A Red to dark-red colour.

P Retinal hemorrhage is seen in trauma, (shaken-baby syndrome).

Optic Disc

E/N/A/P See Chapter 12.

Ears

Auditory Testing

General Approach

Hearing tests are available for children under three years of age. Referral to a local audiology department is made if the family or caretaker of the child responds with a "no" to any of the following indicators:

a. Does the child react to a loud noise?
b. Does the child react to the caregiver's voice by cooing, smiling, or turning eyes and head toward the voice?
c. Does the child try to imitate sounds?
d. Can the child imitate words and sounds?
e. Can the child follow directions?
f. Does the child respond to sounds not directed at him or her?

Perform auditory testing at about age three to four years of age or when the child can follow directions.

External Ear

Inspection of Pinna Position

E/N See Chapter 13.

A The top of the ear is below the imaginary line drawn from the outer canthus to the top of the ear.

P Renal anomalies, Down syndrome.

Internal Ear

Inspection

E 1. A cooperative patient may be allowed to sit for the assessment.

2. Restrain the uncooperative young patient by placing him or her

---

| E Examination | N Normal Findings | A Abnormal Findings | P Pathophysiology |

supine on a firm surface. Instruct the caregiver or assistant to hold the patient's arms up near the head, embracing the elbow joints on both sides of either arm. Restrain the infant by having the caregiver hold the infant's hands down.

3. With your thumb and forefinger grasping the otoscope, use the lateral side of the hand to prevent the head from jerking. Your other hand can also be used to stabilize the patient's head.

4. Pull the lower auricle down and out to straighten the canal. This technique is used in children up to about 3 years of age. Use the adult technique after age 3.

5. Insert the speculum about 6–12 mm, depending on the patient's age.

6. Suspected otitis media must be evaluated with a pneumatic bulb attached to the side of the otoscope's light source.

7. Select a larger speculum to make a tight seal and prevent air from escaping from the canal.

8. Gently squeeze the bulb attachment to introduce air into the canal.

9. Observe the tympanic membrane for movement.

N/A/P   See Chapter 13.

Mouth and Throat

Inspection

Lips

E   1. Follow the same technique described in Chapter 13.
    2. Lip edges meet.
N   The lip edges should meet.
A   The lip edges do not meet.
P   Cleft palates.
A   A thin upper lip.
P   Fetal alcohol syndrome.

Buccal Mucosa

E   Use the same technique as for an adult. If the patient is unable to open the mouth on command, use the edge of a tongue blade to lift the upper lip and move the lower lip down.

N   See Chapter 13.
A   Thick, curdlike coating.
P   Thrush.

Teeth

E/N   See Chapter 13.
A   A lack of visible teeth coupled with roentgenographic findings revealing absence of tooth buds.
P   Genetic causes.
A   Teeth turn brownish black.
P   Caries.

Hard and Soft Palate

E   1. Observe the palate for continuity and shape.
    2. For infants, you will need to use a tongue depressor to push the tongue down. Infants usually cry in response to this action, which allows visualization of the palates.

N   The roof of the mouth is continuous and has a slight arch.
A   Roof of the mouth is not continuous.
P   Cleft palates, unilateral or bilateral.
A   The roof of the mouth is abnormally arched.
P   Trisomy 21, trisomy 18, Noonan syndrome.
A   Epstein's pearls (small, white cysts that feel hard when palpated).
P   Epithelial tissue trapped during palate formation.

Oropharynx

E   See Chapter 13.
N   Up to the age of 12 years, a tonsil grade of 2+ is considered normal. Around puberty, tonsillar tissue regresses. Tonsils should not interfere with the act of breathing.
A   Excessive salivation.
P   Tracheoesophageal fistula.
A   Exudative pharyngitis with fever, sore throat, splenomegaly, petechiae on the palate, and cervical adenitis.
P   Mononucleosis.

E **Examination**   **N** **Normal Findings**   **A** **Abnormal Findings**   **P** **Pathophysiology**

Neck

Inspection

General Appearance

E 1. Observe the neck in a midline position while the patient is sitting upright.

2. Note shortening or thickness of the neck on both right and left sides.

3. Note any swelling.

N There is a reasonable amount of skin tissue on the sides of the neck. There is no swelling.

A Additional weblike tissue found bilaterally from the ear to the shoulder.

P Congenital syndromes (e.g., Turner syndrome).

A Unilateral or bilateral swelling of the neck below the angle of the jaw.

P Parotitis (mumps).

Palpation

Thyroid

E 1. Use the same technique as for an adult with the exception of using the first two finger pads on both hands.

2. Have the younger child who is unable to swallow on command take a drink from a bottle or cup.

N/A/P The normal findings, abnormal findings, and pathophysiology are the same as for an adult.

Lymph Nodes

E 1. Because of the infant's short neck, extend the patient's chin upward with your hand before proceeding with palpation.

2. With the finger pads, palpate the submental, submandibular, tonsillar, anterior cervical chain, posterior cervical chain, supraclavicular, preauricular, posterior auricular, and occipital lymph nodes.

3. Use a circular motion. Note location, size, shape, tenderness, mobility, and associated skin inflammation of any swollen nodes palpated.

N Lymph nodes are generally not palpable. Children often have small, movable, cool, non-tender nodes referred to as "shotty" nodes. These benign nodes are related to environmental antigen exposure or residual effects of a prior illness and have no clinical significance.

A Enlargement of the anterior cervical chain.

P Bacterial infections of the pharynx (strep throat) or viral infections (mononucleosis).

A Enlargement of the occipital nodes or posterior cervical chain nodes.

P Infectious mononucleosis, tinea capitis, acute otitis externa.

Breasts

Inspection of the breasts is performed throughout childhood. Palpation is not usually performed on the patient until puberty, unless otherwise indicated.

Thorax and Lungs

Inspection

Shape of Thorax

E See Chapter 15.

N The infant has a barrel chest; by age 6, the chest attains the adult configuration.

A Abnormal chest configuration.

P Cystic fibrosis.

Retractions

E 1. Evaluate intercostal muscles for signs of increased work of breathing.

2. If at all possible, perform this examination when the patient is quiet because forceful crying will mimic retractions.

N Retractions are not present.

A Retractions can be suprasternal, supraclavicular, subcostal, and intercostal; nasal flaring, stridor, expiratory grunting, wheezing.

| E | Examination | N | Normal Findings | A | Abnormal Findings | P | Pathophysiology |

Nursing Alert

Stridor in Children

Stridor is indicative of upper airway obstruction, particularly edema in children. Inspiration accentuates stridorous sounds. Children who present with stridor should be promptly evaluated to rule out epiglottitis (a medical emergency).

P Abnormal function or disruption of the respiratory pathway or within organs that control or influence respiration; respiratory syncytial virus (RSV).

Percussion

E See Chapter 15.
N Normal diaphragmatic excursion in infants and young toddlers is one to two intercostal spaces.
A/P See Chapter 15.

Auscultation
Breath Sounds

E Use the same assessment techniques as for an adult. Sometimes it is difficult to differentiate the various adventitious sounds because a child's respiratory rate is rapid; for example, differentiating expiratory wheezing from inspiratory wheezing can be difficult. Mastering the technique takes time and practice.
N Bronchovesicular are normally heard throughout the peripheral lung fields up to five to six years of age, because the chest wall is thin with decreased musculature. Lung fields are clear and equal bilaterally.
A Crackles.
P Conditions such as bronchiolitis, CF, bronchopulmonary dysplasia.
A Wheezing.
P CF, bronchiolitis, RSV.

Heart and Peripheral Vasculature
General Approach

1. It is best to perform the cardiac assessment near the beginning of the examination, when the infant or young child is relatively calm.
2. Do not get discouraged during the assessment. The novice nurse is not expected to identify a murmur and location within the cardiac cycle. Be patient because skill will come only with practice.
3. During the assessment, note physical signs of a syndrome such as Down's facies in a child with trisomy 21 or Down syndrome. Many children with Down syndrome have associated atrioventricular (A-V) canal malformations. These defects each involve an atrial septal defect (ASD), ventricular septal defect (VSD), and a common A-V valve.
4. Cardiac landmarks change when a child has dextrocardia. In this condition, the apex of the heart points toward the right thoracic cavity, thus heart sounds are auscultated primarily on the right side of the chest.

Inspection
Apical Impulse

E See Chapter 16.
N In both infants and toddlers, the apical impulse is located at the fourth intercostal space and just left of the midclavicular line. The apical impulse of a child seven years or older is at the fifth intercostal space and to the right of the midclavicular line. The impulse may not be visible in all children, especially in those who have increased adipose tissue or muscle.
A/P See Chapter 16.

Precordium

E Observe the chest wall for any movements other than the apical impulse.
N Movements other than the apical impulse.
A Lifting of the cardiac area.
P Volume overload (CHF); left-to-right shunt defects (VSD).

E **Examination** **N** **Normal Findings** **A** **Abnormal Findings** **P** **Pathophysiology**

Palpation

Thrill

E 1. Palpate as for an adult or use the proximal one-third of each finger and the areas over the metacarpophalangeal joints. Many nurses believe the latter method yields greater sensitivity to the presence of thrills.

2. Place the hand vertically along the heart's apex and move the hand toward the sternum.

3. Place the hand horizontally along the sternum, moving up the sternal border about 1.25 to 2.5 cm each time.

4. When at the clavicular level, place the hand vertically and assess for a thrill at the heart's base.

5. Use the finger pads to palpate a thrill at the suprasternal notch and along the carotid arteries.

N A thrill is not found in the healthy child.

A/P See Chapter 16.

Peripheral Pulses

E 1. Use the same finger to assess each peripheral pulse. The sensation of one finger pad versus another can be different.

2. Use the finger pads to palpate each pair of peripheral pulses simultaneously, except for the carotid pulse.

3. Palpate the brachial and femoral pulses simultaneously.

N Pulse qualities are the same in the adult and the child.

A Brachial-femoral lag.

P Coarctation of the aorta.

Auscultation

Heart Sounds

E 1. Have the child lie down. If this position is not possible, the child should be held at a 45° angle in the caregiver's arms.

2. Use the Z pattern to auscultate the heart. Place the stethoscope in the apical area and gradually move it toward the right lower sternal border and up the sternal border in a right diagonal line. Move gradually from the patient's left to the right upper sternal borders.

3. Perform a second evaluation with the child in a sitting position.

N Fifty percent of all children develop an innocent murmur at some time in their lives. Innocent murmurs are accentuated in high cardiac output states such as fever, stress, or pregnancy. When the patient is sitting, murmurs are heard early in systole at the second or third intercostal space along the left sternal border and are softly musical in quality; they disappear when the patient lies down. Be aware of sinus arrhythmias during auscultation of the heart's rhythm. On inspiration, the pulse rate speeds up, the pulse rate slows with expiration. To determine if the rhythm is normal, ask the child to hold his or her breath while you auscultate the heart. If the pulse stops varying with respirations, then a sinus arrhythmia is present. S_1 is best heard at the apex of the heart, left lower sternal border. S_2 is best heard at the heart base.

A A split S_2 sound.

P Atrial septal defect.

A Systolic ejection murmur.

P Aortic and pulmonic valvular stenosis.

A Holosystolic murmurs heard maximally at the left lower sternal border.

P VSD.

Abdomen
General Approach

1. If possible, ask the caregiver to refrain from feeding the infant prior to the assessment because palpation of a full stomach may induce vomiting.

2. Children who are physically able should be encouraged to empty the bladder prior to the assessment.

3. The young infant, school-age child, or adolescent should lie on the examination table. Have the caregiver hold the toddler

| E Examination | N Normal Findings | A Abnormal Findings | P Pathophysiology |

or preschooler supine on the lap, with the lower extremities bent at the knees and dangling.

4. If the child is crying, encourage the caregiver to help calm the child before you proceed with the assessment.

5. Observe non-verbal communication in children who are not able to verbally express feelings. During palpation, listen for a high-pitched cry and look for a change in facial expression or for sudden protective movements that may indicate a painful or tender area.

Inspection
Contour
E   See Chapter 17.
N   The young child may have a "potbelly."

Peristaltic Wave
E/N   See Chapter 17.
A   Visible peristaltic waves seen moving across the epigastrium from left to right.
P   Obstruction at the pyloric sphincter.

Auscultation
See Chapter 17.

Palpation
General Palpation
E/N   See Chapter 17.
A   Olive-shaped mass felt in the epigastric area and to the upper right of the umbilicus.
P   Pyloric stenosis.
A   Abdominal distension coupled with palpable stool over the abdomen and the absence of stool in the rectum.
P   Hirschsprung's disease.
A   A sausage-shaped mass that produces intermittent pain when palpated in the upper abdomen.
P   Intussusception (intestine prolapses down into the ileum itself).
A   Bowel sounds heard in the thoracic cavity.
P   Diaphragmatic hernia.

Liver Palpation
E   For infants and toddlers, use the outer edge of your right thumb to press down and scoop up at the right upper quadrant.

For the remaining age groups, use the same technique as for an adult.

N   The liver is not normally palpated, although the liver edge can be found 1 cm below the right costal margin in a normal, healthy child. The liver edge is soft and regular.
A   Liver edge palpated more than 1 cm below the right costal margin and full with a firm, sharp border.
P   Hepatomegaly due to viral or bacterial illnesses, tumours, congestive heart failure, and fat and glycogen storage diseases.

Musculoskeletal System
General Approach
1. The extent or degree of assessment depends greatly on the patient's or caregiver's complaints of musculoskeletal problems. Be aware that during periods of rapid growth, children complain of normal muscle aches.

2. Try to incorporate musculoskeletal assessment techniques into other system assessments.

3. Inspecting the musculoskeletal system in the ambulatory child is accomplished by allowing the child to move freely about and play in the examination room while you inquire about the health history.

4. Do not rush through the assessment. Throughout the assessment, incorporate game playing that facilitates evaluation of the musculoskeletal system.

5. Observe range of motion and joint flexibility as the child undresses.

Inspection
Muscles
E   1. Have the child disrobe down to a diaper or underwear.

2. To evaluate the small infant's shoulder muscles, place your hands under the axillae and pull the infant into a standing position. The infant should not slip through your hands. Be prepared to catch the infant if needed.

E **Examination**   N **Normal Findings**   A **Abnormal Findings**   P **Pathophysiology**

3. Evaluate the infant's leg strength in a semi-standing position. Lower the infant to the examination table so the infant's legs touch the table.
4. Place the infant older than four months in a prone position. Observe the infant's ability to lift the upper body off the examination table using the upper extremities.

N Degree of joint flexibility and range of motion are the same for the child as for the adult.
A Increased muscle tone (spasticity).
P Cerebral palsy (CP).
A Inability to rise from a sitting to a standing position.
P Gower's sign occurs in Duchenne's muscular dystrophy (MD).

Joints
E See Chapter 18.
N The infant's spine is C-shaped. Head control and standing create the normal S-shaped spine of the adult. Lordosis is normal as the child begins to walk. A toddler's protruding abdomen is counterbalanced by an inward deviation of the lumbar spine.
A Supernumerary digits, or polydactyly.
P Congenital syndromes (Carpenter, fetal hydantoin, orofaciodigital, Smith-Lemli-Opitz, trisomy 13, VATER).
A Fusion between two or more digits.
P Syndactylism associated with congenital syndromes (Aarskog, Apert, Carpenter, Russell-Silver).

Tibiofemoral Bones
E 1. Instruct the child to stand on the examination table with the medial condyles together.
2. Stand at eye level with the patient's knees.
3. Measure the distance between the two medial malleoli.
4. Measure the distance between the two medial condyles.
N The distance between the medial malleoli is less than 5 cm. The distance between the

medial condyles is less than 2.5 cm. Knock knees, or genu valgum, is common between two and four years of age. Bowleg, or genu varum, is normally present in many infants up to 12 months of age.
A Genu valgum.
P Physiological.
A Genu varum.
P Rickets.

Palpation
Joints
E/N See Chapter 18.
A Palpation of a slight elevation of the tibial tuberosity.
P Osgood-Schlatter disease, caused by repetitive stress.
A Swollen, inflamed, painful joints.
P Juvenile rheumatoid arthritis.

Feet
E 1. Place the patient on the examination table or caregiver's lap.
2. Stand in front of the child.
3. Hold the right heel immobile with one hand while pushing the forefoot (medial base of great toe) toward a midline position with the other hand.
4. Observe for toe and forefoot adduction and inversion.
5. Repeat on the left foot.
N The toes and forefoot are not deviated.
A Toes or forefeet that are deviated.

Nursing Tip

Palpating Muscle Strength in Children

Playing games will assist you if the child is resistant to formal examination. For example, you can test plantar flexion by asking the child to pretend that the feet are pushing the brake on a car while you bear the force with your hands.

| E **Examination** | N **Normal Findings** | A **Abnormal Findings** | P **Pathophysiology** |

P   Metatarsus varus: medial forefoot malignment; abnormal intrauterine position of the fetal foot.

Hip and Femur

Ortolani's manoeuvre is always performed at the very end of the assessment because it may produce crying. The test is performed on one hip at a time. Evaluate the hips up until 18 months of age or until the child is an established walker.

E   1. Place the infant supine on an examination table with the feet facing you.
     2. Stand directly in front of the infant.
     3. With the thumb hold the inner thigh of the femur, and with the index and middle fingers hold the greater trochanter. These two fingers should rest over the hip joint.
     4. Slowly press outward and abduct until the lateral aspects of the knees nearly touch the table. The tips of the fingers should palpate each femora's head as it rotates outward.
     5. Listen for an audible clunk (Ortolani's sign).
     6. With the fingers in the same locations, adduct the hips to elicit a palpable clunk (Ortolani's sign). As each hip is adducted, it is lifted anteriorly into the acetabulum.
     7. Place both of the infant's feet flat on the examination table with the knees together.
     8. Observe the height of the knees. This is called Allis sign.
     9. Turn the infant to a prone position and observe the levels of the gluteal folds.

N   A clunk is not audible or palpated. The knees should be at the same height with the feet on the examination table. The gluteal folds are approximately at the same level.

A   Ortolani's sign, a sudden, painful cry during the test, asymmetrical thigh skin folds, uneven knee level, and limited hip abduction.

P   Developmental dislocation of the hip (DDH) related to familial factors, maternal hormones, breech presentations.

Neurological System
General Approach

1. Some aspects of the neurological assessment are different for the infant and the young child as compared to the adult. An infant functions mainly at the subcortical level. Memory and motor coordination are about three-quarters developed by two years of age, when cortical functioning is acquiring dominance.
2. Incorporate findings for fine and gross motor skills previously tested during the musculoskeletal assessment. Refer to normal developmental milestones (see Chapter 4) and extrapolate warning signs of neurological development lag.
3. Because the infant cannot verbally express level of consciousness, instead assess the newborn's ability to cry, level of activity, positioning, and general appearance.
4. Only reflex mechanisms and cranial nerve testing are described in this section. Refer to the adult neurological assessment for all other testing.

Reflex Mechanisms of the Infant

Neonatal reflexes must be lost before motor development can proceed.

Rooting Reflex

E   1. Place the infant supine with the head in a midline position.
     2. With your forefinger, stroke the skin located at one corner of the mouth.
     3. Observe movement of the head.

N   Up until three or four months of age, the infant will turn the head toward the side that was stroked. In the sleeping infant, the rooting reflex can be present normally until six months of age.

A   An absent rooting reflex from birth through three to four months.

P   Central nervous system disease.

E **Examination**   N **Normal Findings**   A **Abnormal Findings**   P **Pathophysiology**

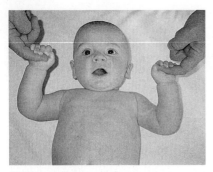

FIGURE 24-3 Palmar Reflex.

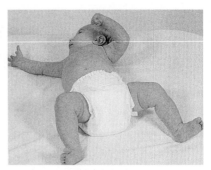

FIGURE 24-4 Tonic Neck Reflex.

Sucking Reflex

E 1. Place the infant in a supine position.
2. With your forefinger, touch the infant's lips to stimulate a response.
3. Observe for a sucking motion.

N The sucking reflex occurs up to approximately ten months.

A Absence of the sucking reflex.

P Prematurity, a breast-fed infant of a mother who ingests barbiturates.

Palmar Grasp Reflex

E 1. Place the infant supine with the head in a midline position.
2. Place the ulnar sides of both index fingers into the infant's hands while the infant's arms are in a semi-flexed position (Figure 24-3).
3. Press your fingers into the infant's palmar surfaces.

N Normally, the infant grasps your fingers in flexion.

A Presence of the palmar grasp reflex after four months of age.

P Frontal lobe lesions.

Tonic Neck Reflex

E 1. Place the infant in a supine position on the examination table.
2. Rotate the head to one side and hold the jaw area parallel to the shoulder.
3. Observe for movement of the extremities.

N The upper and lower extremities on the side to which the jaw is turned extend, and the opposite arm and leg flex (Figure 24-4).

Sometimes, this reflex does not show up until six to eight weeks of age.

A After six months of age, the tonic neck reflex is abnormal.

P Cerebral damage.

Stepping Reflex

E 1. Stand behind the infant, grasp the infant under the axillae, and bring the body to a standing position on a flat surface. Use the thumbs to support the back of the head if needed.

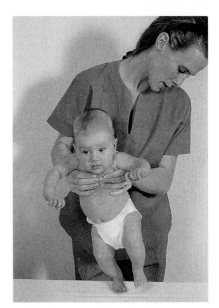

FIGURE 24-5 Stepping Reflex.

E **Examination**   N **Normal Findings**   A **Abnormal Findings**   P **Pathophysiology**

2. Push the infant's feet toward a flat surface and simultaneously lean the infant's body forward (Figure 24-5).
3. Observe the legs and feet for stepping movements.

N Stepping movements are made by flexing one leg and moving the other leg forward. This reflex disappears at about three months of age.

A Presence of the stepping reflex beyond three months of age.

P CP.

Plantar Grasp Reflex

E
1. Position the infant supine on the examination table.
2. Elevate the foot to be examined.
3. Touch the infant's foot on the plantar surface beneath the toes.
4. Repeat on the other side.

N The toes curl down until eight months of age.

A It is abnormal for the plantar grasp reflex to be absent on one or both feet.

P Obstructive lesion (abscess, tumour); CP.

Babinski's Reflex

E
1. Position the infant supine on the examination table.
2. Elevate the foot to be examined.
3. Stroke the plantar surface of the foot from the lateral heel upward with the tip of the thumbnail.

N A child less than 15 to 18 months of age normally fans the toes outward and dorsiflexes the great toe (Figure 24-6).

A After the child masters walking, presence of Babinski's reflex is abnormal.

P Cerebral palsy.

Moro (Startle) Reflex

E
1. Place the infant supine on the examination table.
2. Make a sudden loud noise such as hitting your hand on the examination table.
3. Another technique is to brace the infant's neck and back on the undersurface of your arm while holding the undersurface of the

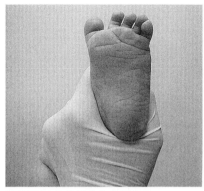

FIGURE 24-6 Babinksi's Reflex.

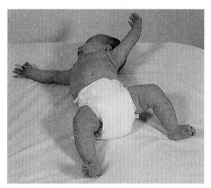

FIGURE 24-7 Moro Reflex.

buttocks with the other hand and then mimicking a falling motion by quickly lowering the infant.

N The infant under four months of age quickly extends then flexes the arms and fingers while the manoeuvre is performed. The thumb and index fingers form a C shape (Figure 24-7).

A Presence of the startle reflex after four to six months of age.

P CP.

Galant Reflex

E
1. Place the infant prone, with the infant's hands under the abdomen.
2. Use your index finger to stroke the skin along the side of the spine (Figure 24-8).

E Examination   N Normal Findings   A Abnormal Findings   P Pathophysiology

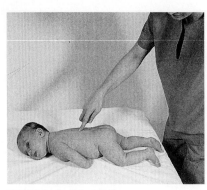

FIGURE 24-8 Galant Reflex.

3. Observe the stimulated side for any movement.

N An infant less than one to two months of age will turn the pelvis and shoulders toward the stimulated side.

A Lack of response from an infant less than two months of age.

P Spinal cord lesion.

Placing Reflex

Do not test the placing and stepping reflexes at the same time because they are two different reflexes.

E 1. Grasp the infant under the axillae from behind and bring the body to a standing position. Use the thumbs to support the back of the head if needed.

2. Touch the dorsum of one foot to the edge of the examination table.

3. Observe the tested leg for movement.

N The infant's tested leg will flex and lift onto the examination table.

A Lack of response.

A It is difficult to elicit this reflex in breech-born babies and in those with paralysis or cerebral cortex abnormalities.

Landau Reflex

E 1. Carefully suspend the infant in a prone position, supporting the chest with your hand.

2. Observe for extension of the head, trunk, and hips.

N The arms and legs extend during the reflex. The reflex appears at about three months of age.

A Presence of the Landau reflex beyond two years of age.

P Mental retardation.

Cranial Nerve Function

A thorough assessment of cranial nerve function is difficult to perform on the infant less than one year old. Difficulty is also encountered with toddlers and preschoolers because they often cannot follow directions or are not willing to cooperate. Testing for the school-age child or the adolescent is carried out in the same manner as for an adult.

Infant (Birth to 12 Months)

E 1. To test cranial nerves (CNs) III, IV, and VI, move a brightly coloured toy along the infant's line of vision. An infant older than one month responds by following the object. Also evaluate the pupillary response to a bright light in each eye.

2. CN V is tested by assessing the rooting or sucking reflexes.

3. CN VII is tested up until two months by assessing the sucking reflex and by observing symmetrical sucking movements. After two months of age, an infant will smile, allowing assessment of symmetry of facial expressions.

4. A positive Moro reflex in an infant less than six months old is evidence of normal functioning of CN VIII.

5. CNs IX and X are examined by using a tongue blade to produce a gag reflex. Do not test if a positive response was already elicited by using a tongue blade to view the posterior pharynx.

6. To test CN XI, evaluate the infant's ability to lift the head while in a prone position.

7. CN XII is assessed by allowing the infant to suck on a pacifier or a bottle, abruptly removing the paci-

---

E   Examination   N   Normal Findings   A   Abnormal Findings   P   Pathophysiology

fier or bottle from the infant's mouth, and observing for lingering sucking movements.

N/A/P   See Chapter 19.

Toddler and Preschooler (1–5 Years)

E   1. The older preschooler is able to identify familiar odours. Most children readily identify the smell of chocolate. Test CN I one side at a time by asking the child to close the eyes and to identify the smell of chocolate. Test each nostril with different substances while occluding the other nostril with your finger. *The use of peanut butter to test the olfactory nerve is discouraged because of the risk of allergic reaction in sensitive children.*

2. Test vision (CN II) using Allen cards.

3. CNs III, IV, and VI are tested in the same fashion as for the infant.

4. CN V is tested by giving the child something to eat and evaluating chewing movements. Sensory responses to light and sharp touch are still not easily interpreted in these age groups.

5. Observe facial weakness or paralysis (CN VII) by making the child smile or laugh. An older preschooler may cooperate by raising the eyebrows, frowning, puffing the cheeks out, and closing the eyes tightly on command.

6. To evaluate CN VIII, ring a small bell out of the child's vision and observe the response to unseen sounds.

7. Test CNs IX and X in the same manner as for the infant.

8. CN XII is difficult to assess in this particular age group.

N/A/P   See Chapter 19.

Female Genitalia

E/N   See Chapter 20.

Perineal Area

E   See Chapter 20.

N   The infant's labia minora are sometimes larger than the labia majora. The hymen is sometimes intact up until the point of sexual activity.

A   A bloody discharge noted at the vaginal opening or on the diaper of a child over two weeks of age.

P   Pseudomenstruation in an infant under two weeks of age due to circulating maternal hormones; discharge beyond two weeks requires further assessment.

Male Genitalia

E/N   See Chapter 21.

A   Urethral meatus behind or along the ventral side of the penis.

P   Hypospadias.

A   Meatal opening on the dorsal surface of the penis.

P   Epispadias.

A   It is abnormal to be unable to palpate the testes.

P   Cryptorchidism, failure of the testis to descend into the scrotal sac.

| **E** **Examination** | **N** **Normal Findings** | **A** **Abnormal Findings** | **P** **Pathophysiology** |

Unit 5

Putting It All Together

25

The Complete Health History and Physical Examination

Performing a complete health history and physical examination is a skill that takes time and practice to develop. It can take between 30 and 90 minutes to conduct a complete health history and physical examination. It is important to develop a routine that is comfortable so that steps in the assessment process will not be overlooked. However, the patient's physical, emotional, or mental state may necessitate a change in the usual progression of the assessment. Clinical judgment and experience will dictate when specific steps should be omitted, deferred, or repeated.

HEALTH HISTORY

Depending on the patient's reason for the visit, this can be the complete, episodic, interval (follow-up), or emergency health history.

◀ NURSING CHECKLIST ▶

General Assessment Reminders

- Understand illness in human terms, not just scientific terms.
- Approach the patient from a holistic viewpoint and try to understand the patient's perspective.
- Remember that nursing is both art and science.
- Follow your judgment; critical thinking incorporates the consideration of objective and subjective data. Always ask, "Why?"
- Act unhurried.
- Act in a professional manner at all times; remember that the patient is simultaneously examining you (mannerisms, facial expressions, hesitations in speech).
- Recognize both the patient's and your potential stressors (work, home environment, schedules) and try to account for them.
- Acknowledge emotional reactions to illness (anger, fear, anxiety, disbelief, confusion, guilt, shame, blame, hurt, and betrayal).
- Embrace sensitivity to cultural and spiritual issues.
- Show respect for the patient and his or her circumstances.
- Possess a sense of self-awareness to guide your actions.

◀ NURSING CHECKLIST ▶

General Approach to the Physical Assessment

- Develop an approach that is logical but allows flexibility.
- Use clinical judgment to modify the examination sequence and adapt to circumstances.
- Allow time at the conclusion of the examination to discuss relevant findings and to allow the patient to ask questions.
- Assist older patients or those with disabilities to focus on how well they can meet the demands of daily life rather than on their limitations.
- Remember that a physical examination can be tiring, both for you and for the patient.

Components of the developmental, cultural, and spiritual assessments are continually evaluated during the course of the patient interaction. Thorough assessments of any or all of these special assessments can be completed as necessary based on the patient's situation. The inspection component of the nutrition assessment is noted during the health history.

PHYSICAL ASSESSMENT

This text has provided a head-to-toe assessment format in order to discuss body systems in their entirety. However, in practice, a head-to-toe assessment combines systems when assessing most body parts. For example, when assessing the hands, components of the skin, musculoskeletal, and neurological assessments are combined. For this reason, the complete physical examination, which demonstrates how to put it all together, reflects this clinical approach. The sample case study at the end of the chapter documents a standard format of the complete physical assessment.

General Survey

The patient's general appearance is assessed during the health history. Incorporate the following into this assessment:

1. Physical Presence
   - Age: stated age versus apparent age
   - General appearance
   - Body fat
   - Stature: posture, proportion of body limbs to trunk

   - Motor activity: gait, speed, and effort of movement; weight bearing; absence or presence of movement in different body areas
   - Body and breath odours
2. Psychological Presence
   - Dress, grooming, and personal hygiene
   - Mood and manner
   - Speech
   - Facial expressions
3. Distress
   - Physical
   - Psychological
   - Emotional
4. Pain

Neurological System

1. Assess mental status: facial expression, affect, level of consciousness, attention span, memory, judgment, insight, spatial perception, calculations, abstract reasoning, thought processes, and content.

After the mental status examination, ask the patient to undress and don an examination gown (underwear may be worn). The patient's bladder should be emptied prior to commencing the assessment process. The urine may be collected for a specimen. Ask the patient to sit on the examination table with the legs hanging over the front. A second drape can be provided to cover the lap and legs. Stand in front of the patient.

Measurements

Record the patient's:
1. Height

2. Weight
3. Temperature
4. Pulse (radial preferred site in adult)
5. Respirations
6. Blood pressure (both arms)
7. Anthropometric measurements (if indicated)

Skin

Throughout the entire head-to-toe assessment, inspect the skin for the following characteristics:

1. Colour
2. Bleeding
3. Ecchymosis
4. Vascularity
5. Lesions

Throughout the entire head-to-toe assessment, palpate the skin for:

1. Moisture
2. Temperature
3. Texture
4. Turgor
5. Edema

Head and Face

1. Inspect the shape of the head.
2. Inspect and palpate the head and scalp.
3. Inspect the colour and distribution of the hair. Note any infestations; palpate the hair.
4. Inspect the face for expression, shape, symmetry (CN VII), symmetry of eyes, eyebrows, ears, nose, and mouth.
5. Instruct the patient to raise the eyebrows, frown, smile, wrinkle the forehead, show the teeth, purse the lips, puff the cheeks, and whistle (CN VII).
6. Palpate the temporal pulses. Palpate the temporalis muscles (CN V).
7. Palpate and auscultate the temporomandibular joints.
8. Palpate the masseter muscles (CN V).

Eyes

1. Test distance vision and near vision (CN II).
2. Test colour vision.
3. Test visual fields via confrontation (CN II).
4. Assess extraocular muscle mobility: cover-uncover test, corneal light reflex, and six cardinal fields of gaze (CNs III, IV, VI).

5. Assess direct and consensual light reflexes and accommodation (CN III).
6. Inspect the eyelids, eyebrows, palpebral fissures, and position of eyes.
7. Inspect and palpate the lacrimal apparatus.
8. Inspect the conjunctiva, sclera, cornea, iris, pupils, and lens.
9. Assess the corneal reflex.
10. Conduct funduscopic assessment: retinal structures, macula.

Ears

1. Test gross hearing: voice-whisper test or watch-tick test (CN VIII).
2. Inspect and palpate the external ear.
3. Assess ear alignment.
4. Conduct otoscopic assessment: EAC and tympanic membrane.
5. Perform Weber and Rinne tests.

Nose and Sinuses

1. Inspect the external surface of the nose.
2. Assess nostril patency.
3. Test olfactory sense (CN I).
4. Conduct internal assessment with nasal speculum: mucosa, turbinates, and septum.
5. Inspect, percuss, and palpate frontal and maxillary sinuses.

Mouth and Throat

1. Note breath odour.
2. Inspect the lips, buccal mucosa, gums, and hard and soft palates.
3. Inspect the teeth; count the teeth.
4. Inspect the tongue; ask the patient to stick out the tongue (CN XII).
5. Inspect the uvula; note movement when the patient says "ah" (CNs IX, X).
6. Inspect the tonsils; note grade.
7. Inspect the oropharynx.
8. Test gag reflex (CNs IX, X).
9. Test taste (CN VII).
10. Palpate the lips and mouth if indicated.

Neck

1. Inspect the musculature of the neck.
2. Inspect range of motion, shoulder shrug, and strength of sternocleidomastoid and trapezius muscles (CN XI).
3. Palpate the musculature of the neck.
4. Inspect and palpate the trachea.

5. Palpate the carotid arteries (one at a time).
6. Inspect the jugular veins for distension; estimate jugular venous pressure (JVP) if indicated.
7. Inspect and palpate the thyroid (use only one approach, either anterior or posterior).
8. Auscultate the thyroid and carotid arteries.
9. Inspect and palpate the lymph nodes: preauricular, postauricular, occipital, submental, submandibular, tonsillar, anterior cervical chain, posterior cervical chain, supraclavicular, and infraclavicular.

Upper Extremities

1. Inspect nailbed colour, shape, and configuration; palpate nailbed texture.
2. Assess capillary refill on nailbed.
3. Inspect muscle size and palpate muscle tone of hands, arms, and shoulders.
4. Palpate the joints of fingers, wrists, elbows, and shoulders.
5. Assess range of motion and strength of fingers, wrists, elbows, and shoulders.
6. Test position sense.
7. Palpate radial and brachial pulses.
8. Palpate the epitrochlear node.

Move behind the patient. Untie the gown so that the entire back is exposed. The gown should cover the shoulders and the anterior chest.

Back, Posterior, and Lateral Thoraxes

1. Palpate the thyroid (posterior approach).
2. Inspect and palpate the spinous processes; inspect range of motion of the cervical spine.
3. Note thoracic configuration, symmetry of shoulders, and position of scapula.
4. Palpate the posterior thorax and lateral thorax.
5. Perform posterior thoracic expansion.
6. Perform tactile fremitus on the posterior thorax and lateral thorax.
7. Percuss the posterior thorax and lateral thorax.
8. Perform diaphragmatic excursion.
9. Palpate the costovertebral angle (CVA); percuss the CVA with your fist.
10. Auscultate the posterior thorax and lateral thorax, perform voice sounds if indicated.

Move in front of the patient. Drape the patient's gown at waist level (females may cover their breasts).

Anterior Thorax

1. Inspect shape of the thorax, symmetry of the chest wall, presence of superficial veins, costal angle, angle of ribs, intercostal spaces, muscles of respiration, respirations, and sputum.
2. Palpate the anterior thorax.
3. Perform anterior thoracic expansion.
4. Perform tactile fremitus.
5. Percuss the anterior thorax.
6. Auscultate the anterior thorax; perform voice sounds if indicated.

Heart

1. Auscultate cardiac landmarks: aortic, pulmonic, mitral, and tricuspid areas and Erb's point.

Ask the female patient to uncover her breasts.

Female Breasts

1. Inspect the breasts for colour, vascularity, thickening or edema, size, symmetry, contour, lesions or masses, and discharge with the patient in these positions: arms at side, arms raised over the head, hands pressed into hips, hands in front, and patient leaning forward.
2. Palpate the breasts with the patient's arms first at her side and then raised over her head.
3. Palpate the brachial, central axillary, pectoral, and subscapular lymph nodes.
4. Teach breast self-examination.

Male Breasts

1. Repeat the sequence used for female breasts. Having the patient lean forward is usually unnecessary unless gynecomastia is present.

Assist the patient into a supine position with the chest uncovered. Drape the abdomen and legs. Stand on the right side of the patient.

Jugular Veins

As the patient changes from a sitting to a supine position for the remainder of the breast assessment, observe the jugular veins when the patient is at a 45° angle. Assess again when the patient is supine.

1. Inspect the jugular veins for distension; estimate JVP if indicated.

Female and Male Breasts

1. Palpate each breast. The arm on the same side of the assessed breast should be raised over the head.
2. Compress the nipple to express any discharge.

Heart

1. Inspect cardiac landmarks for pulsations.
2. Palpate cardiac landmarks for pulsations, thrills, and heaves.
3. Palpate the apical impulse.
4. With the diaphragm of the stethoscope, auscultate the cardiac landmarks; count the apical pulse.
5. With the bell of the stethoscope, auscultate the cardiac landmarks.
6. Turn the patient on the left side and repeat auscultation of cardiac landmarks.

Return the patient to a supine position. Cover the patient's anterior thorax with the gown. Uncover the abdomen from the symphysis pubis to the costal margin.

Abdomen

1. Inspect contour, symmetry, pigmentation, and colour.
2. Note scars, striae, visible peristalsis, masses, and pulsations.
3. Inspect the rectus abdominis muscles (supine and with head raised) and respiratory movement of the abdomen.
4. Inspect the umbilicus.
5. Auscultate bowel sounds.
6. Auscultate for bruits, venous hum, and friction rub.
7. Percuss all four quadrants.
8. Percuss liver span and liver descent; percuss liver with fist if indicated.
9. Percuss the spleen, stomach, and bladder.
10. Lightly palpate all four quadrants.
11. Note any muscle guarding.
12. Deeply palpate all four quadrants.
13. Palpate the liver, spleen, kidney, aorta, and bladder.
14. Assess superficial abdominal reflexes.
15. Perform hepatojugular reflux if indicated.

Inguinal Area

1. Inspect and palpate the inguinal lymph nodes.
2. Inspect for inguinal hernias.
3. Palpate the femoral pulses.
4. Auscultate the femoral pulses for bruits.

Cover the exposed abdomen with the gown. Lift the drape from the bottom to expose the lower extremities.

Lower Extremities

1. Inspect for colour, capillary refill, edema, ulcerations, hair distribution, and varicose veins.
2. Palpate for temperature, edema, and texture.
3. Palpate the popliteal, dorsalis pedis, and posterior tibial pulses.
4. Inspect muscle size and palpate muscle tone of the legs and feet.
5. Palpate the joints of the hips, knees, ankles, and feet.
6. Assess range of motion and strength of the hips, knees, ankles, and feet.
7. Test position sense.
8. Assess for clonus.

Drape the lower extremities. Assist the patient to a sitting position and note the ease with which the patient sits up. Have the patient dangle the legs over the edge of the examination table.

Neurological System

1. Assess light touch: face (CN V), hands, lower arms, abdomen, feet, and legs.
2. Assess superficial pain (sharp and dull): face (CN V), hands, lower arms, abdomen, feet, and legs.
3. Assess two-point discrimination: tongue, lips, fingers, dorsum of hand, torso, and feet.
4. Assess vibration sense: fingers and toes.

5. Assess stereognosis, graphesthesia, and extinction.
6. Assess cerebellar function: finger to nose, rapid alternating hand movements, touching thumb to each finger, running heel down shin, and foot tapping.
7. Assess deep tendon reflexes: biceps, triceps, brachioradialis, patellar, and achilles.
8. Assess plantar reflex and Babinski's reflex.

Ask the patient to stand barefoot on the floor. If the patient is unsteady, use caution when performing these tests. Remain physically close to the patient at all times.

Musculoskeletal System

1. Assess mobility: casual walk, heel walk, toe walk, tandem walk, backward walk, stepping to the right and left, and deep knee bends (one knee at a time). Note any indications of discomfort.

Stand behind the patient.

2. Assess range of motion of the spine.

Open the patient's gown to expose the back. Ask the patient to bend forward at the waist.

3. Inspect the spine for scoliosis.

Close the patient's gown. Stand in front of the patient.

Neurological System

1. Perform the Romberg test; assess pronator drift.
2. Assess the ability to hop on one foot, run heel down shin, and draw a figure eight with foot.

Assist the female patient back to the examination table. Ask her to assume the lithotomy position. Drape the patient. Sit on a stool in front of the patient's legs.

Female Genitalia, Anus, and Rectum

1. Inspect pubic hair and skin colour and condition: mons pubis, vulva, clitoris, urethral meatus, vaginal introitus, sacrococcygeal area, perineum, and anal mucosa.
2. Palpate the labia, urethral meatus, Skene's glands, vaginal introitus, and perineum.

3. Insert the vaginal speculum.
4. Inspect the cervix: colour, position, size, surface characteristics, discharge, and shape of cervical os; inspect the vagina.
5. Collect specimens for cytological smears and cultures.

Stand in front of the patient's legs.

6. Perform bimanual assessment of the vagina, cervix, fornices, uterus, and adnexa.
7. Perform rectovaginal assessment.
8. Palpate the anus and rectum.
9. If stool is on the glove, save it to test for occult blood.

Assist the patient to a sitting position. Offer her some tissues to wipe the perineal area. Ask her to redress. You can answer her questions when she is dressed.

Ask the male patient to stand. Sit on a stool in front of the patient. Have the patient lift the gown to expose the genitalia.

Male Genitalia

1. Inspect hair distribution, penis, scrotum, and urethral meatus.
2. Palpate the penis, urethral meatus, and scrotum.
3. Palpate the inguinal area for hernias.
4. Auscultate the scrotum if indicated.
5. Teach testicular self-examination.

Ask the patient to bend over the examination table. If the patient is bedridden, the knee-chest or left lateral position may be used. Expose the buttocks. Stand behind the patient.

Male Anus, Rectum, and Prostate

1. Inspect the perineum, sacrococcygeal area, and anal mucosa.
2. Palpate the anus and rectum.
3. Palpate the prostate.
4. If stool is on the glove, save it to test for occult blood.

Re-cover the buttocks. Ask the patient to stand up and redress. Offer him tissues to wipe the rectal area. You can answer his questions when he is dressed.

When completing the assessment, ensure that you return the patient to the state you found him or her in at the beginning of the assessment. For example, for the bedridden patient, ensure that the side rails are up (if appropriate) and that the call bell is readily accessible. Ask the patient if there is anything else that can be done to make him or her comfortable.

Document all findings, and thank the patient for his/her time and cooperation.

Appendix

Abbreviations and Symbols

Abbreviations

A, A, & O × 3	awake, alert, & oriented times three (to person, place & time)	AWMI	anterior wall myocardial infarction
a	before	ax	axillary
AB	abortion	bid	twice a day
abd	abdomen; abdominal	bil	bilateral
ABG	arterial blood gas	BKA	below the knee amputation
Abx	antibiotic	BP	blood pressure
ac	before meals	BPH	benign prostatic hypertrophy
AC>BC	air conduction is greater than bone conduction	BPM	beats per minute
		BS	bowel sounds; breath sounds
AC<BC	air conduction is less than bone conduction	b/t	between
		BSE	breast self-examination
ACL	anterior cruciate ligament	BUN	blood urea nitrogen
AD*	right ear	bx	biopsy
ADL	activities of daily living	C	Celsius, centigrade
AEB	as evidenced by	c	with
AFI	amniotic fluid index	CA	cancer
AGA	appropriate for gestational age	CABG	coronary artery bypass graft
AIDS	acquired immunodeficiency syndrome	CAD	coronary artery disease
		CBS	capillary blood sugar
AKA	above the knee amputation	CC	chief complaint
ALS	amyotrophic lateral sclerosis	cc*	cubic centimeter
ant	anterior	CCD	congenital cardiovascular defect
AOM	acute otitis media	CHD	childhood diseases; congenital heart disease
AP	apical pulse; anteroposterior		
A&P	anterior & posterior; auscultation & percussion	CHF	congestive heart failure
		CHI	closed head injury; creatinine height index
ARMD	age-related macular degeneration		
		Cl	chloride
AROM	active range of motion; artificial rupture of membranes	cm	centimeter
		CMT	cervical motion tenderness
AS	aortic stenosis	CMV	cytomegalovirus
AS*	left ear	CN I–XII	cranial nerves I–XII
ASA	acetylsalicylic acid	CNS	central nervous system
ASD	atrial septal defect	c/o	complaining of; complaints of
Atb	antibiotic	CO_2	carbon dioxide
AU*	both ears	COA	coarctation of the aorta
AV	arteriovenous	COPD	chronic obstructive pulmonary disease
A-V	atrioventricular		
A&W	alive & well	CP	chest pain; cerebral palsy

*The Institute for Safe Medication Practices (ISMP) considers these abbreviations dangerous because of possible misinterpretation. For additional information, see Appendix E: ISMP List of Error-Prone Abbreviations, Symbols, and Dose Designations.

CPD	cephalopelvic disproportion	GI	gastrointestinal
creat	creatinine	GU	genitourinary
CRC	colorectal cancer	GYN	gynecologic
C/S	cesarean section delivery	H/A	headache
CT	computerized tomography	HCG	human chorionic gonadotropin
CV	cardiovascular	HDL	high-density lipoprotein
CVA	costovertebral angle;	HEENT	head, eyes, ears, nose, throat
	cerebrovascular accident	HELLP	hemolysis, elevated liver
CVP	central venous pressure		enzymes, low platelets
CVS	chorionic villi sampling	H/H	hemoglobin & hematocrit
CXray	chest X ray	Hib	Haemophilus influenza b
cx	cervix	HIV	human immunodeficiency virus
d	day(s)	hl	health
DBP	diastolic blood pressure	HNP	herniated nucleus pulposus
d/c*	discontinue; discharge	h/o	history of
D&C	dilation & curettage	HOB	head of bed
DDST II	Denver Developmental	HPI	history of present illness
	Screening Test II	HPV	human papillomavirus
DES	diethylstilbestrol	HR	heart rate
DM	diabetes mellitus	hs*	at bedtime
DOA	dead on arrival	HSV	herpes simplex virus
DOB	date of birth	HT	height
DOE	dyspnea on exertion	HTN	hypertension
DRE	digital rectal examination	hx	history
DTR	deep tendon reflex	IADL	instrumental activities of daily
DUB	dysfunctional uterine bleeding		living
DVT	deep vein thrombosis	IBW	ideal body weight
dx	diagnosis	ICP	intracranial pressure
dz	disease	ICS	intercostal space
EAC	external auricular canal	IDM	infant of diabetic mother
EDC	expected date of confinement	IICP	increased intracranial pressure
	(delivery date)	I&O	intake & output
EDD	estimated date of delivery	IOP	intraocular pressure
EEG	electroencephalogram	IPPA	inspection, palpation,
EENT	eyes, ears, nose, throat		percussion, auscultation
EFM	electronic fetal monitoring	IUD	intrauterine device
EKG	electrocardiogram	IUGR	intrauterine growth retardation
ENAP	examination, normal findings,	IUP	intrauterine pregnancy
	abnormal findings,	IUPC	intrauterine pressure catheter
	pathophysiology	IV	intravenous
EOM	extraocular muscle	IWMI	inferior wall myocardial infarction
ESR	erythrocyte sedimentation rate	JVD	jugular venous distension
ETOH	ethyl alcohol	JVP	jugular venous pressure
FAS	fetal alcohol syndrome	K+	potassium
Fe	iron	kg	kilogram
FHH	family health history	KOH	potassium hydroxide
FHR	fetal heart rate	KUB	kidneys, ureters, bladder
FHT	fetal heart tone	L	liter
FLM	fetal lung maturity	Ⓛ	left
FM	fetal movement	LAD	left anterior descending
FOB	father of baby		(coronary artery)
FOBT	fecal occult blood test	lat	lateral
FROM	full range of motion	LBP	low back pain
FSH	follicle-stimulating hormone	LCM	left costal margin
FTT	failure to thrive	LDL	low-density lipoprotein
fx	fracture	LE	lower extremity
Ⓖ	gallop	lg	large
GC	gonorrhea and Chlamydia	LGA	large for gestational age
GCS	Glasgow Coma Scale	LH	leutinizing hormone
GDM	gestational diabetes mellitus	LLE	left lower extremity
GERD	gastroesophageal reflux disease	LLL	left lower lobe (of lung)

LLQ	left lower quadrant (of abdomen)	OOB	out of bed
LLSB	left lower sternal border	OPV	oral polio vaccine
LMD	local medical doctor	OREF	open reduction with external fixation
LMP	last menstrual period		
LOC	level of/loss of consciousness	ORIF	open reduction with internal fixation
LSB	left sternal border		
LUE	left upper extremity	OS*	left eye
LUL	left upper lobe (of lung)	OTC	over the counter (medications)
LUQ	left upper quadrant (of abdomen)	OU*	both eyes
		0	no, none
Ⓜ	murmur	oz	ounce
MAC	mid-arm circumference	p	after
MAL	midaxillary line	Pap	Papanicolaou
MAMC	mid-arm muscle circumference	pc	after meals
MCL	midclavicular line	PDA	patent ductus arteriosus
MD	muscular dystrophy, doctor	PE	physical examination, pulmonary embolus
Mec	meconium		
MF	milk fat	PERRLA	pupils equally round, reactive to light and accommodation
MGR	murmur, gallop, rub		
MI	myocardial infarction	PFT	pulmonary function test
MMR	measles, mumps, rubella	PHH	past health history
MMSE	Mini Mental State Exam	PID	pelvic inflammatory disease
MN	midnight	PIH	pregnancy-induced hypertension
MRI	magnetic resonance imaging		
MS	multiple sclerosis	PLT	platelets
MSAFP	maternal serum alpha-fetal protein	PMH	past medical history
		PMI	point of maximal intensity or impulse
MSM	men who have sex with men		
MVA	motor vehicle accident	PMS	premenstrual syndrome
MVI	multivitamin	PND	paroxysmal nocturnal dyspnea
mets	metastasis of malignancy	po	by mouth
ml	milliliter	post	posterior
mm Hg	millimeters of mercury	PP	patient profile
mo	month(s)	PPD	purified protein derivative; packs per day
mod	moderate		
mvt	movement	PPH	postpartum hemorrhage
NA	not applicable	prn	as necessary
Na+	sodium	PROM	passive range of motion; premature rupture of membranes
NaCl	sodium chloride		
NAD	no acute distress		
NCP	nursing care plan	PS	pulmonic stenosis
NGT	nasogastric tube	PT	physical therapy
NKA	no known allergies	pt	patient
NKDA	no known diagnosed or drug allergies	PTA	prior to admission (arrival)
		PTV	prior to visit
nl	normal	PUD	peptic ulcer disease
NPO	nothing by mouth	PVC	premature ventricular complex (or contraction)
NS	normal saline		
NSAID	nonsteroidal anti-inflammatory drug	PVD	peripheral vascular disease
		q	every
NSR	normal sinus rhythm	qd*	every day
NSVD	normal spontaneous vaginal delivery	qh	every hour
		qid	four times a day
N&V	nausea & vomiting	qod*	every other day
N, V, D	nausea, vomiting, diarrhea	Ⓡ	right; rectal
O_2	oxygen	r	rectal
OB	obstetrics	RCA	right coronary artery
OD*	right eye	RCM	right costal margin
OM	otitis media	RHD	rheumatic heart disease
OME	otitis media with effusion	RLE	right lower extremity
		RLL	right lower lobe (of lung)

RLQ	right lower quadrant (of abdomen)	TENS	transcutaneous electrical nerve stimulation
RML	right middle lobe (of lung)	THA	total hip arthoplasty
ROM	range of motion	THR	total hip replacement
ROS	review of systems	TIBC	total iron binding capacity
RR	respiratory rate; red reflex	tid	three times a day
RSB	right sternal border	TKR	total knee replacement
RT	related to, radiation therapy	TLC	total lymphocyte count
RTC	return to clinic	TM	tympanic membrane
RUE	right upper extremity	TMJ	temporomandibular joint
RUL	right upper lobe (of lung)	TORCH	toxoplasmosis, other (syphilis,
RUQ	right upper quadrant (of abdomen)		hepatitis B), rubella, cytomegalovirus, herpes simplex
Rx	prescription drug	TPR	temperature, pulse, respirations
rx	reaction	tr	trace
s	without	TSE	testicular self-examination
SAB	spontaneous abortion	TSF	triceps skin fold
SBE	subacute bacterial endocarditis	TVH	total vaginal hysterectomy
SBP	systolic blood pressure	tx	treatment
SCA	sickle cell anemia	u/a	urinalysis
SDH	subdural hematoma	UC	uterine contraction
SEM	systolic ejection murmur	UCHD	usual childhood diseases
SEMI	subendocardial myocardial infarction	UE	upper extremity
SGA	small for gestational age	URI	upper respiratory infection
SH	social history	U/S	ultrasound
SIDS	sudden infant death syndrome	UTI	urinary tract infection
sgy	surgery	UUN	urine urea nitrogen
sl	slight; slightly	VBAC	vaginal birth after cesarean
SLE	systemic lupus erythematous	VE	vaginal examination
SOB	shortness of breath	VS	vital signs
s/p	status post (after)	VSD	ventricular septal defect
SQ*	subcutaneous	VSS	vital signs stable
SROM	spontaneous rupture of membranes	VTX	vertex
s/s	signs & symptoms	WBC	white blood cell
SSCP	substernal chest pain	WD	well developed
ST	sore throat	wk	week
STI	sexually transmitted infection	wkend	weekend
sx	symptom	WN	well nourished
sz	seizure	WNL	within normal limits
T&A	tonsillectomy & adenoidectomy	WSW	women who have sex with women
TAB	therapeutic abortion	WT	weight
TAH	total abdominal hysterectomy	x	except
TB	tuberculosis	X	times
		yo	year old (age)
		yr	year(s)

Symbols

~	similar	=	equals	♀	female
≅	approximately	#	pounds	♂	male
@	at*	>*	greater than	△₁△₂△₃	trimester of pregnancy (one triangle for each trimester)
✓	check	<*	less than		
△	change	%	percentage	$\overline{1}$	one
↑	increased	+ or ⊕*	positive	2°	secondary
↓	decreased	− or ⊖	negative		

Index

Note: Page numbers in **bold type** refer to boxed text, figures, and tables

F

face, 125, 368
  expressions, 86, 126, 264
  inspection, 130–31
face shields, **74**
facial nerve (CN VII), **260**, 277–78
family health history, 20–21, 343. *See also* health history
  anus, rectum, and prostate, **314**
  breasts, **171**
  female genitalia, **287**
  male genitalia, **304**
  neurological system, **261**
  and pregnancy, **326**
fasciculation, **247**
fat
  body, 85
  dietary, 56
feet, 255–56, 358–59
females. *See also* pregnancy
  reproductive system, **27**, 288–90
femur, 359
fetus
  heart rate, 332
  movement count, **339**
fibrillation, **247**
fistula, anorectal, **317**
focusing (in interviews), 9, 11
fontanel, 341, 349
fornices (vaginal), 300
fremitus, tactile, 197, **198**
Freud, Sigmund, 34
friction rub
  abdominal, 230
  pericardial, 218, **219**
  pleural, 202, **204**
frostbite, **108**

G

gait, 244, **245–46**
Galant reflex, 361–62
gastrointestinal system, **27**. *See also* abdomen; rectum
gaze, cardinal fields of, 144–45
genetic testing, **338**
genitalia, female, 286–302, 343
  anatomy and physiology, 286–88
  assessment, **289**, 290–302, 371
  bimanual examination, 299–301
  external, 290–92
  inspection, 290–92
  internal, 294–96
  nutritional status and, **62**

palpation, 292–94, **301**
  in pregnancy, 325, 331–32
  rectovaginal examination, 301–2
  speculum examination, 294–96
genitalia, male, 303–12, 343
  anatomy and physiology, 303–4
  assessment, 305–12, 371
  auscultation, 310
  inspection, 305–7
  palpation, 307–10
genogram, **21**
glabellar reflex, 284
glands. *See specific glands*
Glasgow Coma Scale, 267–68
glaucoma, **139**
glossopharyngeal nerve (CN IX), **260**, 278–79
gloves, **73, 74,** 76
glucose, 68
gonococcal cultures, 298
graphesthesia, 274
grooming, 262–64
gums (gingivae), 154, 166–67

H

hair, **26**
  anatomy and physiology, 105
  care, **106**
  inspection, 118–22, 348–49
  nutritional status and, **62**
  palpation, 122–23
  of pediatric patients, 340, 348–49
  in pregnancy, 324, 329
  pubic, 290, 305
hands, 252–53
  washing, **73, 74, 75**
head. *See also specific structures*
  anatomy and physiology, 125–26
  assessment, 129, 368
  inspection, 129, 349–50
  nutritional status and, **62**
  palpation, 129, 131–32, 349–50
  in pediatric patients, 341, 346–47, 349–50
  in pregnancy, 330
  shape, 129, 349
headaches, **127, 128**
health, 12, 25
health care, **49–52**
health history, 12–28, 366–67. *See also* family health history; medical history; surgical history
  concluding, 28
  head and neck, **127**
  information for, 12–13